The Lactation Consultant in Private Practice

The ABCs of Getting Started

LINDA J. SMITH

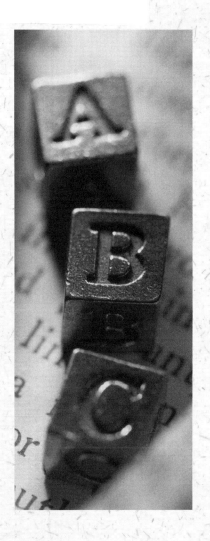

JONES AND BARTLETT PUBLISHERS
Sudbury, Massachusetts
BOSTON   TORONTO   LONDON   SINGAPORE

World Headquarters
Jones and Bartlett Publishers
40 Tall Pine Drive
Sudbury, MA 01776
978-443-5000
info@jbpub.com
www.jbpub.com

Jones and Bartlett Publishers Canada
2406 Nikanna Road
Mississauga, ON L5C 2W6
CANADA

Jones and Bartlett Publishers International
Barb House, Barb Mews
London W6 7PA
UK

Library of Congress Cataloging-in-Publication Data

Smith, Linda J.
    The lactation consultant in private practice: the ABCs of getting started / Linda J. Smith.
        p. cm.
    Includes index.
    ISBN 0-7637-1037-7
        1. Lactation. 2. Breast feeding. I. Title.

RJ216 .S563 2002
618.7'1—dc21   2002025667

Acquisitions Editor: Penny M. Glynn
Production Manager: Amy Rose
Associate Production Editor: Tara McCormick
Editorial Assistant: Karen Zuck
Production Assistant: Karen C. Ferreira
Marketing Associate: Joy Stark-Vancs
Manufacturing & Inventory Coordinator: Amy Bacus
Composition: Jackie Davies
Text Design: Anne Flanagan Graphic Design
Cover Design: Kristin E. Ohlin
Printing and Binding: Courier Stoughton
Cover Printing: Courier Stoughton

This book was typeset in Quark 4.1 on a Power Macintosh G3. The font families used were Garamond and Myriad.

Printed in the United States of America
06 05 04 03 02   10 9 8 7 6 5 4 3 2 1

Dedication

I would like to gratefully dedicate this book to Kay Hoover, Chris Mulford, Teriann Shell, and Kym Smythe.

Kay and Chris started the very first conference for Lactation Consultants in Private Practice, held in March 1990 in Philadelphia, PA. I've attended almost every year, and every time I've come away with new information and ideas, and—more importantly—new friends and colleagues. We roll up our sleeves, share what we're learning from mothers and babies, and dig into business and clinical topics in great detail. The seeds of several important documents and research have been sown at this conference, most notably *Candidiasis and Breastfeeding* by Lisa Amir, Kay Hoover, and Chris Mulford.

After 10 years, Teriann took over sponsorship of the conference with Kym Smythe's able assistance. Teriann has started and run private practices in two states, including her current practice in rural Alaska. I am inspired by Teriann's growth as a lactation consultant in private practice and by her continued dedication to the profession and to mothers.

Space does not permit me to acknowledge and thank the many other private practice lactation consultants (PPLCs) that I interviewed for this book. I feel very fortunate to count many PPLCs as my friends, peers, and colleagues. Thank you all for your support, ideas, strength, courage, and skill.

May our safety net continue to grow and be strong for our literal and figurative children and grandchildren all over the world. ■

Contents

12 Information Resource Management, Computers and the PPLC   133
Dennis L. Smith

13 Promotion and Marketing   157
Debi Page Ferrarello

14 Pitfalls Related to Business   165
Linda J. Smith

Introduction

So, you think you want to be a lactation consultant, open a private practice, and earn a good living by helping mothers and babies breastfeed? This book will help you crystallize your decision. It is designed to present a serious orientation and guide to the lactation consultant profession as manifested by the private practice lactation consultant (PPLC).

The ABC sequential format for establishing a private lactation practice presented in this book parallels my ABC Protocol™ for approaching clinical problems. The book is divided into three parts: Attitude, Business Skills, and Clinical Skills. Each part begins with an overview and includes a "pitfalls and problems" chapter. Each part also includes two examples of successful private practices.

Part A (Attitude) explores what it takes to be a PPLC, including how to acquire the LC role through education, apprenticing, and self-study. The goal is to help potential PPLCs understand what's involved and to describe the context of the PPLC in the community. Successful attitudes will also be evident in other sections of the book and in the stories of successful practices.

Part B (Business) addresses the business, marketing, and legal aspects of operating your private practice. The detailed and practical instructional chapters highlight the personal experiences of the contributing authors, all of whom currently operate successful private practices.

Part C (Clinical Practice) guides you through the process of functioning as a lactation consultant in private practice, focusing on the clinical issues falling within the scope of practice of the PPLC. This chapter provides a framework for applying your clinical skills and knowledge. Some sample clinical forms and handouts are included in the appendices.

You may notice that in some places, several contributing authors address similar principles or concepts. This repetition is deliberate, underscoring the importance of these concepts and allowing each chapter to stand alone. Some of the core concepts will also emerge in the words of the LCs who describe their private practices. Although most of the contributing authors live and practice in the United States, we have tried to speak to universal principles that are adaptable in many cultures, countries, and communities. The descriptions of one remarkable woman's practice in Zimbabwe and another's amazing political advocacy in Mexico help this book maintain an international focus.

Six real private practices are included to illustrate the flexibility, creativity, ingenuity, and adaptability needed for this work. Written by the owners, the stories and details of their private practices differ from each other, and may even differ markedly from suggestions in the body of the book. These stories are examples of how the book's principles evolved, were implemented, or have been adapted in real communities.

This book is primarily aimed at those individuals who want to operate a full-time, profitable, and long-term private lactation consultant practice. Others may find the information useful for other purposes or in other settings.

Throughout, we have assumed that the PPLC is female, because the vast majority of International Board Certified Lactation Consultants are women. This assumption is not meant to diminish the accomplishments of our male colleagues who hold the IBCLC credential.

Every effort has been made to make this book as complete, timely, and accurate as possible. However, the information is provided "as is." No warranty or responsibility for the use of this information is implied or intended. In other words, don't blame us if your practice doesn't succeed, you make a bad clinical or business decision, or we left out something you wish you'd known.

We offer this information in a spirit of sharing, collaboration, and support for our colleagues and the families we serve.

Foreword

Economics, Breastfeeding, and Policy: The Value of the PPLC

Kevin Frick, PhD

P rivate practice lactation consultants have many issues to consider on a daily basis. You must consider whether your business is profitable. To maintain profitability, you must provide services that are desirable, of high quality, and well-received by patients. You must track the equipment that you rent to patients and make sure that they return the equipment. You must keep up with the latest evidence on breastfeeding promotion. These issues, in combination with the level of activity that most American adults find themselves managing today, will give you little time for thinking about policy issues regarding your profession and the feeding practices that you are promoting. While you—as an individual lactation consultant—may not feel that you can make a difference, policy making in America often depends on the time and energy invested by a small number of individuals who gather information, speak out, and make well-articulated points.

Further, the profession as a whole cannot ignore policies that are being discussed and made at all levels around them. In the past several years, three very important documents have been released that have a bearing on lactation consultants. The first document, *HHS Blueprint for Action on Breastfeeding*, was released by the Surgeon General of the United States in October 2000. It makes a number of references to lactation consultants, in particular suggesting that the services provided by lactation consultants to new mothers be culturally appropriate. Such suggestions will affect the training of future lactation consultants, as well as the type of care that is expected from those who are already acting as lactation consultants.

The second of these documents was a monograph released by the American Association of Health Plans (a group of managed care organizations) and the Department of Health and Human Services in July 2001, titled *Advancing Women's Health: Health Plans' Innovative Programs in Breastfeeding*. It describes efforts to promote breastfeeding by eight health plans. Some health plans provided extensive programs to their employees in addition to programs for their enrollees. Many of these strategies incorporate the services of lactation consultants. Given the degree to which managed care organizations dominate health care financing in the United States at this point in time, you could benefit from taking a strong interest in a document like this one. As an individual lactation consultant or in a group with your colleagues, you can help to influence managed care organizations at a local or national level.

The third document, which was released in 2001 by the United States Breastfeeding Committee, is entitled *Breastfeeding in the United States: A*

National Agenda. This strategic plan reiterates the need for culturally appropriate lactation services, suggests that third-party payers finance lactation services, points to the need for evidence-based lactation care, and recommends a seamless interaction between hospital-based and community-based lactation care. This ambitious agenda sets very high goals that can contribute to breastfeeding promotion and that are likely to directly affect the lactation consultant profession and individual lactation consultants who need to increase their knowledge, work with other providers, and interact directly with insurers.

These three documents provide important examples of the way in which breastfeeding has attracted the attention of policy makers at the highest levels of the public health and health care systems. Given this fact, you could benefit from arming yourself with information to take to policy makers to make the case for reimbursement, for educational requirements contributing to your professionalization, and for other issues related to breastfeeding promotion.

Economics provides one set of tools for policy analysis to help you make your case on these issues. Many policy makers subject new policies and policies regarding new interventions to cost-benefit and cost-effectiveness analyses. These analyses, in turn, provide information about the economic efficiency of programs. Economic efficiency is a measure of whether society as a whole is improved by the introduction of a new policy or intervention. Economic analyses can, but often do not, describe distributional issues—that is, does a new policy make every individual better off or does a policy that benefits society as a whole make some people better off and others worse off? Further, politicians often ignore measures of economic efficiency to favor one group over another because of personal interests or because of the ability of a particular group to make its voice heard the loudest. Thus economics does not provide all the tools necessary for policy making, but it does offer a useful set of tools that can help make points that will attract the attention of many policy makers.

Before discussing what is known and what is not known from cost-benefit and cost-effectiveness analyses of breastfeeding and breastfeeding promotion, it is important to define two terms. Cost-benefit analysis measures the costs and benefits of an activity (such as breastfeeding) or an intervention (such as breastfeeding promotion). This type of analysis not only assesses the *costs* in dollars, but also quantifies the *effects* in dollars. Some effects can easily be measured in dollars (e.g., medical care savings), whereas others are more difficult, if not impossible, to measure in dollars (e.g., the value of the bonding that occurs between mother and child). Economists have developed techniques to place dollar values on less tangible benefits, but the validity of their results has inspired debate. Some people's uneasiness with the concept of placing a dollar value on health or other intangible effects of interventions makes cost-benefit analyses that include measures other than medical care savings difficult for some policy makers to accept. The advantage of these analyses derives from their ability to compare any type of program with any other type of program, because everything is measured in dollars. In contrast, cost-effectiveness analyses include a nonmonetary measure of effectiveness. While some researchers have attempted to construct a single nonmonetary measure of effectiveness, this type of analysis is best suited for comparing alternatives with the same outcome.

So the question remains: How can lactation consultants and those with whom they collaborate in the policy process use economic tools to further the cause of breastfeeding or breastfeeding promotion? It is useful to begin with a phrase commonly used in breastfeeding promotion: "Breast is best." Lactation consultants work with all types of mothers, including those who believe in this statement and who need help to continue breastfeeding, and those who are looking for information to determine how true this statement is and how to make breastfeeding work for themselves and their children. This statement is even believed by many mothers who choose not to breastfeed. Still, despite the seemingly self-evident nature of this statement and its applicability to a comparison of the health effects of breast milk versus formula, this does not necessarily mean that policy makers will find it economically efficient to make regulations or fund programs that promote breastfeeding.

The first element of a discussion of the economic benefits of breastfeeding is a review of the health benefits for which an economic value can be applied. We can find examples of how breastfeeding has positive short-term effects for the mother, such as a more rapid contraction of her uterus and a more rapid return to pre-pregnancy weight. Likewise, we can point to examples of long-term benefits for mothers, such as a reduced risk of breast cancer. We can identify examples of health benefits for breastfed children, including less gastrointestinal disease, less otitis media, and less diarrhea. Each of these health benefits can affect medical care utilization. Lower medical care utilization leads to lower expenditures. These benefits might accrue to the mother, to her insurer, or to a government program such as Medicaid. Regardless, the changes in health that result from breastfeeding promotion will be an important consideration in economic evaluation of a breastfeeding promotion program.

Breastfeeding also has effects on the convenience of feeding the child that are generally positive, although the effects may be mixed. While the food for the baby is always readily available as long as the mother is present or has provided pumped breast milk, the mother has reduced flexibility because of the need for her presence or the need for her to express breast milk.

Finally, breastfeeding has the potential to affect mother–child bonding, and mothers who breastfeed may have either positive or negative feelings about breastfeeding in general. Other effects, such as greater intelligence, have also been attributed to breastfeeding, although these are not universally accepted.

The positive benefits result from breastfeeding in general. For the women whom you help to continue breastfeeding, these positive benefits increase as a result of your assistance. Your support comes in many forms. You can help the mother with her own technique or her child's technique. You can help by providing information and supplies. You can provide pumps for mothers who want to pump and link mothers to other services when necessary (e.g., send mothers back to their pediatricians or to pediatric otolaryngologists when a child has tongue-tie). Your assistance can help mothers to become more efficient at breastfeeding. All of these positive benefits would be compared with the costs of promoting breastfeeding. While your services are not very expensive, neither are they free.

Mothers who choose to pay for lactation consultant services have made their own "cost-benefit" decision in favor of lactation consultants. The key policy question is whether this decision should simply be left to each mother using her own resources to obtain lactation consultant services or whether policy should officially encourage the use of lactation consultant services. The latter policies might include training lactation consultants and paying for lactation consultant services on the mother's behalf.

Now that you are aware of how to frame the issues related to the economic evaluation of breastfeeding promotion, you may wonder what data exist to help to answer the range of questions raised here. Several researchers have analyzed the costs and benefits of breastfeeding, and these studies have been reviewed recently in the literature. The basic conclusion of these studies and an additional formal analysis that accompanied one of the reviews is that breastfeeding has the potential to save enormous amounts of resources related to medical care and substantial resources in food costs, as the costs of the dietary supplements necessary for a mother are quite limited in comparison to the costs of formula. The analyses performed to date have made projections to (1) the small populations that were directly studied, (2) the entire population of mothers of newborns in the United States, or (3) the additional mothers who would breastfeed if the prevalence of breastfeeding changed from previously low rates to the rates that have been set as goals in *Healthy People 2000* and *Healthy People 2010*. In spite of the strong case that can be made for a positive net benefit of breastfeeding itself (i.e., the benefits outweigh the costs), very limited evidence supports the economic efficiency of breastfeeding promotion activities. Indeed, this field represents a fertile area of research for the lactation consultant profession. You may be able to play an important role in this research.

All of this discussion about the economic evaluation of breastfeeding promotion is important because in some instances you may need to communicate about the costs and benefits of breastfeeding promotion. Consider a business plan that you take to potential lenders when you are starting or expanding your business. In this case, it would be important to make clear to the lender that the individual mothers making cost-benefit decisions would choose to use your services. This type of discussion would focus on all of the individual benefits that were discussed previously.

For discussions with corporate, managed care, or government decision makers, the discussion would need to focus on the costs and benefits of providing lactation consultant services to a population. The population will vary with the audience, of course. A managed care organization might want to make sure that what it pays for your services is less than the benefits it receives from having mothers breastfeeding longer (i.e., medical benefits). A corporation might be interested in knowing that the costs of your services are offset by a variety of savings, including potentially lower medical care premiums (which are most easily realized if the employer self-insures), lower worker absence rates, and higher worker satisfaction that could contribute to improved job performance and employee retention. Finally, the government would be interested in knowing that the costs of your services are offset by decreased medical expenditures and potential savings on WIC and other programs.

The costs of your services may be paid for entirely by the managed care organization, corporation, or government, or they may be shared by these organizations and the mother. You will need to discuss both the costs and benefits of your activities and help policy makers to see that the benefits outweigh the costs in which they are interested. Again, this discussion does not guarantee that a policy maker will agree to pay for your services, but it does help make your case.

As mentioned earlier, economic analysis does not always demonstrate the distribution of costs and benefits. In addition to some people being winners and others being losers because of a certain policy, some levels of government (e.g., local as compared with federal) may be winners and others may be losers. Similarly, some agencies (e.g., WIC as compared with Medicaid) may be winners and others may be losers. It is quite possible that one government program or level of government will benefit from an intervention to promote breastfeeding, even as others incur higher costs as a result of a new effort to promote breastfeeding. This trade-off requires that you or the entire group of lactation consultants with whom you are working discuss the issues with multiple decision makers and help them to see the entire set of results of the program to understand that it makes society as a whole better off.

In summary, private lactation consultants should either occasionally or regularly consider the larger issues that affect themselves, their profession, and the natural form of feeding children that they promote. The policy-making process can affect all of these considerations. The policy-making process will continue to move ahead whether you take an active or a passive role. Taking an active role will position you to better anticipate and make the most of new opportunities and new constraints. Economic tools are not the only ones needed to approach the policy-making process, and much work needs to be done to enhance the use of these tools in this arena with specific reference to breastfeeding. Nevertheless, having a basic understanding of the tools will better prepare you to take an active role in the policy-making process.

REFERENCES

U.S. Department of Health and Human Services. *HHS Blueprint for Action on Breastfeeding*. Washington, DC: U.S. Department of Health and Human Services, Office on Women's Health, 2000.

United States Breastfeeding Committee. *Breastfeeding in the United States: A National Agenda*. Rockville, MD: U.S. Department of Health and Human Services, Health Resources and Services Administration, Maternal and Child Health Bureau, 2001.

American Association of Health Plans. *Advancing Women's Health: Health Plans' Innovative Programs in Breastfeeding Promotion*. Washington, DC: American Association of Health Plans, 2001.

Preface

Thoughts on Private Practice

Barbara Wilson-Clay, BSEd, IBCLC

Thanks to my mother's example, I always knew I would breastfeed. To this day, my experiences nursing our three children remain among my life's sweetest memories. How I became an LC is rather more complicated. When I got pregnant with my first child in 1978, I was working in a community mental health setting, doing outreach with Appalachian children from neglectful and abusive homes. In the three years prior to my pregnancy, I had been a Child Protective Caseworker. That job involved investigating complaints filed against parents who lived in shacks in impoverished hollows where children played barefoot in the snow. Misery, alcoholism, poverty, and stress contributed to violence, and much of the violence was aimed at children and even babies. Although I tried my best to help these families, it was clear to me, even as a very young woman, that what was wrong in these families would defy fixing.

When I became pregnant, I devoured books by Frederick Lamaze and Grantly Dick-Reed, and pondered their theories about birth. Then I discovered Karen Pryor's book, *Nursing Your Baby*. Fascinated by her insights, I began to think and read more widely about bonding. I wondered: Would a mother who was deeply attached to her child permit or participate in violence toward that child? As I nursed my own baby, it became clear to me there was a biological component to bonding. I suspected then, as I do to this day, that attachment begins and proceeds optimally with supported childbirth and successful breastfeeding. I decided to put my energies toward *prevention* of child abuse by investing in the establishment of a strong mutual maternal–child bond via these mechanisms.

When I became an accredited La Leche League (LLL) Leader in 1981, I quickly became involved in the Professional Liaison Department. This cadre of Leaders works to build bridges between LLL and the professional community. These leaders also serve mothers who experience special circumstances and need information or assistance that may be outside the scope of the local group Leaders. I loved being of service to these mothers, women who often faced enormous challenges. I loved the detective work and intellectual stimulation involved in helping them discover solutions that allowed them to reach their breastfeeding goals. When I mentioned that a group of individuals was trying to establish a profession of lactation consultants, my husband was dubious. "Who would pay for a service like that?" he asked me repeatedly. But *my* first thought was: "Sign me up!"

I feel proud to have contributed in a small way to the formation of the profession, and I am grateful that I have been able to continuously work as a private practice LC (PPLC) since my certification as an IBCLC in 1987. As a pioneer in the field, my conscious intention was to impart to my community what an LC is and does. This effort involved setting high standards for my conduct at a time when the standards weren't even written down. I deliberately wanted to set my bar high, because pioneers always have a lot to prove, and we have a responsibility to pave the way for those who come after us. From the first, I have cared passionately about the work, and I want others to respect it and value it as I do.

I've had a wonderful time, but being in private practice carries a price and isn't for everyone. It can be a very lonely business. For me, it was often frightening. I believe I spent the first several years in practice living in a state of terror. People showed up in my office every day with problems that were too big for me to manage. I was seeing things in person that I had seen only in books (if I was lucky!). People paid me to solve their problems, and I honestly felt as if I was taking their money under false pretenses.

The fact that their doctors hadn't been able to help these women either provided no consolation. I was afraid I would miss something or harm someone. Most nights found me poring over journal articles, Ruth Lawrence's book, or on the phone to my PPLC friend in Dallas, Judy Eastburn. Why did those mothers *still* have sore nipples? *Why* wouldn't that baby nurse? *Where* was that milk supply? The truth is that no one with an easy-to-fix problem *needs* a PPLC. Instead, the PPLC gets the "train wreck" cases. Lactation is such a robust biological process that it provides the novice mother and her new baby lots of wiggle room. By the time a mother consults a PPLC, all fail-safe mechanisms have failed and at least two things are going wrong simultaneously.

A case study I often share demonstrates this fact. This first-time mother had a long, difficult labor. When forceps failed to deliver her baby, an emergency cesarean section was performed under general anesthesia. The first breastfeeding was delayed for 24 hours due to both maternal and infant stress. The baby was deeply suctioned after meconium aspiration, and had a raspy cry indicating some damage to the vocal cords and, likely, a very sore throat. Even with help from the nurses, the baby couldn't latch. The young mother, who lived in a rural area, was discharged home bottle-feeding. Luckily, she had good family support. On day 7 postpartum, she was readmitted to the hospital for emergency gallbladder surgery. I saw the mother and baby on day 15. The poor woman had three separate gauze bandages taped to areas of her abdomen, and she couldn't tolerate holding the baby in the cradle position. With help from her sister, she had been able to maintain a milk supply by pumping, but she attributed the baby's continued rejection of the breast to nipple confusion from all the bottles. Upon assessment, I discovered that in addition to all of these problems, the mother had inverting nipples *and* the baby was tongue-tied!

Family members and physicians often look at such a complicated situation and assume it cannot be resolved. They give the mother "permission to wean" rather than sort it out. But it is the role of the PPLC to do precisely that: Sort it out. This kind of case walked through the door from the first week I practiced. I've learned first-hand that it is called *practice* because if you do it long enough, you might get good at it.

Today, I no longer panic when I encounter train wrecks. I've had enough experience to have seen most everything at least once before, and I still read everything I can get my hands on. This approach allows me to draw from research evidence and from past successes and failures to come up with a plan. Looking back, however, I think that my initial terror was appropriate. In fact, given the absence of standardized LC preparation, I suspect that any new PPLC who *isn't* terrified probably lacks enough self-awareness to trust with the job.

Many PPLCs, in my opinion, practice similarly to a nurse practitioner (NP)—that is, independently of direct physician supervision. Like the NP, these PPLCs make clinical decisions and recommendations based on clinical assessment. While some very fine PPLCs have skills that allow them to function in this way, it concerns me (given our lack of comprehensive training) that this approach may not be appropriate.

From the first, I have acknowledged that my work with mothers and babies must be viewed in the context of a *team* of care providers. Every mother and baby pair I see generates a report to a physician—either the mother's or the baby's, and sometimes both. In a brief report, seldom more than two paragraphs, I describe the presenting problem, my assessment, and my suggestions. Often I refer back to the pediatrician to discuss consultation with another specialist. When I first began my practice in 1987, the physicians probably wondered who I was and what I was doing. Now they have come to rely on my assessments, and today most of my referrals come from physicians. They appreciate my cooperative approach, my detective work on their behalf, and my acknowledgment that it is their role to provide the medical supervision. It's a relief to me to have that relationship with the physicians because it protects the mother and the baby. But it must always be understood that they did not invite me into the relationship—I essentially forced the relationship with the tool of the report. Once the report is delivered, the communicated information becomes the link that forges a relationship. For that reason, learning to write diplomatic and informative reports is a critical skill.

I mentioned before that being a PPLC is lonely. Private practice is also very competitive. In my experience, this environment translates into a reluctance to share information and tricks of the trade. The LCs who advised and supported me emotionally typically practiced in other cities. When I first began practicing, I had a partner. Her friendship and companionship meant a great deal to me. When our partnership dissolved under the stress of two very different views of what we wanted from the practice, the experience was as painful to me as a divorce. I worked solo for many years afterward because I never wanted to go through such an experience again. My advice to anyone thinking of a partnership is to spend time in advance making sure that your views of the business and of the profession are compatible. Keep the financial contributions absolutely equal so that no unequal power relationships arise. Have regular partner meetings and discuss problems as they occur so they don't fester into resentments.

Whether you practice solo or in partnership, are affiliated with a doctor's office or home health organization, it is important to join your ILCA affiliate. Networking with other LCs, particularly PPLCs, helps the profession—even if it doesn't always result in personal friendship or mutuality.

Whenever anyone asks me how I would have done things differently, I am forced to admit that I *couldn't* have gone about it otherwise because there was no better training available at the time. It concerns me that in many areas ace   xxiii

of the country this reality still prevails. I am firmly convinced that we have to change the way LCs are educated so that our first years in practice aren't so terrifying for us and so potentially risky for our clients! Progress is being made, and I applaud the many lactation courses under development. However, because of the types of problems the PPLC encounters, I believe she should be a graduate of a four-year course of study (or a master's program) that provides the appropriate training background for the type of problems she must assist.

Given the rich contributions made by non-nurse members of the LC profession, I hesitate to call for all PPLCs to be nurses. I've always visualized the clinically competent LC as having an interesting amalgam of skills drawn from several diverse areas. I think she should be well trained in counseling techniques. She must understand infant oral-motor anatomy and physiology. She should know about medications and breast milk. It is critical that she understand both infant behavior and adult education theory. The PPLC must demonstrate sophisticated skill in the use of equipment. To communicate effectively with other health care professionals, she must understand medical terminology. She needs to be able to write a report, testify in court, and maintain accurate charts and records. She must be able to identify a child who needs immediate medical care and to recognize red flags for breast cancer. Some of what she needs to know is found in the dental literature. Other information resides in plastic surgery, child neurology, speech pathology, ENT, and psychology texts. She needs to know her Code of Ethics and her Scope of Practice, and she needs to understand lactation science like the professional we hope she is.

To stay economically viable, many PPLCs have relied heavily upon retail sales of breastfeeding-related products. This strategy carries a risk of failing to look and act ethically. This potential conflict of interest is not discussed as much as it should be, and the profession has not codified proper conduct in this area as diligently as needs to be done.

The PPLC still operates out in front of the pack. While the vanguard is a thrilling place to be in many respects, it places a burden on the individual, who is very visible, to constantly uphold the high standards our new profession professes. If we don't deliver, it makes all of us look bad. As individuals we don't have much power beyond the power of example, but collectively we can continue to move our profession forward. We must join together in our professional organization to press for accreditation of LC training programs and we must support the IBCLC credential. We need to do this to make sure that the next generation of mothers will be able to obtain help from skilled LCs. We also need to make sure women in the next generation have the opportunity to become skilled LCs, and, hopefully, to make a living doing what they love.

About the Authors

Linda J. Smith, BSE, FACCE, IBCLC

Linda Smith has been helping breastfeeding women since 1974. She has started and operated private lactation practices in four cities, including her current practice in Dayton, Ohio. She has been a La Leche League Leader for 28 years in nine cities and two countries, practiced as a childbirth educator for 20-plus years, worked in a three-hospital system in Texas and a public health agency in Virginia, and served as breastfeeding coordinator for the Ohio Department of Health.

Linda is the author of *Comprehensive Lactation Consultant Exam Review; Coach's Notebook: Games and Teaching Strategies for Lactation Education; Core Curriculum for Lactation Consultant Practice*, Chapters 5 and 9; and the video, *A Healthier Baby by Breastfeeding*. She is a founder of IBLCE and founder and past board member of ILCA. She currently sits on the United States Breastfeeding Committee representing the Coalition for Improving Maternity Services (CIMS).

Linda and her husband Dennis own and operate the Bright Future Lactation Resource Center in Dayton, Ohio, whose mission is "Supporting the people who support breastfeeding" with lactation education programs, consulting services, and educational and promotional resources. The center can be reached via the Internet at www.BFLRC.com.

CONTRIBUTING AUTHORS (IN ORDER OF THEIR CHAPTERS)

Barbara Wilson-Clay, BSEd, IBCLC

Austin Lactation Associates, http://www.lactnews.com

Barbara Wilson-Clay lives and works in Austin, Texas, where she and her husband raised their three daughters. Barbara helped pass legislation to protect the rights of breastfeeding women in Texas, helped found the Texas Chapter of Healthy Mothers/Healthy Babies, and is a co-founder and board member of the Mothers Milk Bank at Austin. She has been instrumental in her community in assisting corporate clients in developing on-site breastfeeding support for working mothers. She is a well-known lecturer and author, whose research and commentaries have appeared in the *Journal of Human Lactation, Current Issues in Clinical Lactation, Birth Issues*, and *ICEA Journal*. Barbara helped develop and contributed to the book *Core Curriculum for Lactation Consultant Practice*. A La Leche League Leader since 1981, Barbara served as Area Professional Liaison for Texas and helps develop material for LLLI. She reviewed and abstracted articles for *Breastfeeding Abstracts*, and served on the editorial review board of the *Journal of Human Lactation*. She is a contributing editor of *Current Issues in Clinical Lactation*. Barbara served a term as the ILCA delegate to the Board of Directors of the International Board of Lactation Consultant Examiners. With Kay Hoover, she is the author of *The Breastfeeding Atlas*, a lactation management text containing 230 clinical photographs.

Kevin D. Frick, PhD

Assistant Professor, Johns Hopkins Bloomberg School of Public Health
Department of Health Policy and Management
Health Services Research and Development Center
Johns Hopkins University, Department of Economics

Dr. Frick has been involved in studying the cost-effectiveness of a number of community-based interventions. In one pilot program, a community health nurse and peer counselor encouraged an increased duration of breastfeeding among low-income women who had decided to breastfeed prior to the intervention. Dr. Frick always makes an effort to make his economic analyses relevant for and accessible to policy makers and individuals delivering health care. He is also the father of two children. Each was breastfed exclusively for approximately six months and continued nursing until the age of two. Lactation consultants assisted in the process of initiating breastfeeding for both children.

Carol A. Ryan, RN, BSN, IBCLC

Carol A. Ryan has been an IBCLC since 1987 and is the Coordinator of Parenting and Lactation Services at Georgetown University Hospital in Washington, D.C. She has been in private practice for 19 years. She is a highly respected speaker and lecturer. Carol was the Vice President for Operations of ILCA during 1995–1998 and serves as Vice President for Professional Development, ILCA, during 2000–2002. She is a contributing author to the *Core Curriculum for Lactation Consultant Practice* and AWHONN's *Standards & Guidelines for Professional Nursing Practice in the Care of Women and Newborns*, 5th edition. She serves as a member of the U.S. Breastfeeding Committee. Her three adult children were breastfed.

Diane Wiessinger, MS, IBCLC

Diane Wiessinger received her master's degree from Cornell University in 1978. She has been an IBCLC since 1990 and a La Leche League Leader since 1985. Her special interests are the mechanics of latch-on, the language used to promote breastfeeding, and the importance of mother-to-mother contact in supporting breastfeeding. She has operated a home-based private practice in Ithaca, New York, since 1992, and self-publishes breastfeeding handouts under the name *Common Sense Breastfeeding* (www.wiessinger.baka.com).

Debi Page Ferrarello, RN, BSN, MS, IBCLC

Debi is president of Breastfeeding Resources, Inc., a company providing in-patient lactation consultation, breastfeeding classes for expectant parents, and in-service education for health care professionals. She maintained a private practice for 11 years, before specializing in contracting lactation services to hospitals and education for health care professionals. She and a colleague have recently formed a nonprofit corporation whose mission is to provide lactation services to breastfeeding families regardless of their ability to pay, and to provide opportunities for clinical experience to aspiring lactation consultants and other health care professionals.

Debi completed her bachelor's degree in 1984 and received a master's degree in Community Health Education in 2001. She is married to a man who knows more about breastfeeding than any other English teacher in the greater Philadelphia area, and is the mother of two boys at an age where they won't tell anyone what she does for a living, and a daughter who has successfully breastfed a variety of stuffed animals.

Debi can be reached at her address of 1059 Clemens Avenue, Abington, Pennsylvania, 19001-4003, by phone at (215) 886-2433, or by e-mail at imibclc@cs.com.

Elizabeth C. Brooks, JD, IBCLC

Elizabeth works as a lactation consultant in her home-based private practice, and at Chestnut Hill Hospital (in Philadelphia, Pennsylvania). She is an at-home mother to three school-aged children. Earlier, she practiced law as a prosecutor with the District Attorney's Office in Philadelphia and as a federal civil litigator in Washington, D.C.

Diane DiSandro, BA, IBCLC

Diane has been helping mothers breastfeed since 1980. She opened her full-time private lactation practice in January 1991 on a shoestring, and has been operating in the "black" since March 1991. So far, this shoestring business has sent two children to college and renovated her house. She has a home office where she sees most of her clients, staffed by herself and her office manager, Miss Manage. She sees an average of 15 mothers and babies per week, and has a group of independent contractors who answer her phones and help with filing, mailing, sorting, organizing. She could not have grown her business without the love and support of her husband Ray and her four children, Liz, Ray, Patrick, and Michael. Diane's address is 688 Sunnyside Avenue, Audubon, Pennsylvania 19403-1739.

Jane A. Bradshaw, RN, BSN, IBCLC

Jane lives in Lynchburg, Virginia. She graduated from the University of Vermont with a bachelor of science degree in nursing in 1972. She worked as a hospital and Public Health Nurse before beginning her education in breast-feeding, taught primarily by her three children. By working part-time with her husband in his busy veterinary practice, she learned many business skills that became useful when she later started her own practice. She became a La Leche League Leader in 1981 and a certified IBCLC in 1986. In addition to lac-taction consulting services, her practice has grown to include professional and clerical employees and a variety of classes and services for expectant and new parents. She works part time as a lactation consultant at Bedford Memorial Hospital, as an Instructor for Lactation Education Resources and professional speaker for lactation conferences. She was an Associate Editor for the *Journal of Human Lactation* from 1989 to 1997. Her main goals are to work to increase breastfeeding knowledge among professionals and provide the support mothers need to be able to breastfeed as long as possible.

Dennis L. Smith, MS

Dennis L. Smith is the Chief Information Officer for the Bright Future Lactation Resource Center. He followed Linda Smith as she progressed from a "League Mom" in Maryland, through being a "Leader" in San Antonio, Texas, an "Educator" in Ottawa, Ontario, Canada, became an IBLCE and ILCA Founding Board member in Washington, D.C., to becoming a lecturer and author in Dayton, Ohio. Along the way he donated the International Lactation Consultant Association's first database design and was involved in a variety of military information management efforts, including keeping track of airplanes and their parts, and some military hospital information management activities. He chaired the Department of Defense Computer Institute's Computer Security Department and later its Information Resource Management Department and retired from the U.S. Air Force Material Command as a Colonel responsible for Information Systems Architecture. He currently consults on institutional Web site development within the Lactation Consultant community and is designing and assembling an economical but enveloping personal flight simulator. More information about the author and perhaps even more timely advice on information resource management for the lactation consultant in private practice may be found at www.BFLRC.com/DLS.

MODEL PRIVATE PRACTICES (IN ORDER OF THEIR APPEARANCE)

Kay Hoover, MEd, IBCLC

Home-based office, home visits—Philadelphia, Pennsylvania

Kay has operated a part-time private practice in the suburbs of Philadelphia for 16 years; she is also a part-time consultant to the Philadelphia Department of Public Health Division of Early Childhood, Youth and Women's Health. Her job is to help the hospitals in the City of Philadelphia to be more supportive of breastfeeding. She has held two jobs as a hospital lactation consultant. Kay co-authored *Candidiasis and Breastfeeding*, Unit #18 of the *Lactation Consultant Series* published by La Leche League International in July 1995. She also self-published *The Link Between Infants' Oral Thrush and Breast and Nipple Pain in Lactating Women*, first edition, March 1995; second edition, August 1996; third edition, May 1998; and fourth edition, January 2001. With Barbara Wilson Clay, Kay co-authored *The Breastfeeding Atlas* (1999) and *The Diaper Diary* (2001).

Diane Wiessinger, MS, IBCLC

Home-based office, mixed visits—Ithaca, New York.

See biography above.

Eve Moeran, RN, IBCLC

Storefront/retail store plus consultancy—San Diego, California

Eve Moeran is a Registered Nurse from New Zealand and has held RN degrees from Australia, the United Kingdom, and the United States. She graduated as a

Midwife from the Royal Women's Hospital in Melbourne Australia and earned her IBCLC in 1999.

Roberta Graham de Escobedo, BA, IBCLC

Workplace support—Merida, Yucatan, Mexico

Supporting breastfeeding mothers since 1982, Roberta has been in private practice since 1995 in Merida, Yucatan, a city of almost one million people. She is currently the only IBCLC within a 600-mile radius. Originally from the Chicago area, she has lived in Yucatan for almost 30 years with her husband Alfonso and their two breastfed children. About 85% of her consults are house calls or hospital visits and the corporate lactation segment of her practice is expanding rapidly. Roberta also teaches at the University of Yucatan's School of Nursing and also at the School of Education. She can be contacted in Yucatan at Calle 3 #227 (32A-34) Col. Pensiones, Merida, Yucatan Mexico 97219 or by phone and email at 52 999 925-1844, roberta@ecoyuc.com.

Patricia Lindsey, IBCLC

Medical Office and Private Practice—Orlando, Florida

Pat Lindsey began helping breastfeeding mothers in 1977 when she became an accredited volunteer breastfeeding counselor for La Leche League. In the early 1980s, Pat worked in a volunteer pilot program at Florida Hospital where La Leche League Leaders went on the maternity floor and gave on-hand assistance to breastfeeding mothers during their hospital stay. In 1991, Pat worked for the Seminole County Women, Infant and Children (WIC) department where she implemented their Breastfeeding Peer Counselor Program. Pat began working in the office of Pediatrics Plus as a lactation consultant intern in 1995 and became IBCLC in 1996. In 1997, Pat established a private practice (Pat Lindsey, IBCLC—Lactation Services http://www.PatLC.com) in addition to continuing as Pediatrics Plus' lactation consultant (http://www.pedsplus.com). Pat's volunteer and employment background has provided her with a broad scope of breastfeeding experience as she has worked with thousands of mothers and babies in a variety of settings. Pat has developed and markets Lactation Visit Receipt, a lactation superbill with instructions on filing for third-party reimbursement. She lives in the rural community of Chuluota, Florida with Butch, her husband of 34 years. She is the mother of two adult children and the grandmother of a grandson.

Pamela Morrison, IBCLC

Developing country, isolated LC—Harare, Zimbabwe

Pamela grew up in East Africa and moved to Zimbabwe in 1971. She lives with her husband and three sons in Harare, where she has worked as a lone lactation consultant in private practice with mothers from all racial and ethnic groups for the past 11 years. She is a former La Leche League Leader, served as an assessor and facilitator for the WHO/UNICEF Baby Friendly Hospital Initiative, and was a legal secretary. Pam's address is 10 Camberwell Close, Borrowdale, Harare, Zimbabwe, telephone 263-4-883500, e-mail Pamela@ecoweb.co.zw.

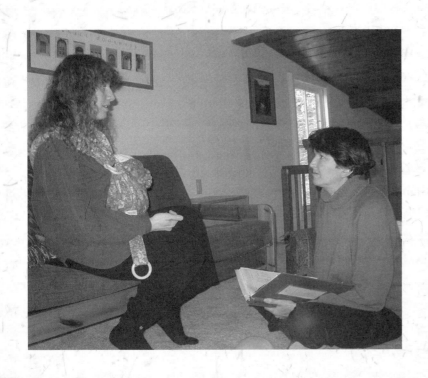

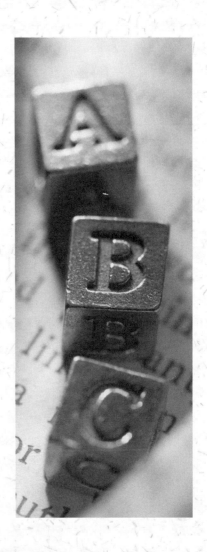

Attitude and Acquiring the Lactation Consultant Role

Do You Have What It Takes?

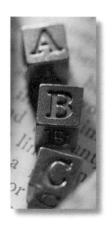

1 Overview of Successful Attitudes and Abilities

Linda J. Smith, BSE, FACCE, IBCLC
Diane Wiessinger, MS, IBCLC

Do you have what it takes to be a successful private practice lactation consultant (PPLC)? In Part A—Attitude—we explore attitudes and abilities that you'll need to make this work become your career.

First, to be a successful PPLC, you need to become a very, very good lactation consultant—which in itself is a worthy goal in any practice setting. You need commitment, consistency, and compassion to be able to help mothers all day, every day, on a full-time basis. To be a successful PPLC, you also need to become a competent businesswoman. You need persistence, professionalism, and planning to turn your passion into your livelihood.

Let's stop and define "success." Does success mean your lactation-related business brings in enough money to support yourself and your family? Or do you want to make only enough money to cover outside expenses? Do you define success as being able to competently help mothers all day, as your humanitarian mission, with monetary income irrelevant to your goals? In this book, *we take the position that "success" means that your lactation practice is your livelihood.* The practice brings in enough income to cover its own business expenses, provides an adequate and appropriate income to you and your employees, if any, and operates in compliance with all professional, legal, and community laws and standards.

✔ I have the desire to succeed as a private practice lactation consultant in every possible way—professionally, financially, emotionally, and psychologically.

✔ I want to be in this work as a full-time career—not as a hobby, not as something I do in my spare time between driving car pool and fixing meals, and not because it sounds like a quick and easy way to make money.

✔ I am willing to invest time, energy, and money to become an excellent lactation consultant.

✔ I believe in and act on the premise that the breastfeeding mother–baby dyad is an inseparable unit.

✔ I understand and adhere to the Code of Ethics and other published policy documents for lactation consultants.

✔ I am comfortable doing clinical breastfeeding support work as a business.

A SUCCESSFUL ATTITUDE FOR A LACTATION CONSULTANT

People seem to enter the field of human lactation for one of two reasons: either they wanted badly to do so, or someone else wanted badly for them to do so. That someone else is usually an institution that decides it can have an IBCLC on staff without adding an employee. An institution may assume it can get double duty that way—the same amount of work from the same number of people with the added "cachet" of having an IBCLC on staff. That approach rarely succeeds, of course. Lactation consultants who actually work as lactation consultants have quite enough to do working exclusively with breastfeeding; expecting them to also perform as nurses is neither to expect nor desire a change in breastfeeding satisfaction among the population served.

The people who went through the credentialing process for someone else are unlikely to enter private practice unless they "catch the fervor" and self-ignite. The work is too exacting and the pay too poor for an IBCLC to strike out on her own for reasons other than passion. Some women who are not yet IBCLCs may still decide to work in private practice. That's a mistake, unless circumstances prevent the person from working effectively toward IBLCE certification in any other way. To deliberately stop short of becoming an IBCLC and yet establish a career as a "private practice lactation consultant" deceives the public and tarnishes the image of the entire profession. It's dishonest. Fortunately, it's also rare.

A variation on this theme is the non-IBCLC who sets up private practice as a doula or childbirth educator. It's incumbent on these women to find the nearest, best breastfeeding help available to their clients, and to make use of it—always learning more themselves, but also making very sure that they never act as dead-ends in a mother's search for good breastfeeding help because they were sure they knew enough. Just as an IBCLC without certification in childbirth services needs to refer her clients to the best help she can find for those seeking such services, the non-IBCLC needs to remember that a vast body of breastfeeding knowledge and resources exists that her clients can best access through an IBCLC.

These non-IBCLC childbirth care providers may still believe that having nursed one or more children themselves and having read the most common lay texts have given them most of the necessary information. That may (or may not) be true when the only issue is helping a mother establish breastfeeding. If the path is full of stones, the non-IBCLC needs to be very careful that she doesn't wear the mother out before passing her along to someone with more current information and specialized skills. Being well-meaning is not the same as being well-trained.

Many IBCLCs enter the field because they want it for themselves. It's a long road—at least several years of work with breastfeeding mothers before being eligible even to sit for the exam. It's not unusual for us to get calls from women who nursed a child themselves, helped a few neighbors, perhaps have a background in professional nursing already, and now want to become lactation consultants.

I always take these requests seriously. We can't afford to lose any good people, and the process is self-selecting; the woman who doesn't stay the course simply doesn't become an IBCLC. It's not a decision I have to—or ought to—make before she even investigates the possibility. But I have seen only one such caller actually become certified. Most had no idea there was so much work involved or so vast a body of knowledge to learn.

The great majority of us enter private practice either because that was always our goal as we worked toward certification, or because we became disillusioned with the depth of breastfeeding help we were able to offer in our institutional settings and want to do better. We are, in a word, passionate.

THE MOTHER–BABY RELATIONSHIP

A fundamental attitude for the PPLC is to *believe* in the concept of the mother-baby dyad as an *inseparable unit*. Believe in this concept deeply—down to your toes—and act in support of this principle in everything you do and say. The dyad concept is unique in health care. Fragmentation of the dyad—that is, separating the mother and baby—has led to or been at the root of many of the problems we encounter daily!

The mother and baby are each separate systems, and together they form another interactive and interrelated system.[1] The mother-baby relationship is more than the sum of its parts. The mother is the gatekeeper and interpreter for her child; the child is part of her environment. The child is an active participant in all aspects of breastfeeding, and is the leader in this delicate dance. The mother is the baby's *entire* environment. We support, promote, and protect practices that acknowledge the *motherbaby*[2] as a unit.

THE "RULES" FOR SUCCESSFULLY PROVIDING BREASTFEEDING CARE

Why does the Attitude section include five "rules"? These concepts represent the cornerstones in the foundation of breastfeeding support work. If you have a problem with any of them, you will probably have a problem providing professional breastfeeding care. You may even be working *against* breastfeeding in overt or covert ways. These rules have evolved over the course of nearly 30 years of volunteer support of mothers and babies. They form a short list—others could probably add more core concepts.

Rule 1: Feed the Baby.

The child is the most vulnerable member of the breastfeeding team, and babies are trying to double their birth weight in the first four to six months of life. Therefore, a successful attitude means paying close attention to the baby's nutritional status. Hunger does not help the baby develop feeding skills. Underfeeding compromises the baby's health, undermines the mother's confidence, and wounds the child's soul. Whatever else we do, we always make sure the baby is getting enough to eat.

Rule 2: The Mother Is Right.

Supporting the mother—empowering her, encouraging her, validating her—is a fundamental attitude. In fact, this support may be even more important in the long run than "fixing" a specific breastfeeding problem. Research shows that when someone has a good experience, they tell three or four people. If they have a bad experience, they tell 10! Our compassion, our paying attention, our *listening* is vital to the mother's self-esteem, regardless of the outcome of the breastfeeding situation. Tailoring our suggestions to the mother's reality is essential. Even our use of the term "suggestions" instead of "advice" or "recommendations" or—even worse—"instructions" speaks to this attitude. The mother is right. Period.

Rule 3: It's Her Baby.

The mother owns her breasts, birthed (or adopted) the baby, and is always right (see Rule 2). Acknowledging, reinforcing, fostering, and developing the mother's intuition about her baby is another vital attitude. We can never, *ever* do or suggest anything that would pit the mother against her baby, or the baby against the mother. The dyad is an inseparable unit, remember? This attitude emerges in our interactions with mothers and babies, in our political and advocacy work, and in our educational activities.

Rule 4: Nobody Knows Everything.

We won't ever have all the answers. Knowing our own personal and professional limits is part of this attitude. Knowing that *there's more to be known* is vital! Cooperating and collaborating with others is also part of this aspect of attitude. There's always someone who sees a situation through a different pair of eyes, has different clinical skills, or connects with the mother in a unique way. Part of our role is to help the mother find other resources to help her family and work collaboratively as a member of the health care team. We do not "own" any mother-baby dyad—see Rules 2 and 3. This attitude is part of the science of breastfeeding care.

Rule 5: There's Another Way.

Staying current, doing our homework, going to conferences and seminars, reading journals, participating in local coalitions, and keeping our minds open to new ideas are all part of a successful attitude. Lactation consultant skills continually evolve, and new research changes our knowledge and skill base every year. The half-life of breastfeeding information seems to be about five years: What we "know" today is significantly different than what we "knew" only a few years ago. This rule also applies to individual clients: There's usually no *one* perfect suggestion or plan of care for an individual mother–baby dyad. This attitude is the core of the *art* of helping mothers breastfeed.

Both business and professional rules govern the PPLC. Being a PPLC may be a somewhat scary proposition because of the enormous, complex matrix of skills and knowledge needed. We're not all nurses, yet we assist mothers and babies in vulnerable times. We're not all dietitians, yet we're expected to know about the nutrititive properties of human milk, appropriate early complementary foods for children, and the role of maternal nutrition during breastfeeding. We're not all pharmacists, yet we're expected to have general knowledge of how drugs transfer into milk and where our role begins and stops in helping mothers who need pharmaceutical therapy. We're not all child development specialists, yet we need to thoroughly understand children's behaviors during breastfeeding throughout their first two years of life or longer. We're not all experienced mother-support group leaders, yet we're expected to have intimate and thorough knowledge of the breastfeeding relationship extended over years (not days or months). We're not all social workers or professional counselors, yet we must be able to listen effectively to mothers and help them sort out their feelings about breastfeeding. We're not necessarily the same age, ethnic background, or from the same culture as the

RULES AND SCOPE OF PRACTICE

mothers we help, yet we're expected to understand each mother-baby dyad as they interact within their own cultural milieu. We're not all accountants, yet we are expected to maintain accurate financial records for our practices. And we're not all marketing experts, yet we must competently market our practices, our profession, and our passion—breastfeeding.

Some of the guidelines for being a PPLC include the following:

- We don't give medical advice.
- We don't give drug advice, and we don't prescribe.
- We don't diagnose or treat medical conditions.
- We don't give legal opinions.

On the other hand,

- We recognize normal breastfeeding and abnormal conditions affecting the breastfeeding mother, breastfed baby, or their relationship.
- We collaborate and cooperate with medical care providers.
- We identify options for the mother and baby.
- We understand milk synthesis and infant suck very thoroughly.
- We understand and support the concept of the mother-baby dyad.
- We stay current on the published professional literature relevant to our clients.
- We support others who provide care to the mother, baby, and family.
- We support, promote, and protect breastfeeding in a wide variety of contexts.

THE IMPORTANCE OF BREASTFEEDING

This point bears repeating. If you are not passionate about the importance of breastfeeding, you will probably not enjoy or succeed in this work. To illustrate the importance of breastfeeding, here's a story from Rachel Myr, a talented midwife from Kristiansand, Norway:

A colleague wrote on the topic of why breastfeeding seems to be exempt from the general trend toward using evidence-based practice in maternity care. The flip side of this attitude is the emotional strength with which maternity staff members defend their positions in regard to breastfeeding. If you doubt that this is peculiar to breastfeeding, think back to the last time you heard a really heated discussion about how frequently a mother's fundus should be palpated postpartum, and what the appropriate fundal height is on the second postpartum day. Or what color lochia should be by day 5, or what is the right amount. Or what is the best procedure for bandage changes after a cesarean, or cord care. Been a while, eh?

Now think back to the last discussion about how to help a mother breastfeed who is experiencing some difficulty with latch. The entire tone is different; the temperature rises and so does the pulse and blood pressure of all participants.

I use this now to illustrate how *important* breastfeeding is, since it seems to hit us so squarely where we live, regardless of what our own personal experience was. It took me about 10 years of distressing conversations with my colleagues to see it this way. It wasn't until the day one of my colleagues started yelling at me "You think it's all so easy, well it's NOT, and I breastfed for a MONTH and never had more than an ounce of milk, and it was REALLY HARD...," and then started to cry, that I came to my current realization. What made it all the more convincing was that the baby she breastfed is now a man of 40, she is retired, and recalling her experience can still reduce her to a quivering mass. Do we need stronger arguments for why women deserve good help to succeed at breastfeeding? Wouldn't the world be better without all this anguish?

MOTIVATION AND COMMITMENT

Why do you want to do hands-on clinical breastfeeding support all day? Are you angry because a health care professional gave you incorrect information or unhelpful advice, or no advice at all during your own breastfeeding experience? Are you a volunteer mother-support group leader or counselor who now wants to do "the same kind of work" for pay? Have you really enjoyed nursing your own baby, and now want to help other mothers? Are you a nurse or other health care provider who wants to branch out or expand your practice? Do you see this field as a quick, lucrative shortcut to a health-related occupation? Take some time to explore why you want to enter private lactation practice. You might even want to lurk on *Lactnet* (Lactation Information and Discussion, LactNet@peach.ease.lsoft.com) for a few weeks, following several discussion threads. Lactation consultants are far more than cheerleaders, which will quickly become obvious.

Your motivation needs to support a long-term commitment to this work. Otherwise, you risk burnout, boredom, and frustration—not to mention wasted time and money.

TIME

Starting a new business takes an enormous amount of time and energy. My mother Dorothy Dahlstrom once said, "I used to think there were only 24 hours in a day, until I went into business for myself." Do not underestimate the amount of time needed to establish a private lactation practice. You should count on committing full-time (40–60 hours per week or more) to this venture for at least a few years. Most of us with families find this aspect particularly difficult, especially over the long term.

If you truly believe in the importance of the mother–baby relationship—which is a core principle of lactation consultants—be prepared to live this principle in your own life. To preach, "Babies and mothers should be viewed as an inseparable dyad," but leave your infant in day care many hours each day is hypocritical at best. We fit our practices around our families' needs. Sometimes that means relying on hired help for parts of the business or for household chores. At other times we deliberately shift the business to the "back burner" while we deal with family crises. Although some business tasks can be done in waiting rooms or during soccer or choir practice, a large part of the work requires large blocks of uninterrupted time.

Another side of the time issue is the principle that *work expands to fill the time available to do it.* You will need to become very skilled at setting boundaries, using little chunks of time productively, and multitasking. You must learn to take care of yourself, or you will be of no help to others. Boundary setting also applies clinically: A reasonable approach is to match your level of commitment to the mother's level of commitment.

Yet another time issue is this: Breastfeeding care proceeds at the baby's pace and the mother's pace. Depending on your own personality, this process can be intensely frustrating or beautiful to watch as it unfolds. If your personality type thrives on closure, wrapping things up neatly, or clearly scheduled activities, you may quickly become dissatisfied with this aspect of PPLC work. The converse is also true: If you prefer to "go with the flow," take each day as it presents itself, and chafe against schedules and deadlines, then you may have trouble handling the business aspects of your practice.

MONEY

This issue has probably divided more breastfeeding supporters than any other. Charging money to help women breastfeed is repugnant to some, yet completely and obviously appropriate for others. No one hesitates to pay an auto mechanic, catering service, or photographer for his or her expertise or time. Yet many people repair cars, cook delicious meals, or take great photographs as a hobby. Breastfeeding and human lactation is both a life-skill that every mother should be able to do easily and a complex behavior involving two (or more) individuals that challenges the best scientific, behavioral, and medical minds in the world.

Money fights can divide the lactation consultant from her family and friends. Money issues have split up more than a few breastfeeding-related businesses. As you consider how your practice will look, think about the money at every turn. Hire good financial advisors, plan thoroughly, reevaluate your plan frequently, and research how money affects all aspects of your practice. If you don't want to think about money, you may want to reconsider even starting a private practice.

IMAGE

I don't know where, or how many times, I've heard it: If you want to change someone's mind about something, be like that person in every respect except the area in which you want to create change. Dress the same, talk the same, read the same books, go to the same movies. Dramatically outdressing your clients will add to their discomfort more than it will add to your credibility. A friend taking a childbirth class from a particularly attractive instructor once told me, "I had only one complaint about the class. We all sat around looking like beached whales, and she waltzed in looking like a fashion model." We don't need to be fashion models, but we do need to be clean and neat, with teeth freshly brushed. Be remembered more as an attitude than as a personality. How wonderful for a mother to be able to say to her friends, "I don't really remember much about the lactation consultant, but now I know I can do this."

We need to ensure privacy. Many of us use our own homes, but our clients are probably unfamiliar with nursing toddlers, and I haven't yet met the client's husband to whom lactating breasts are commonplace. Clients aren't interested in having your family participate in the visit. Find a way to keep your family out of sight, if not out of earshot. A firmly closed door is important. Unplanned evidence of our families is best kept out of the way as well. While a framed picture of a preschooler may be appealing, a half-eaten graham cracker underfoot is not. At the same time, there's much to be said for a homelike atmosphere. "I'm just like your neighbor," it says. "It's okay. It's safe. I'm not sitting in judgment."

We need to tread carefully and respectfully in suggesting changes in a woman's parenting. Something as simple as asking "Did that feel right to you?" may open the way for her to change directions. I may show mock indignation followed by a bit of information: "Now why would anyone call that gas? You bet that's a smile! And they do it only when they feel good inside. He may not smile *at* you yet, but he does smile *because* of you." Or I may wax enthusiastic about a bit of information that's new to me or to the field: "Have you ever heard of cholecystokin? I hadn't either, until just a couple years ago." I want the mother to feel smart, interested, interesting, and competent.

I don't think I've ever seen a truly yucky baby. Virtually all of them are gorgeous, or have a beautifully shaped head, or marvelous hands, or a wonderful smile, or behave in a way that is bright, or strong, or remarkable. I never feel I'm shading the truth when I remark on a baby's wonderfulness, and any mother loves to hear about it. How you feel about her baby affects how she feels about you. Aren't we lucky that babies are so easy to feel good about! But it's her baby (Smith's Rule 3). No touching until your hands are washed and you've received permission. No taking over the diaper change to save time. No gratuitous holding, no matter how delectable the baby. You'll just have to hope that the mother needs to go to the bathroom (and there had better be a very clean one nearby for her to use), in which case you may be allowed to commune with her little one until she returns.

It's not uncommon for a mother to report that she has left her doctor's office in tears. That should never, never happen with her lactation consultant. She should leave me feeling supported, empowered, listened to. She should feel relieved that a plan is in place, even if we agree that it's a temporary plan. She should feel that she decided on the plan and that it's phrased in ways that make sense to her and adapted to her particular needs. She should feel a weight lift from her own shoulders, without either of us feeling that it has transferred to mine. Rather, she should feel strong enough and supported enough to carry her own burden more easily. How we dress, the settings we choose, our approaches to a consult will all vary from person to person. The lifting of a weight from a client's shoulders, however, should be common to all PPLCs.

SUMMARY

A successful private practice lactation consultant has a deep commitment and desire to succeed in helping women breastfeed and is dedicated to excellent practice in every possible way—professionally, financially, emotionally, and psychologically. A successful PPLC starts with becoming an excellent lactation consultant through formal and continuing education, experience working with mothers, and passing the IBLCE examination. The successful PPLC follows sound business practices in establishing and running her practice as a career—not as a hobby, not as something to do in her spare time, and not because it sounds like a quick and easy way to make money. If you want to help breastfeeding mothers in a less intense way, many breastfeeding advocacy activities and organizations would welcome your involvement. A successful attitude includes cooperation, collaboration, and consultation with other professionals, volunteers, and agencies that interact with mothers and children.

Maybe this section on attitude is really more about how we want the client to *feel* as we say good-bye, rather than about what we want her to *see* when we say hello. Mother Teresa said, "Let no one come to you without leaving better and happier." This is an excellent mission statement for a lactation consultant in private practice!

NOTES

1. Karen Kerkhoff Gromada, RN, MSN, IBCLC, personal communications.

2. I first heard *motherbaby* used as one word by Audrey Naylor, MD, DPH, of Wellstart International.

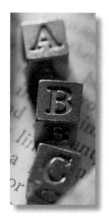

2 Role Clarification

Linda J. Smith, BSE, FACCE, IBCLC

This chapter clarifies the differences and similarities between International Board Certified Lactation Consultants (IBCLCs)[1] and other breastfeeding care providers. This information is provided to help the IBCLC accurately describe her professional qualifications to parents and professionals, possibly seek employment, negotiate third-party reimbursement for her services, and other purposes.

INTRODUCTION

Many different titles and terms are used for those who provide breastfeeding care, or *breastfeeding care providers*. This chapter[2] describes the evolution of breastfeeding care providers and clarifies the differences in training, experience, and competency assessment among them. Breastfeeding care providers addressed here include health care providers who have obtained special education in breastfeeding, La Leche League Leaders,[3,4] breastfeeding peer couselors[5] and helpers, and International Board Certified Lactation Consultants.[6]

BACKGROUND OF PROFESSIONAL LACTATION EDUCATION AND ASSISTANCE/SUPPORT

Effective professional breastfeeding support in the United States has dual roots in medical education and mother-to-mother support. In the 1920s, Dr. Julius P. Sedgwick ran a demonstration project in Minneapolis, Minnesota and concluded that the vast majority of mothers can breastfeed their babies if they have the strong support of their physicians. He advocated for medical faculty to "devote more time to observing and studying this natural function, and less to the study of artificial feeding and formula making." Soon after, Dr. Florence McKay and the Brooklyn Pediatric Society replicated the Minneapolis study in Nassau County, New York and concluded that "Breastfeeding . . . was a matter of medical education and lay instruction." Two decades later, Dr. Edith Jackson observed that in her Rooming-In project in New Haven, Connecticut, "breastfeeding was often 'contagious' because one mother successfully nursing would encourage others to try."[7] Appendix B contains a chronology and a more thorough discussion of the development in the United States of professional lactation education and support from these dual roots.

Lactation Education and Training Programs

There are numerous providers of lactation education programs. Many breast-feeding care providers have obtained their special knowledge through programs listed in the International Lactation Consultant Association's[8] (ILCA) *International Directory of Lactation Management Courses and Programs.*[9] Others have acquired their knowledge through attendance at conferences, workshops, or symposia; by extensive self-study; and from on-the-job experiences in paid or volunteer work. ILCA actively supports the development of varied educational programs in lactation management.

Education and Certification

Taking a course or enrolling in an educational program is an excellent way to obtain knowledge and skills. In addition to education, the principle of passing a standardized criterion-referenced examination as a demonstration of knowledge and competence is well established in the health professions. If completion of an educational program was the sole requirement for demonstrating acquisition of skills and knowledge, licensing and certification boards would not exist. As the Virginia Board of Health Professions states, "Mere participation in an educational activity, no matter how well structured, does not constitute acceptable evidence that competence has been acquired."[10]

Some educational programs offer completion certificates or titles. "Certified Lactation Consultant" and "Certified Lactation Educator" are the most common completion "titles."[11] These completion titles are not equivalent to certification by the International Board of Lactation Consultant Examiners (IBLCE).[12]

The U.S. Department of Health and Human Service (DHHS) sponsored the development of the National Commission on Health Certification Agencies (now NCCA) in 1977. NCCA sets standards for certification agencies. Following NCCA guidelines, the IBLCE developed its international examination in lactation in 1985. IBLCE is accredited by the NCCA.

ILCA is currently developing an international program to accredit educational programs in lactation management. The criteria established for courses listed in ILCA's *International Directory of Lactation Management Courses and Programs* represent a limited, interim step toward international guidelines for lactation education. For further information, see ILCA's *The International Board Certified Lactation Consultant: Scope of Practice and Education Guidelines* in this book's appendices.

OVERLAPPING FUNCTIONS OF BREASTFEEDING CARE PROVIDERS

There is overlap among breastfeeding care providers and other health care providers who supply care and services to the mother–infant dyad. This overlap[13] is in the best interest of mothers and babies because of their many different needs and situations. Overlap generally increases care options for clients and results in better standards of care. The scopes of practice[14] of various breastfeeding care providers compared in this document also overlap in some areas.

Comparison of Functions of Breastfeeding Care Providers

The three most common types of breastfeeding care providers in the United States are peer counselors, La Leche League Leaders,[15] and IBCLCs.[16] This comparison represents the typical functions of the *average* individual breastfeeding care provider in each category.[17] The designations and frequency of performance reflect the minimum expectations for each. Each category will always encompass a range of abilities and skills, from the novice to the expert. The tables in this chapter focus on the services available to mother–baby dyads by breastfeeding care providers. Some are qualified to perform more than one set of functions. Because of the diversity of situations involving breastfeeding care providers, these definitions should be considered guidelines, rather than strict regulations or directives. An individual in a specific setting may also perform functions other than those listed and still be working appropriately and within her respective scope of practice.

Designations and Abbreviations Used in Tables[18]

Italics = Mandatory, primary, or major function. These are core competencies, expected of all in this category.
Regular type = Permitted, possible, or contributing
CE = Continuing Education
MD, RN, RD = Medical Doctor, Registered Nurse, Registered Dietitian
LC = Lactation consultant (IBCLC)
> = greater than
< = less than

Promotion of Breastfeeding and Breastfeeding Services to the Public

The larger role of promoting breastfeeding to the general public and professional community is addressed by ILCA, La Leche League, and many other organizations in a rich variety of ways. Both ILCA and LLLI have many more services available to their members and the general public than are described in this document. Information on these services and programs is available from each organization.

> Responsibility for health promotion is shared by the individual, the family, the community, health professionals, the media, and governments.[33]

Comparison of Typical Scopes of Practice

Breastfeeding care is *part* of the scope of practice for physicians, midwives, nurses, dietitians, and other health care providers. Breastfeeding care is the *entire* scope of practice of lactation consultants. If a lactation consultant (or other breastfeeding care provider) is credentialed in another field, she may provide other kinds of care or services *in addition* to breastfeeding care. Table 2.5[34] compares the various published scopes of practice of three common providers: Registered Nurses (RN), Registered Dietitians (RD), and International Board Certified Lactation Consultants (IBCLC).

TABLE 2.1 Scope of Practice

Scope of Practice	Peer Counselor	LLL Leader	IBCLC
Education and training	*Personal experience >3 months* *Training by agency* Conferences/workshops	*Personal experience >12 months* *Apprenticeship 12+ months* *Directed reading* *Accept LLL principles* Conferences/workshops Self-directed reading	4-year degree 2500+ hours contact with mothers *Specific CE programs* Personal experience Specific courses Apprenticeships/mentorships Conferences/workshops Self-directed reading Specific alternate pathways
Competency assessment	*Agency requirements*	*LLLI requirements* *Evaluation panel*	*IBLCE requirements* *Criterion-referenced exam*
Continuing competency	Agency requirements	CE encouraged	*Recertification by exam every 10 years* CE option every other 5-year period
Supervision	Agency rules	*LLLI structure*	*Standards of Practice* *Code of Ethics* Agency rules
Availability	On schedule	As time permits	*On schedule*; coverage must be arranged
Compensation	Agency policy	Volunteer	Agency rules Client payment Third-party payment
Discipline and accountability	*Agency requirements* Personal liability	*LLLI Procedures Handbook* Deaccreditation *LLLI insurance* Personal liability	*IBLCE discipline panel* Decertification *Malpractice insurance* Agency/employer actions Termination Personal liability
Scope of practice	*Agency policy* Some state agencies have policies[19]	*LLLI Leader Handbook* *Breastfeeding Answer Book*	*Standards of Practice for Lactation Consultants* Agency rules

TABLE 2.2 Educational/Promotional Functions

Function	Peer Counselor	LLL Leader	IBCLC
Contact initiated by	Agency	Mother	Agency, MD[20] or client, other providers
Influence the decision to breastfeed	Frequent	Sometimes	Sometimes
Conduct support groups	Sometimes	*Primary*	Rare
Teach/conduct formal classes	Sometimes	Rare[21]	*Primary*
Phone help to mother	Frequent	*Primary*	Frequent
Long-term breastfeeding	Frequent	*Primary*[22]	Frequent
Explain normal breastfeeding	*Primary*	*Primary*	Frequent
Social issues	*Primary*	*Primary*	Frequent
Encouragement	*Primary*	*Primary*	Frequent
In-service, professional education	Rare	Sometimes	*Primary*

TABLE 2.3   One-to One Clinical and Practical Support

Function	Peer Counselor	LLL Leader	IBCLC
First feedings	Rare[23]	Rare[24]	*Primary*[25]
Minor breastfeeding problems	Frequent	Frequent	Frequent
Breastfeeding crisis intervention	Sometimes; refers to LC and primary providers	Sometimes; works mainly with mother[26]	*Primary*[27]; works with mother and primary provider
Major breastfeeding problems	Sometimes; works with LC and primary providers	Sometimes; works mainly with mother	*Primary*; works with mother and primary provider
Physical contact with mother and baby	Rare	Sometimes	*Primary*
Breast assessment	No	Rare[28]	*Primary*
Baby oral assessment	No	No	*Primary*
Weigh baby	Rare	No	Frequent
Dispense equipment	Sometimes	Sometimes	*Primary*
Hospital visits	Sometimes	Rare	*Primary*
Office visits	Frequent	Rare	*Primary*
Home visits	Frequent	Sometimes	*Primary*

TABLE 2.4   Administration, Documentation, and Other Functions

Function	Peer Counselor	LLL Leader	IBCLC
Written documentation	Frequent Agency policy	*Primary* LLLI guidelines	*Primary* Detailed documentation
References used	Agency policy	LLLI guidelines	Professional sources
Written care plans	Rare	No	*Primary*
Written information on problem	To mother only	To mother primarily	To mother and primary provider
Direct contact with MDs	No	Rare[29]	*Primary*
Referrals; many mothers self-refer to breastfeeding counselors	*Agency policy* To LC To supervising MD, RN, RD, other To LLL groups	*Leader Handbook* LLLI policy[30]	*Written/oral reports to primary provider* *Mother and baby must have primary provider* Agency rules To MD To other LCs To other allied professionals To LLL, peer counselor, groups
Research	Rare	Rare[31]	Frequent
Policy formation	Sometimes	Sometimes	Frequent
Materials development	Sometimes	Sometimes[32]	Frequent

TABLE 2.5   Providers' Scopes of Practice

Nurse (RN)	Dietitian (RD)	Lactation Consultant (IBCLC)
Performs physical assessment	Assesses nutritional status of clients	Assesses the breastfeeding process and mother and baby related to breastfeeding
States nursing diagnoses	Designs diets for special needs	Generates lactation/breastfeeding analysis
Writes nursing care plan	Writes nutritional care plan	Writes lactation/breastfeeding care plan
Provides comprehensive health teaching for all aspects of maternal and child care	Provides nutrition education on values of certain foods, age-appropriate diet, textures, and progression	Provides theoretical and practical breastfeeding education to parents, public, and professionals
Completes necessary documentation	Completes nutritional documentation	Completes lactation documentation
Assesses client against health norms, identifies deviations, and generates referrals	Assesses client against nutritional norms, identifies deviations, and generates referrals	Assesses client against lactation norms, identifies deviations, and generates referrals
Assists in initiating breastfeeding	Encourages human milk feedings	Assists in initiating breastfeeding
Evaluates effectiveness of care plan strategy implementation and modifies it as needed	Assesses intakes, evaluates nutritional value of foods, and makes recommendations	Evaluates breastfeeding process and makes modifications as needed
Addresses physical and psychosocial issues affecting human system	Addresses nutritional needs of mother, partially breastfed babies, and breastfed babies with problems	Addresses all physical and psychosocial issues affecting breastfeeding
Provides anticipatory guidance and takes measures to assure follow-up	Provides anticipatory guidance, encourages continued breastfeeding, and discourages inappropriate supplemental and complementary feeds	Provides long-term follow-up and assistance through entire continuum of breastfeeding, from prenatal care through weaning

The rationale for all professional credentialing is public protection. The United States has a myriad of regulatory processes, including accreditation, certification, and licensure. "Healthcare credentialing is important because it is central to the core issues facing the healthcare system today: competition, specialization, quality, cost-effectiveness, access to care, and management of legal risks Accreditation, certification, and other credentials may be more essential in healthcare than in any other field. This is because in no other field do consumers care so much about the quality of services and yet have so little ability to judge that quality themselves."[35] Competence in the skills and knowledge known as lactation management is subject to the same discussions as competence in other subjects. The "determination of professional competence in the United States is based on complicated and interrelated processes of education, licensing, certification, and recredentialing."[36]

Concerns have been raised that only licensed health professionals are appropriate providers of lactation management services or lactation counseling. This controversy appears to be based on the following suppositions:

1. *Licensure provides a mechanism to remove the incompetent or unethical practitioner.*

   Although this is true for general incompetency or lack of ethics, no licensing boards thoroughly examine competency or ethics related to breastfeeding management. Both LLLI and IBLCE provide disciplinary measures

EDUCATION, TITLES, AND CREDENTIALS

to remove an incompetent or unethical practitioner, or a practitioner who is working outside their clearly defined scopes of practice.

IBCLCs and LLL Leaders have professional liability insurance available to them for their work as breastfeeding care providers. LLLI provides liability insurance for Leaders working as volunteers within LLL's guidelines. In its 40 years of experience, LLLI has never had a liability suit charged against a representative. Professional malpractice insurance is available to IBCLC's through several private agencies that also insure nurses, dietitians, certified childbirth educators, and other allied health professionals (see Appendix A for insurance information).

2. *Licensure provides assurance of clinical judgment.* This idea is sometimes stated as a concern that *only licensed care providers can recognize illness in the mother or baby.*

Clinical judgment has been described as the ability to differentiate normal from abnormal. According to many professionals, clinical judgment is not acquired from taking any particular course, but rather from seeing many examples of both abnormal and normal.

Many of the issues addressed by breastfeeding care providers involve identification and explanation of normal behaviors. When the unusual or abnormal situation presents itself, it is obviously not the norm and is appropriately referred. Procedures for referral and collaboration, and their roles as members of the health care team, are clearly defined in Scope of Practice documents of LLL Leaders and IBCLCs.[37] Recognition of obvious infant or maternal illness is expected of all breastfeeding care providers.

PUBLIC PROTECTION IN LACTATION MANAGEMENT

There are two legally protected, copyrighted titles referring to breastfeeding care providers:

• International Board Certified Lactation Consultant (IBCLC)
• La Leche League Leader (LLL Leader).

Holders of these copyrighted titles share three characteristics:

• Clearly defined, published scopes of practice
• Disciplinary requirements intrinsic to certification
• Extensive experience in working with normal lactation

HEALTH GOALS

More than decade ago, *Healthy People 2000: National Health Promotion and Disease Prevention Objectives* included the following goal: "Increase to at least 75% the proportion of women who breastfeed their babies in the early postpartum period, to 50% the proportion who continue breastfeeding until their babies are 5-6 months old." The *National Objectives* for 2010 include "increase to 25% the proportion who continue breastfeeding for 12 months." Breastfeeding success has two basic facets: (1) the decision to initiate breastfeeding, and (2) continuance until the mother reaches her self-set goal.[38] Breastfeeding promotion alone is not enough to meet the *Year 2010* goals;[39] it is also necessary to create a safety net for mothers who initiate breastfeeding.[40] The United States joined 29 other nations in declaring that "All women should be enabled to practice exclusive breastfeeding and all infants should be fed exclusively on breastmilk until 4–6 months of age. Thereafter, children should continue to be breastfed, while receiving appropriate and adequate complementary foods, for up to two years of age or beyond."[41] WHO's current (2001) population-based infant-feeding recommendation reads: "To achieve optimal growth, development and health, infants should be exclusively breastfed for the first six months of life. Thereafter, to meet their evolving nutritional requirements, infants should receive nutritionally adequate and safe complementary foods while breastfeeding continues for up to two years of age or beyond." Meeting these goals will require a concerted and joint effort from all care providers. A crucial factor will be the availability of sufficiently skilled, timely, and cost-effective breastfeeding help to all mothers. This information is provided to assist agencies, employers, and other providers in tailoring a local breastfeeding support network to meet specific community needs.

SUMMARY

IBCLCs are first and foremost professional breastfeeding care providers. Some IBCLCs also hold credentials as registered nurses, pharmacists, La Leche League Leaders, midwives, childbirth educators, or other health-related professions.

All breastfeeding care providers are, by definition, dedicated to helping mothers breastfeed their babies. For breastfeeding to succeed, the mother and baby must function smoothly as a team. A mother must learn to read and respond to her infant's cues with appropriate actions. Likewise, for breastfeeding assistance to succeed, breastfeeding care providers need to work as a team. They respond to mothers' needs with appropriate actions. For every mother who is helped by one kind of assistance, another needs something totally different to fulfill her breastfeeding goals. Appropriate referrals and collaboration go both ways: True teamwork exists when volunteer counselors work closely with paid providers, physicians work closely with allied health professionals, and mothers and babies benefit from the help that best suits them in their unique situations. In this manner will breastfeeding become the community norm.[42]

NOTES

1. *Lactation consultant:* A health care professional whose scope of practice is focused on providing education and management to prevent and solve breastfeeding problems and encouraging a social environment that effectively supports the breastfeeding mother–baby dyad. "ILCA acknowledges the IBLCE examination as the professional credential for lactation consultants."

2. Much of this information was prepared for the Ohio Department of Health and the U.S. Department of Health and Human Services (1991–1993) in response to confusion about various titles and credentials of breastfeeding specialists and counselors.

3. La Leche League International (LLLI) was founded in 1956 to give information and encouragement, mainly through personal help, to all mothers who want to breastfeed their babies. While complementing the care of the physician and other health care providers, it recognizes the unique impor-

tance of one mother helping another to perceive the needs of her child and to learn the best means of fulfilling those needs. LLLI is an independent corporation.

4. La Leche League International has published standards for their accredited Leaders. Other breastfeeding mother-support groups may have published standards for their affiliated group leaders, and should be contacted directly for that information.

5. *Peer counselor:* An individual whose most relevant qualification is her own personal experience in breastfeeding her baby. She provides assistance to breastfeeding mothers by active listening, asking questions, and giving information and suggestions regarding the normal course of breastfeeding. She is supervised according to the rules of the agency for which she works as a volunteer or paid peer counselor.

6. An International Board Certified Lactation Consultant is a person who has passed the examination sponsored by the

International Board of Lactation Consultant Examiners. Pathway A Eligibility criteria include a baccalaureate (four-year) degree or higher, minimum 2500 hours practice as a breastfeeding consultant, and minimum 30 hours of continuing education related to breastfeeding within the three years before sitting for the exam. Since its inception in 1985, IBLCE has always recommended a four-year degree as a basic entry criterion but had no legal basis for requiring it. Beginning with the 1988 exam, sufficient data had been compiled to legally defend that criterion and the alternate pathways. According to the National Commission for Certifying Agencies, all entry barriers, including academic requirements, must be legally defensible and based on rigorous job relevancy criteria. Recertification by examination is mandatory at least every 10 years; this process ensures continued competency in basic skills and knowledge. Recertification by continuing education is acceptable for one five-year period between recertifications by examination; this ongoing effort helps expand the knowledge and skill base of the practitioner.

7. Lawrence, Ruth. *Breastfeeding, A Guide for the Medical Profession*, 4th ed., p. 634. St. Louis: C.V. Mosby, 1994.

8. International Lactation Consultant Association is a worldwide association for health professionals with special interest in breastfeeding. ILCA has developed and published *Standards of Practice for Lactation Consultants*, which provides guidelines for practice.

9. Available from ILCA and on ILCA's Internet site, www.ILCA.org.

10. Commonwealth of Virginia Revised Code, sec. 54.1-100.

11. None of the unprotected "titles" has any disciplinary requirement associated with use of the title. None of these programs requires personal breastfeeding experience.

12. International Board of Lactation Consultant Examiners was established to develop and administer a voluntary certification program for lactation consultants that includes a recertification process. The exam is offered in several languages in many sites around the world.

13. Stromberg, Clifford. *Healthcare Credentialing: Implications for Academic Health Centers*. Washington, DC: Report to the Association of Academic Health Centers, 1991, p. 3.

14. Formalized scope of practice documents for breastfeeding care providers are being developed. Scope of practice documents for licensed health care providers may not address breastfeeding or lactation.

15. A La Leche League Leader is an accredited breastfeeding care provider representing La Leche League International. LLL Leaders are mothers who have fulfilled LLLI's requirements for Leadership and been accredited by LLLI. Volunteer LLL Leaders are experienced breastfeeding mothers and are familiar with research and current findings dealing with breastfeeding. They offer practical information and moral support to nursing mothers through monthly meetings and telephone help.

16. The information in this section is derived from a Key Informant Survey I performed in 1991. Twenty-six breastfeeding care providers from 15 states, representing a broad diversity of backgrounds, provided data for this comparison.

17. I originally prepared this chart for ILCA and LLLI. It was submitted jointly for DHHS's Role Delineation Project in 1993 but was not used in the final document.

18. References used for Peer Counselor activities: *Peer Counselor Training Manuals* from Washington, D.C., Tennessee, Texas, Illinois, and Mississippi. References for LLL Leader activities: *The New LLLI Leader's Handbook*, LLLI 1989, and *The Breastfeeding Answer Book*, LLLI 1991. References for IBCLC activities: *Recommendations and Competencies for Lactation Consultant Practice*, ILCA 1991, and recommended by IBLCE; *Exam Blueprint/Task Analysis* data, IBLCE 1985; *Standards of Practice for Lactation Consultants*, ILCA 1995.

19. *Breastfeeding Support Policies for the Ohio Department of Health WIC and CFHS Programs*, 1993.

20. May include any primary care provider: MD, DO, CNM, advanced practice nurse.

21. LLL developed a Breastfeeding Class program that has been implemented in some geographic areas. Teaching classes is an optional role of the LLL Leader.

22. Natural, baby-led weaning and supporting the mother's choice of long-term breastfeeding are especially well supported by LLL Leaders.

23. Not required, but if present in the first few hours and days, may assist.

24. Not expected, but if present may assist.

25. Very frequent, unless LC works only in outpatient setting.

26. LLL's Professional Liaison Department, Medical Associates Program, and the Professional Advisory Board are important resources for the LLL Leader. All materials published by LLLI are carefully reviewed by the Professional Advisory Board.

27. LCs are expected to work collaboratively with the primary provider as part of a team approach.

28. Permitted, but rarely done; only by very experienced Leaders.

29. LLL strongly encourages the mother to stay in contact with and dialogue with her primary care provider(s) regarding the situation; rarely does the Leader contact the physician directly. A Leader may contact a physician without referencing a particular mother.

30. LLL's Professional Liaison Department, Medical Associates Program, and the Professional Advisory Board are important resources for the LLL Leader. All materials published by LLLI are carefully reviewed by the Professional Advisory Board.

31. Service provided by LLLI.

32. Service provided by LLLI.

33. Sharbaugh, Carolyn S., ed. *Call to Action: Better Nutrition for Mothers, Children, and Families*. Washington, DC: Maternal and Child Health Interorganizational Group, sponsored by the Maternal and Child Health Bureau, HRSA, Public Health Service, U.S. Department of Health and Human Services, 1990.

34. Developed in early 1993 from interagency and interdisciplinary resources.

35. Stromberg, Clifford. *Healthcare Credentialing: Implications for Academic Health Centers*. Washington, DC: Report to the Association of Academic Health Centers, 1991, p. 1.

36. Martini, C. Evaluating the competence of health professions. *JAMA* 260:1057-1058 (1988). Quoted by Stromberg, p. 1.

37. *The New LLLI Leader's Handbook*, 1989; *The Breastfeeding Answer Book*, 1991; both published by LLLI. *Standards of Practice for Lactation Consultants*, 1995. *Code of Ethics for International Board Certified Lactation Consultants*, 1995. IBLCE requires candidates to provide character and competency information in their applications for IBLCE Certification Examination.

38. Inch, Sally. Antenatal preparation for breastfeeding. In *Effective Care in Pregnancy and Childbirth, Vol 1: Pregnancy*. Oxford University Press, 1989.

39. Baer, E. C. Promoting breastfeeding: A national responsibility. *Studies in Family Planning* 12:198, 1981.

40. McIntyre, E. Breastfeeding management: Helping the mother help herself. *Breastfeeding Review*, July 1991, 129-131; Botroff, Joan L. Persistence in breastfeeding: A phenomonological investigation. *Journal of Advanced Nursing*, 12:201-209, 1990; Auerbach, Kathleen G. Guilt, grief, and maternal regret. *Journal of Human Lactation*, March 1986, 70-71; Verronen, P. Breastfeeding: reasons for giving up and transient lactational crises. *Acta Paediatrica Scandia*, 71:447-450, 1982; DaVanza J., et al. Do women's breastfeeding experiences with their firstborns affect whether they breastfeed their subsequent children? *Social Biology*, 37:223-232, 1990.

41. Innocenti Declaration on the Protection, Promotion, and Support of Breastfeeding, 1990, signed by Dr. Audrey Nora on behalf of the United States.

42. Koop, C. Everett. U.S. Surgeon General. *Report of the Surgeon General's Workshop on Breastfeeding and Human Lactation*, 1984.

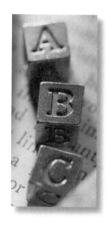

3 Becoming a Lactation Consultant

Carol Ryan, RN, BSN, IBCLC
Linda J. Smith, BSE, FACCE, IBCLC

If you're going to do it, do it right.

The journey to becoming a lactation consultant demands dedication and commitment to the work and energy involved in attaining this goal. The profession of lactation consultation brings an awesome sense of responsibility; tending to the health and welfare of mothers and their infants carries the specter of mature, responsible practice of breastfeeding management. It cannot be taken lightly, nor is it a quick way to make extra or a lot of money.

We use the term *lactation consultant* to mean an International Board Certified Lactation Consultant (IBCLC)—an individual who obtains and maintains certification through the International Board of Lactation Consultant Examiners (IBLCE). No other "title" provides the same degree of public protection as this international criterion-referenced credential.

The three requirements for certification are academic preparation, specific education in lactation, and experience helping breastfeeding mothers. This chapter describes these requirements, then concludes with a brief overview of the professional responsibilities of lactation consultants.

ACADEMIC PREPARATION

Becoming a professional lactation consultant is roughly equivalent to getting a master's degree in a health field. More than 80 percent of currently certified lactation consultants have bachelor's degrees in a health-related profession, and the majority of those are registered nurses or licensed midwives. Others have degrees in nutrition/dietetics, physical or speech therapy, or allied health fields. A growing number of physicians are validating their special knowledge of breastfeeding by taking the IBLCE exam, and even a few pharmacists have joined the ranks of IBCLCs.

To provide breastfeeding support as a professional, you will need at least a baccalaureate degree, preferably in a health-related field. If your degree was obtained in an unrelated field, plan to take additional social and physical science courses related or relevant to breastfeeding, nutrition, counseling, research, and human development. Starting in 2003, coursework in anatomy and physiology, sociology, psychology or counseling, child development, nutrition, and medical terminology will be a prerequisite to taking the exam (see *www.IBLCE.org* for more details).

Part of your education must include developing effective counseling skills. By this, we do not mean "counseling" as a politically correct way of telling a mother what she should do. Rather, it means being able to really listen to her (or a colleague) to identify and validate the other person's feelings and needs during an interaction, before attempting to problem-solve. La Leche League's *Human Relations Enrichment* course and training manual is one excellent way to learn listening and communication skills specific to lactation.

If you do not have a health-related degree or have no college education, seriously consider enrolling in a professional nursing or midwifery program. Begin from the ground level and build upon your education. A baccalaureate or master's degree program is ideal. Pursuing a two- or three-year RN program is the minimum preparation if you have some college background in another field. Realistically, a nursing license will open many doors for you because hospitals and health agencies often require a nursing license in addition to IBCLC certification. At this writing, the few non-nurse IBCLCs employed by hospitals or health agencies are either licensed in a related allied health field (speech therapist, registered dietitian, and so on) or were long-term volunteer breastfeeding counselors in mother-support groups (such as La Leche League or Nursing Mothers Councils) with literally decades of experience.

SPECIFIC EDUCATION IN LACTATION

Read (and preferably purchase) several professional texts in lactation. (See Appendix B or visit http://www.iblce.org/suggested_reading_list.htm.) There is simply no substitute for becoming intimately familiar with the published literature and evidence-based research relevant to breastfeeding and human lactation. An excellent overview and summary of the body of knowledge is the *Core Curriculum for Lactation Consultant Practice* (http://www.ilca.org/pub.html). Membership in the International Lactation Consultant Association (ILCA) will provide the networking system, annual conferences, and, most importantly, the *Journal of Human Lactation*.

Starting in 2003, there will be requirement of a minimum of 45 documented clock hours of specific education in lactation, reflecting the Exam Content Outline (http://www.iblce.org/exam_blueprint.htm), in the three years immediately preceding sitting for the certification examination. We strongly recommend taking a comprehensive lactation management course, or even several of these courses. Most of the lactation management courses currently offered do not require any prerequisite other than interest, time, and money. Some courses are taught through colleges or universities, while private companies or individuals sponsor others. Distance-learning programs and Internet-based courses are available if you cannot travel to take a course. As of this writing, two U.S. universities offer degree programs related to human lactation: The Union Institute in Cincinnati, Ohio, and Pacific Oaks College in California (see Appendix B for details). The ILCA maintains an updated list of educational programs on its Web site (http://www.ilca.org/courses.html). In the future, preparation courses will be accredited through the International Lactation Education Accreditation Council.

Counseling skills are crucially important to lactation consultant practice. One of the best avenues to learn these skills is through La Leche League's Human Relations Enrichment (HRE) course and workbook. Even if you have taken other courses in counseling, the HRE program is valuable as it focuses on breastfeeding issues (see www.lalecheleague.org).

If you are just beginning your education, you may be overwhelmed by the breadth and depth of the material covered in a comprehensive lactation management course. Stick with it! In addition to pursuing your targeted study, attend meetings of breastfeeding coalitions and as many continuing-education seminars and conferences as possible.

BREASTFEEDING MANAGEMENT EXPERIENCE

Breastfeeding management experience is probably the most difficult, and yet the most important, area of preparation. Academic preparation and lactation-specific education involve studying breastfeeding "from the outside, looking in." You also need to fully grasp what breastfeeding is *like* for the mother–baby dyad—"from the inside, looking out." The only effective way to do so is by listening to many, many breastfeeding mothers and the day-to-day, hour-to-hour issues that concern them. Attending several extended series of mother-support group meetings is one excellent way of learning breastfeeding from the inside out (see Shadowing Guidelines, Appendix B).

Listen to your friends who are breastfeeding. Ask your mother, aunt, grandmother, sister, and/or cousin what breastfeeding was (or is) like for them—the good parts and the bad parts; what they liked and what they didn't like; who and what helped; and what hurt or caused a problem. Attend breastfeeding mother-support groups in your area—a lot of them, over a lengthy period of time. Read books on breastfeeding that are written for mothers, by mothers. Do not analyze or try to solve anyone's problems at this point—just listen. Focus on the experience of the *mothers*.

You most definitely need to connect with mothers to succeed in lactation consultant practice. This means you must be able to listen to and validate their concerns at all contact points—before trying to help solve their problems, during the consult, and as part of follow-up—interspersed throughout all your interactions with them. To achieve this goal, you may need help working through your *own* personal breastfeeding experience(s) or lack thereof. This statement is especially true if your own experience was less than "ideal" or less than you wanted it to be. Whether you work alone or with one or more trusted colleagues or professional counselors who are sensitive to the importance of breastfeeding, take the time to figure out what you did right, what went wrong, who supported you and who didn't, what kind of support you valued most, what you needed and received (or didn't get), and other emotionally charged issues. Keep working through your own experience(s) until you are at peace with all of your feelings about your own personal breastfeeding experience(s).

IBLCE requires 2500 hours of "breastfeeding consultancy" as a prerequisite to taking the exam. In other words, you need to be the "helper," directly in contact with breastfeeding dyads—in either a paid or a volunteer position. However, there's a risk to mothers and babies if totally unprepared people start giving breastfeeding advice. We strongly advise you to locate and work closely with a mentor, guide, or teacher who has been an IBCLC for at least five years. Be prepared to volunteer your time and/or pay your mentor. It takes time for a mentor to supervise a novice, and the mentor's time is very valuable.

We also urge you to accumulate your experience hours in a wide range of situations and settings. Try to work with and learn from premature babies through toddlers, mothers from different religions and cultures, rich and poor women, young and mature mothers, healthy and sick women, mothers of first babies, and mothers of multiples. Ideally, you should spend a substantial amount of time (measured in months or years, not days) in a group setting where you can discuss your work with other colleagues. Even though you will probably end up practicing in your own neighborhood, breastfeeding transcends age, nationality, and culture. Take your time—rushing this process does not work well, and it is good practice toward learning to work at the baby's pace.

Anyone can claim to be a "lactation consultant" and hang out a private practice shingle, but only IBCLCs have the highly respected IBLCE credential to support their practice. The IBCLC designation is legally defensible. Parents demand the right to protection and care that is focused on their health and welfare. IBCLCs are legally responsible for the care they give, and they are members of a medical health care team centered on the needs and concerns of the individual families they serve.

PROFESSIONAL RESPONSIBILITIES

Professional Credentials

The International Board of Lactation Consultant Examiners (IBLCE) is the official certification board for lactation consultants (see Appendix A). This body was established in 1985 by a small group of very experienced La Leche League International (LLLI) leaders dedicated to the realization that specific standards and requirements were needed by those assisting mothers and babies with breastfeeding needs and concerns above and beyond the basics of breastfeeding support. IBLCE is a nonprofit corporation fully accredited by the U.S. National Organization for Competency Assessment (NOCA).

Several professions are uniquely intertwined in the common goal of lactation management. To ensure consistency among practitioners, IBLCE has set very specific standard requirements for all those choosing to sit for its certification examination. Although the majority of IBCLCs are Registered Nurses (RN), other professions are represented as well: nutritionists; medical doctors; anthropologists; occupational, speech, and physical therapists; childbirth educators; researchers; volunteer breastfeeding support group counselors; and maternal child health advocates. The contributions and focus of these varied professionals add to the common goal of providing the best evidenced-based information, support, and encouragement of breastfeeding.

Due to the worldwide recognition of the IBCLC credential, international, national, and governmental bodies alike welcome and respect the inclusion of IBCLCs as allied health care providers within their scopes of service. As more health care providers and third-party payers recognize the value and contributions of IBCLCs, it is understandable that their numbers are growing in tandem.

Professional Association

Every profession of note has its own professional organization. The International Lactation Consultant Association (ILCA) serves more than 4000 IBCLCs, allied health professionals, medical personnel, breastfeeding and human milk advocates, and breastfeeding volunteers worldwide. ILCA was incorporated in 1985 with the purpose of establishing a professional network to support, protect, and promote breastfeeding. It has established guidelines for competent, ethical, evidenced-based lactation consultation practice.[1] It has fostered development of professional standards and ethical practice for lactation consultants (see Appendix A). It has developed materials to inform all health care professionals of the importance of human milk and breast-feeding and the consequences and risks of not breastfeeding.[2] Research in all aspects of lactation, human milk, and infant feeding are supported as well. ILCA stands firm in its support of the *International Code of Marketing Breast Milk Substitutes* and its subsequent resolutions. (See Appendix A for a brief summary of the *Code* and details of how to get more information.)

ILCA supports its global membership through its peer-reviewed, scientific *Journal of Human Lactation*; a Web-based newsletter, the *ILCA Globe*; and the published *Standards of Practice*, which contributes to ethical private practice. ILCA has also published numerous position papers, sponsors an annual international conference, bestows research grants, awards scholarships for the annual conference, has innumerable volunteer positions for active member participation, lists affiliate and sister groups, and provides access to Independent Study Modules for continuing education (CERP) credits. ILCA participates within a global forum with nongovernmental organization (NGO) status with both UNICEF and the World Health Organization (WHO). Its official memberships in other organizations include the World Health Assembly, Codex Alimentarius, the International Board of Lactation Consultant Examiners, the U.S. Breastfeeding Committee, Healthy Mothers/Healthy Babies Coalition, the USDA Breastfeeding Promotion Consortium, and the Healthy People 2000/2010 Coalition (see www.ILCA.org and Appendix A).

Just as the IBCLC credential enhances your creditability as a private practice lactation consultant, so membership in the ILCA enhances your creditability as a professional. Listing the credential and professional organization on a résumé adds to your desirability when seeking employment and especially when marketing your practice. Your IBCLC and ILCA connections speak volumes about your commitment and dedication.

You're Visible Now

Everyone is noticing; everyone is watching. Whether you like it or not, you are continually advocating and modeling your profession, breastfeeding, human milk use, and mothers and their children. The way in which you conduct yourself in public, your work setting and environment, your dress, your attitude, your manner of speaking, your treatment of others (whether other LCs or professional workers), your interpersonal relationships, even the presentation of your health care provider reports speak loudly and clearly about you and what you represent! IBCLCs are becoming more prominent in the health care environment. And people are noticing!

This public scrutiny is not new: Every new profession pays its dues. Advocacy is one vital component of what lactation consultants do. Actively participating in task forces, joining committees on all levels, letter writing, keeping current on local and national events, and working for global support when and where applicable are the driving forces that contribute to the growing awareness and acceptance of breastfeeding and human milk for human infants and children (see Part C). Do consider the consequences of isolation common to private practice. Step outside the box, and move forward one small step at a time to do your part by sharing your passion and dedication. Consider the beneficiaries!

Stay Connected

Establish and maintain a cordial working relationship with your community, specifically local mother–baby breastfeeding support groups. If the private practice lactation consultant is respectful of the groups' intent, shows and offers gracious acceptance, and makes herself available, then harmony usually follows. The training and level of professional responsibility in these groups may be different from yours, but the goal of breastfeeding mothers and infants is the same. Availability and willingness to assist when asked, to support with current materials, and to provide referrals all help share the task of promoting, supporting, and protecting human milk for human infants one community at a time. Life is too short, time too precious, and babies too dear to be territorial.

AFTER CERTIFICATION, THEN WHAT?

You're not finished—in fact, you are just getting started. Continue to gain experience, preferably in several different settings and with a variety of colleagues. Read the other parts of this book, and keep planning. The rest of Part A explores the personal side of PPLC work, including options for supporting breastfeeding in other venues.

SUMMARY

Becoming a competent professional lactation consultant calls for college-level academic preparation, specific education in breastfeeding and human lactation, substantial experience helping breastfeeding mothers, certification by the International Board of Lactation Consultant Examiners, and ongoing maintenance of skills and knowledge through continuing education and other self-directed learning experiences.

NOTES

1. *Evidence-Based Guidelines for Breastfeeding Management During the First Fourteen Days*. Raleigh, NC: International Lactation Consultant Association, 1999.

2. *Summary of the Hazards of Infant Formula*. Raleigh, NC: International Lactation Consultant Association, 1991.

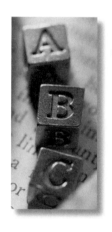

4 Pitfalls Related to Attitudes

Diane Wiessinger, MS, IBCLC

Every profession, however wonderful, has its pitfalls. Some of the pitfalls, like the grime on the car mechanic's hands, are a function of the actual work. Others, like the mechanic's frustration with the manufacturer and the issues covered in this chapter, derive more from attitude. Lactation consultants (LCs) in private practice are susceptible to loneliness, over-involvement with their clients, and a tendency to see the abnormal in the normal. Sadly, we also have a tendency to see and work with the abnormal. We are lured by the promise of a quick fix and easy money if we use certain technologies, and like members of many other professions we endure personality clashes and professional disagreements. Unlike many other professionals, however, we don't have large salaries to compensate for our troubles. But there are coping techniques. And there are rewards—oh yes, there are rewards.

ISOLATION

There are three groups of workers I envy. One is the group whose co-workers grow older along with them. That description fits just about anyone who works in a traditional workplace. You start fresh out of school, get a few promotions, and rub elbows with colleagues of assorted ages at each level, but generally you can find peers of your own age. You don't find yourself entering menopause while every client with whom you work is entering parenthood.

The second is the group whose work isn't important. Everyone's work is important, of course, but if you make quilts, and someone doesn't buy your quilt, his IQ doesn't drop as a result. His risk of contracting a host of illnesses doesn't rise. His relationship with his mother doesn't change. If you go on vacation and lose some business, the only one who loses, really, is you.

The third group I envy is the group whose members do their work with co-workers nearby. I'm sure the cubicle employees envy me my solitude and flexibility, but oh, to be able to chat with another human without having to pick up the phone or arrange a lunch date!

LCs in private practice are isolated temporally, emotionally, and physically. We are isolated temporally in that we start out helping women who share our stage of life. We may demonstrate positioning using our own baby or model the simplicity of breastfeeding just by inviting a mother over to our house for an hour. For a long time, I saw myself as a fellow-traveler on my clients' road. Gradually, I realized that they probably saw me as comparable to a much older sister. It's only now beginning to dawn on me that I could be their mother. The grandmothers and I share more cultural history than the mothers and I do. When did this transition happen? How many years has it been since my shirt got damp when I demonstrated hand expression? In the past, it wasn't unusual to have a lasting friendship grow out of a long and complicated client situation or to find a real soul mate among the local La Leche League Leaders. I'm not sure that such events will happen much any more. In my transient college community, as my old friends leave, where will my new friends come from?

The emotional isolation comes from our inability to share the passion, the interest, or even the nuts and bolts of this profession with most people. When a woman says she's a schoolteacher, her partner in conversation can continue with, "Oh really? Which school? What grade? What's your opinion of the latest school referendum? Do you know Sally Ann?" When a woman says she's a lactation consultant, she must first explain what that means, then conversation is likely to stop. Almost as painful, she may have to listen to why her partner in conversation was unable to breastfeed or hear misinformation presented in such a way that there's no tactful way to offer corrections. If asked to elaborate on what she does, she may find herself groping for some cocktail party-level description of a field that encompasses women's rights, child development, history, politics, medicine, human relations, and economic forces. At least she can treat herself to some extra hors d'oeuvres afterward, on the grounds that explaining what she does uses more calories than the schoolteacher's explanation requires.

The physical isolation comes from not having a fellow private-practice IBCLC within 20 miles, or 100. Most of the other health care workers in town disagree with her, if not fundamentally then certainly in the details, making relationships with them just another form of work. Sharing a practice can be difficult, except in larger communities, and a large number of us work alone. That's part of what makes conferences so wonderful. The friends that we make through e-mail come alive for us at conferences. We chatter, we sparkle, we laugh. The air at breastfeeding conferences fairly crackles with energy. And then we get on the planes—a handful of us on each one, reminiscing at the gate. Then we change planes, and only one of us is left at the next gate. The good news is that bits of the energy we generated are carried in every direction, sometimes halfway around the world. The sad news is that, by the time that energy has been diluted by all those miles, there's still only one private-practice LC in town, and her nearest fellow PPLC is 20 miles away, or 100.

At first, the LC's passion for her profession is likely to carry her along, and it may be years before she realizes that she needs to hoard her emotional resources. Taking care of herself involves a multitude of little indulgences. The checklist on the following page includes some possibilities.

HOW TO CONSERVE YOUR EMOTIONAL RESOURCES

✔ Allow the answering machine to take phone calls.

✔ Trade days with another LC so that one of them takes no new clients on Mondays and the other takes no new clients on Fridays.

✔ Eat lunch out (or in) once a week with either the same friend or various friends.

✔ Find an exercise or walking partner, and help each other stick with it.

✔ Develop another specialty utterly unrelated to breastfeeding, and practice it. It might be coaching a sport, making placemats for the local fair, or refinishing furniture. If possible, have this new interest area include other people. Whatever you choose, give it serious time.

✔ Keep chocolate in the house.

✔ Set aside time to read professional material, and set aside time to read for fun.

✔ Buy expensive bath soap, or give yourself an extra minute in the shower just to soak.

✔ Go outside mid-day, put your shoulders back, and look UP. Take a deep breath and register the weather, good or bad, before going back to work.

✔ Do facial stretches that involve using the muscles that say "N-o-o-o-o-o-o." Do them publicly, as often as needed.

✔ Once in a while, say "Yes."

IDENTIFYING TOO CLOSELY

I take my clients "to bed" with me. I can't help it. And it has been one of the most difficult parts of a solo private practice. If my clients are all struggling, my sense of humor wanes, I feel I should stay close to the phone, and my work life overwhelms my personal life. If my clients are doing well, the world is bright even if it rains, and I have the energy and enthusiasm for play. There are two obvious solutions to my problem—become such a perfect LC that everyone always does well, or remember that it's *her* baby, not mine.

LCs enter this profession because we care. But the reality is, we can't live a mother's life for her. Many of the situations we see wouldn't happen to us in the first place. We'd pump more often, or really do skin-to-skin, or refuse to wean. We'd give breastfeeding a higher priority, or we'd have a more supportive partner, or we'd change doctors. But heaven forbid the world should be filled with little clones of Marvelously Maternal Me and You. Each of the women with whom we work has her own priorities and her own important place in the world. Our job is to help that mother find a balance that works for *her*. That balance may or may not include breastfeeding the way we would do it, and it may or may not include breastfeeding at all.

Sometimes I envision our profession as helping a woman understand the food on her plate. She is a juggler with a stick, with a plate of food to balance on the end of that stick. No two meals are alike, so each plate has a different balance point. As we help her get a feel for her own plate, she realizes she needs to shift the stick a little to the left, up a little, just a tad to the right . . . ah, now it balances. And she leaves us happily balancing that plate all by herself. It's her baby, her plate, her life. It's her plate whether she ever finds a way to balance it—and some never do. But yes, I do sleep better when my clients are thriving.

My father-in-law is a doctor. In the early years of my marriage, every time he saw me, he asked, "Are you all right?" and meant it. When he talked with my husband, he asked, "Is Diane all right?" At the time, I had a minor health problem and feared that my father-in-law knew something terrible about my prospects that I did not. Over the years, I have learned that he was simply being his version of a doctor: He saw illness and calamity around every corner.

It would be easy to fall into the same trap as an LC. If every mother and baby you see has difficulty, it must be because breastfeeding is inherently difficult. Thank goodness the world has you to save it!

That's where mother-to-mother support groups come in. Almost every month, I go to a local La Leche League meeting. The mothers there nurse without pain, with terrible positioning, without my wisdom. Their skinny babies fatten up, their fat babies slim down, they nurse toddlers and preschoolers and twins. They lead normal, varied, active lives. And they help keep me grounded in the reality that breastfeeding is a normal biological relationship. It's imperfect, it's inconsistent, it's adaptable, and It Tends to Work. If it's not working for a client of mine, there's almost always a way to make it work to her satisfaction! Breastfeeding Tends to Work.

Seeing so many varied normal babies helps in spotting abnormal, too. One of my earliest clients had a baby who just didn't seem "right." Something about the way he used his hands bothered me. But he was being seen regularly by a pediatrician, so I dismissed my inexpert worries and concentrated on helping them with breastfeeding. Eventually I persuaded the mother to come to a La Leche League meeting. One of the Leaders at the meeting spent 15 seconds with the baby, looked at me wide-eyed, and said, "There's something wrong with that baby!" "Oh, I know what you're seeing," I told her, "but the doctor doesn't seem to think there's a problem." The baby was diagnosed a few months later with neurological problems. The mother was relieved that they were spotted "so early, so we can start working on them before they get worse." I wish I could say I helped her to that early intervention. It's been said that, when we hear hoofbeats, our first thought shouldn't be zebras. Going to La Leche League meetings helps me see lots of horses. But it helps to know that zebras exist, and to keep a watchful eye out for them as well.

ZEBRAS VERSUS HORSES; WE DON'T SEE NORMAL ANY MORE; OVERREACTING TO NORMAL

Our profession is full of vivid imagery. As one LC described us, we are the downstream villagers who pull poor drowning souls out of the river. Our job is also to determine why they keep falling in upstream and to help prevent it from happening in the first place. In the meantime, we sometimes have to deal with "train wrecks"—those situations where everything that can go wrong, has. The train-wreck baby was born by cesarean at 37 weeks and was given formula in the hospital for mildly elevated bilirubin. His mother wasn't told to pump, her unrelieved engorgement led to mastitis, the baby has

EMOTIONAL ASPECTS, INCLUDING TRAIN WRECKS

thrush and is refusing to nurse because her supply is low, the bottle works for him, and his mouth hurts. Her partner has just moved out, her incision is infected, she's poor and has a broken arm from the car accident that killed her dog, she's slated for a breast biopsy tomorrow and has a doctor with minimal English language skills who's doing research for a formula company. . . .

That woman exists. She's out there. And you're going to have multiple chances to work with her over the years.

Perhaps Lactnet was invented because of train wrecks. Maybe it sprang, fully formed, from Zeus's forehead (or, more accurately, from the wonderful minds of two lactation consultants in private practice, Kathleen Bruce of Vermont and Kathleen Auerbach of Washington). However it came into being, you need it. E-mail could have been invented solely for our profession. We're far-flung and eager for answers. Lactnet, an e-mail group for breastfeeding specialists around the world, offers a chance to bounce questions off 2000 colleagues and tap into their collective wisdom. Not the least of its benefits is the discovery that not all great minds think alike. You may get four or five reasonable answers to a given situation. Most of the time, no one Truth exists. Even so, sharing the puzzle with so many excellent people will help you find an approach that may work for your client.

Lactnet and other established breastfeeding Web sites and groups need not be your only sources of e-salvation. Even in Lactnet's early days of smaller enrollment, I could see that I'd be too embarrassed to ask lots of questions. I inquired whether some others would like to form a small subgroup—what I came to think of as "my e-mail group practice." Ultimately nine of us across the United States joined together to chat as often as we like about whatever we like—not always related to breastfeeding. We complain about a bad pump or a broken washing machine. We rejoice in a baby who is finally nursing or a child who is coming home from college. We pick one another's brains for help in writing protocols, puzzling out unusual client situations, deciding whether to take that hospital job. We became fast friends before most of us actually met, and now count any conference as successful if two or more of us have a chance to get together there. Sometimes we go several days without "talking." More often, I find a note from one or more of our group members every time I check my mail during the day. As important as Lactnet has been to my business, I would give it up in a heartbeat before I would give up the eight wise women who have become such an essential part of my life.

ETHICAL ISSUES, INCLUDING OVERUSE AND UNDERUSE OF EQUIPMENT

A few years ago, a study found that doctors recommended X-rays more often when they had a financial stake in the radiology department. The doctors themselves believed they were making their decisions in exactly the same way, regardless of financial reward. In fact, they were influenced by their wallets. It's a lesson LCs need to take to heart.

Our primary goal is not to help mothers provide human milk for their babies. Our primary goal is to facilitate breastfeeding. Occasionally the provision of human milk other than at breast is all a woman is able to achieve, and equipment may help her do so. More often, equipment is used to facilitate breastfeeding. When overused by us, either use of equipment becomes a wedge between mother and baby that we were responsible for creating. Yet, for many of us, pumps and other equipment represent our largest source of revenue. To use it wisely, we must walk a very careful tightrope. I stock equipment for two reasons. First, I like being able to equip a mother immediately if she needs it. Second, pumps represent a very large share of my income. Here are my guidelines, which may differ from those of other LCs.

I try my best to distrust the pump and equipment companies. I take no free equipment, candy, or conference goodies. I forge no relationships, dealing with anonymous clerks at the main office rather than with an area representative. I use thoroughly cleaned demonstration equipment to help a mother decide whether she wants to invest, and I keep an inventory of parts to keep her replacement costs low. I keep my profit margin on equipment as low as the company allows. I make sure my clients have the names and phone numbers of other places where they can buy or rent equipment, and I direct phone callers elsewhere if time is critical and another source is located closer to them. When a client wants to buy a sling from me, I first show her how simple it is to make one. I try to look at every purchase through her eyes: How long will she use it? What would be the least expensive approach that would still meet her needs? And then, of course, I happily tuck her check into my wallet and add her sum to my month's total. Do I fall into the same category as those doctors who thought they weren't being influenced? How could I possibly know for sure?

At the same time, I try to distinguish between gadgets and tools. A *gadget* is anything in my life that makes a simple job more difficult. It may be a spring-loaded jar opener, a combination measuring spoon and paring knife, or the latest breast pump or nipple shield. A *tool* is something that helps make a difficult job simpler. Sometimes the only way to decide whether the latest breastfeeding gizmo is a gadget or a tool (or both, depending on circumstances) is to buy it and experiment with it. I always try to keep those experiments in line with a mother's emotional reserves, and I don't charge a mother for any new style of equipment about whose value I remain undecided. The sample of the latest pump technology goes—free of charge—to the second-time working mother who knows how a pump should perform, not to the mother of premie twins who needs the best performance I can give her. Knowing what's new on the market may help my clients, but I try not to learn about it at their expense.

As private practice LCs, we are rarely the first breastfeeding specialists a mother has seen. She had a breastfeeding class with her childbirth instructor; she received help in the hospital; her pediatrician, mother-in-law, and sister have given her advice; and she comes to us awash in conflicting recommendations. In part, she is asking, "Have I done all right so far?" To criticize the information sources she has used is to criticize her care of her baby. It doesn't help anyone. The most effective book I have read on dealing with children, clients, and colleagues is *How to Talk So Kids Will Listen and Listen So Kids Will Talk*. Learning to speak the words that you would like to hear if you were the other person is a dual-personality technique that pays huge dividends; the fewer bridges we burn in our relations with colleagues, other health professionals, and clients, the faster our profession will gain recognition.

One of our most effective tools in helping a mother sift through the information she has been given is helping her uncover her own feelings about a

CLINICAL CONFLICTS WITH PROVIDERS, MOTHER SUPPORT GROUPS, AND OTHER SOURCES OF BREASTFEEDING SUPPORT

particular path. A gentle, "Does that make sense to you?" may be all it takes for a woman to realize that some of what she has been told is silly.

Having something available on paper as soon as—or even before—a client asks for it is a potent way to override other misinformation. Its presence means that you have seen her issues before, that specific answers or at least a partial understanding of how to deal with them exists, and that you understood her situation well enough to anticipate many of her questions. When I gave a simple sheet on jaundice to a woman of middle-school literacy, she was extremely grateful. "No one gave me any information before," she said. Emboldened with that piece of paper, she felt better able to advocate for her baby. Paper is power. At the other end of the spectrum was my home visit to a young pediatrician. For nearly every question she asked, I was able to pull from her client folder a handout addressing the issue. We got to giggling about it. Even though she was a physician, she learned that her questions were the questions of every uncertain new mother. She also learned that I knew my stuff.

Perhaps my most effective tool in working with physicians whose information is outdated or lacking has been my doctor reports. I don't contradict what the doctor told the mother, I just give him copies of the handouts and articles I gave the mother, occasionally with especially pertinent (but not knife-twisting) parts highlighted: "Enclosed is the information I shared with this mother." This approach gives the doctor the option, at least, of educating himself or herself. Most of the time, I suspect these reports are not read, but by the time a doctor has received the umpteenth copy of Dr. Jack Newman's sheet on using fluconazole, the tide seems to turn. Change is rarely immediate, but it is always possible.

Surprisingly, the health care professionals most willing to accept new information from us may be those with a less direct interest in breastfeeding—anesthesiologists, oral surgeons, neurologists, occupational therapists, and endocrinologists. Something about infant feeding seems to bring out the worst in many otherwise excellent obstetricians and pediatricians. Tread gently, and take your time.

It is important to spend some time delineating in your own mind how the local breastfeeding coalitions and mother support groups fit into your life. They are your friends—not your competition or your enemy. They play a complementary, not a competing, role. If you are seen as competition or an untrustworthy source of help, work diligently to dispel that notion. This tiny beginning of a breastfeeding culture that we're nurturing remains far too fragile to withstand in-fighting. Find common ground. If it doesn't exist, create it. Mothers can only gain from your efforts.

Formula representatives are famous for their food. While we may be tempted to rely on information, they rely on marketing research that says, "Forget the facts. Offer food." When I meet with other breastfeeding supporters, I tend to bring journal articles. Formula reps, in their greater wisdom, would bring jelly doughnuts. I suspect that the breastfeeding specialists who make a point of eating with their colleagues are more likely to resolve any differences amicably—provided, of course, that someone at the table has read *How to Talk so Kids Will Listen and Listen so Kids Will Talk*.

There are many solid reasons for not entering private practice lactation consultant work: The pay is low, the responsibility is great, the emotional investment is substantial, the potential for overwork is large, the sense of swimming against the current is unavoidable. Why do we do it? How many reasons would you like?

Most women in our culture have had one of life's greatest pleasures and most fundamental relationships stolen from them. It was stolen so long ago and so cleverly that they don't even recognize the loss. Their expectations for their children's well-being are so low that the differences between breast-feeding and formula feeding are expressed in terms of advantages of breast-feeding, with no recognition of the damage done by formula feeding. We have a chance to give a huge and lifelong gift to our clients, their children, and the generations to follow—a chance to do work that really, truly matters on multiple levels. (Yes, I listed the importance of our work as a potential pitfall, but it is also one of the glories.) We can work in a field that uses our individual talents in fresh and exciting and changing ways, and we can ally ourselves with an outstanding group of women around the world. We can proceed at our own pace, expanding and even shrinking our business to suit ourselves. We can, single-handedly, effect a significant change in our local, regional, or global culture. We can model the importance of this piece of our biological heritage for our children, long past their own weanings. We can share the joy we've experienced in breastfeeding and help bring that joy to life in other women's eyes. We can die satisfied with ourselves for the contribution we've made to the world. If these are riches, then the lactation consultant in private practice is a rich woman indeed.

YOU WON'T GET RICH AS A LACTATION CONSULTANT

SUMMARY

Lactation consultants in private practice are susceptible to loneliness, over-involvement with their clients, and a tendency to see the abnormal in the normal because we spend much of our time seeing the abnormal. We are lured by the promise of a quick fix and easy money if we use certain technologies, and like members of many other professions we endure personality clashes and professional disagreements. Unlike many other professionals, however, we don't have large salaries to compensate for our troubles. Yet, the rewards are awesome and richly satisfying, empowering to our clients and ourselves, and—one mother and baby at a time—effecting a significant change in our local, regional, or global culture.

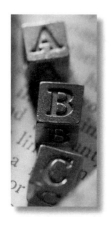

5 Advocacy for Breastfeeding

Linda J. Smith, BSE, FACCE, IBCLC

While IBCLCs are expected to do more than just clinical support work (see Chapter 23), "many hands make light work" of the larger goals of promoting and protecting breastfeeding. If you want to help mothers in a less intense way than providing direct hands-on (clinical) care as an IBCLC, we encourage you to become involved in one or more advocacy or promotional activities. This chapter describes some of your options.

PROMOTION

Breastfeeding promotion means identifying breastfeeding as the best way to feed babies to those who are undecided, believe formula feeding is just fine or the norm, or simply do not know the facts. The U.S. Breastfeeding Committee recently recommended a national media campaign to promote breastfeeding as one of its top five strategies for implementing *Protecting, Promoting, Supporting Breastfeeding in the United States: A National Agenda*.[1]

There is probably not one "right" way to promote breastfeeding, and certainly different audiences will respond to different messages about breastfeeding. Transforming breastfeeding into the normative, natural, and achievable behavior will require the efforts of many creative and talented people with skills in social marketing, research, media use, psychology, and other areas.

Breastfeeding promotion can include a wide range of activities, many of which are described in the World Breastfeeding Week (WBW) action kits developed by the World Alliance for Breastfeeding Advocacy (WABA).[2] Past themes for World Breastfeeding Week have been:

- 1992: Baby-Friendly Hospital Initiative
- 1993: Mother-Friendly Workplaces
- 1994: Making the Code Work
- 1995: Breastfeeding: Empowering Women
- 1996: Breastfeeding: A Community Responsibility
- 1997: Breastfeeding: Nature's Way
- 1998: Breastfeeding: The Best Investment
- 1999: Breastfeeding: Education for Life
- 2000: Breastfeeding: It's Your Right
- 2001: Breastfeeding in the Information Age
- 2002: Breastfeeding: Healthy Mothers and Healthy Babies

World Breastfeeding Week commemorates the signing of the Innocenti Declaration (see Appendix A) on August 1, 1990. The Declaration was signed by representatives of many nations (including the United States), and includes four specific targets designed to enable women to exclusively breastfeed their babies for six months and continue breastfeeding, with appropriate complementary food, for two or more years:

OPERATIONAL TARGETS: All governments by the year 1995 should have:

- Appointed a national breastfeeding coordinator of appropriate authority, and established a multisectoral national breastfeeding committee composed of representatives from relevant government departments, non-governmental organizations, and health professional associations;

- Ensured that every facility providing maternity services fully practices all ten of the *Ten Steps to Successful Breastfeeding* set out in the joint WHO/UNICEF statement (World Health Organization, Geneva, 1989), "Protecting, promoting and supporting breast-feeding: the special role of maternity services";

- Taken action to give effect to the principles and aim of all Articles of the International Code of Marketing of Breast-milk Substitutes and subsequent relevant World Health Assembly resolutions in their entirety; and

- Enacted imaginative legislation protecting the breastfeeding rights of working women and established means for its enforcement.

Obviously, many nations did not meet these targets by 1995, and many have not even come close as of this writing (early 2002). Plenty of opportunities remain for promotion of breastfeeding in general, and any of these goals or other goals in particular.

Promotion can also include small, short-term, or community-based actions. Even a simple action such as putting a breastfeeding-theme bumper sticker on your car or wearing a breastfeeding-theme T-shirt to a sports event is a positive, proactive step that raises awareness of the issues. Everyone can find opportunities to carry the "breastfeeding is important" message forward—it requires only a clear intent and awareness of opportunities.

PROTECTION

Protection refers to laws, policies, and programs that enable a mother who has decided to breastfeed to do so. Examples include legislation that protects a woman's right to breastfeed her baby in public; hospital and clinic policies that support breastfeeding; and work-site lactation programs. Protective activities also include monitoring and enforcing the *International Code of Marketing of Breastmilk Substitutes* (see Appendix A) periodically. For example, during the international *Code* monitoring project conducted in summer 2000, I attended a several-day training session and spent nearly three weeks traveling around my geographic region to observe, interview, and collect information. Many opportunities exist for those interested in this kind of activity. In-depth lactation management experience is not required—just a curiosity and interest in the issues and a willingness to learn and participate.

GLOBAL AND NATIONAL INITIATIVES AND ORGANIZATIONS

You might want to get involved with one or more of these global or national organizations:

- World Alliance for Breastfeeding Advocacy (WABA) or its regional affiliates
- International Baby Food Action Network (IBFAN)

- International Women Count Network
- La Leche League International (LLLI: www.lalecheleague.org)
- Australian Breastfeeding Association

INCLUDING BREASTFEEDING IN OTHER SOCIAL OR POLITICAL AGENDAS

If you (or a family member or close friend) are active in any civic or other organizations, you could investigate whether breastfeeding should or could be included in that organization's agendas. Examples include but are not limited to:

- Kiwanis (has worked with LLLI to produce an excellent poster)
- Rotary International
- Service organizations
- Religious organizations
- Day-care provider networks
- Workplace organizations or trade unions
- Civil rights groups (especially relevant for "breastfeeding in public" issues)
- Health organizations (some cancers, respiratory illness, poor vision, and other health problems are associated with artificial feeding)
- Women's issues or women's rights activities

Whether you continue on your journey to be a lactation consultant in private practice, or keep your "day job" and do breastfeeding support, protection, or promotion work in the nooks and crannies of your life, remember that every little bit helps. Here are two examples of catching the little victories:

> One Sunday evening I was shopping with my son in the auto parts section of a large, multiproduct store, wearing one of my breastfeeding-theme T-shirts. A shy young male clerk approached me and asked if he could ask a question about breastfeeding. He said, "My sister is pregnant and wants to breastfeed, but she's heard that breastfeeding really hurts." I reassured him that breastfeeding is supposed to be as pleasant and comfortable as a kiss, and if it isn't, there are lots of us in the city who know how to help her. I gave him my business card, along with phone numbers for the local La Leche League warm line, the public health prenatal clinic, and the WIC[3] breastfeeding clinic. He smiled broadly, clearly very relieved.
>
> Some time later, the same son was the senior lifeguard at a municipal pool. One day a young high-school age lifeguard approached him and said in a somewhat alarmed voice, "Carl, there's a mother over by the bleachers who is—um—*breastfeeding her baby* in one of the deck chairs." Carl's response was an elegantly simple, "So? We allow eating on deck. Leave her alone—breastfeeding is great for her and her baby." In those three short sentences, a problem was avoided, a mother supported, and a high-school student learned a lesson in normal infant feeding. Three victories!

The point of these stories: you never know when or where opportunities to promote breastfeeding will occur!

SUMMARY

Advocacy activities are ideal for those who want to help mothers in a less intense way than providing direct hands-on (clinical) care as an IBCLC. Many opportunities exist for protecting and promoting breastfeeding in a wide variety of settings.

NOTES

1. Visit www.USBreastfeeding.org to obtain a copy of this document.

2. World Alliance for Breastfeeding Action (WABA), Penang, Malaysia: 1992–2002. Action kits for WBW are available from INFACT Canada, La Leche League International, and ILCA. See Appendix B for addresses.

3. Supplemental Food Program for Women, Infants and Children, a program of the U.S. Department of Agriculture. WIC clinics strongly support breastfeeding mothers with education and tangible assistance.

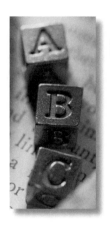

6 Realities of Private Practice

Kay Hoover, M.Ed., IBCLC
Diane Wiessinger, MS, IBCLC

KAY HOOVER,
M.Ed., IBCLC

I had been a La Leche League Leader for 14 years when the first certifying exam was given in 1985. My co-LLL Leader Chris Mulford was a nurse. We both took the exam, we both passed, and together we started a private practice, Breastfeeding Consultants, Inc. First, we contacted the state government to make sure it was legal to start such a business in Pennsylvania. Next, we bought liability insurance from the one company we could find that was insuring our new allied health care profession. Then, we incorporated. In January 1986, we saw our first client. In our first year, we saw 12 mother–baby pairs.

As members of the first exam cohort, we had few opportunities to learn *how* to practice as LCs. Chris was a hospital maternity nurse, so she and I went on consults together, and I learned my clinical skills from her. Neither of us was business-oriented. We each put up about $3000 to start the practice. Over the six years of our business we paid ourselves back the money we had invested, and we paid for our expenses and continuing education out of our earnings. At the end of the total of our six years as Breastfeeding Consultants, Inc., we each earned about $2000. We dissolved our corporation when we were both hired to set up a breastfeeding center at a hospital. We remained there for four years before hospital cutbacks sent us back to private practice. At that point we decided to each be solo proprietors and refer to each other.

When Chris and I started, we charged $25 per visit. Our clients had to tell us we were not charging enough. Anyone who wants to make money to support herself as a lactation consultant needs to have a better business sense than we had. It has been exciting to be a pioneer in a new field, but I could not have managed without the financial support of my husband.

Here is one way to know whether you have set your fees high enough: If a mother calls and you do not want to see her, you are not charging enough.

LC business is sporadic; it is not an ongoing service. A private practice lactation consultant (PPLC) constantly needs to find new clients. After attending a marketing seminar, I realized that PPLCs need to advertise to the people from whom they need to get referrals—pediatricians, nurse practitioners, midwives, obstetricians, family practice doctors, hospital lactation consultants, breastfeeding support group leaders, and pump rental locations.

One challenge in operating a part-time private practice is being available when a mother in crisis needs you. I have not figured out how to "have a life" and be in private practice. Now, as a solo practitioner, I need to arrange coverage for times I will be out of town. I am glad we have a network of PPLCs, because we are there for one another.

I am also glad I had a business partner at the beginning. When we started, I told Chris I was concerned that entering into business together would ruin our friendship, but it did not. It always felt good to be able to support and be supported by each other. I remember going out on a consult together in that first year and wondering whether we would be able to help the mother, then agreeing as we drove home that we *had* helped her.

Occassionally I spent the night with a family. It would begin with a late evening consult. The baby was so-so at the breast, and I felt if I could help them a few more times they would have it. So I slept on the sofa and got up for each feeding. I had breakfast with the family in the morning, headed home for a shower and a change of clothing, and then went off to work for the day.

Sometimes I do a free consult when I know the mother cannot afford my services. Sometimes I barter. Chris bartered her first overnight visit with a couple who lived on a horse farm. She slept in a recliner with their Maine coon cat on her lap, and went back the next afternoon to pick up a load of manure for her garden.

Once when I did a visit on my own, I remember my legs shaking as I knocked on the door. During the consult, the baby "shut down" and I wondered if he was okay. "Is the baby breathing?" I thought to myself. I tried not to react and worry the parents and, indeed, he was fine. Later as I saw other babies respond in the same way, I no longer worried as much. Now when it happens, I place my hand on the baby's chest to confirm that the baby is breathing. But just in case, I also took an infant CPR course.

At first every consult seemed like such a different scenario. Now they all seem alike. Bottom line—is the baby getting enough to eat?

In fall 1989, I spent a month in California at the Lactation Institute. After four years of experience in our private practice, I had seen about 70 families. Once I had the opportunity to watch Chele Marmet work intensively with many families, I came home with more confidence. After that experience Chris and I rarely did visits together.

In the early years, Chris would say to a client, "You know, we are just making this up as we go along." When I think of those first clients on whom I was learning, remember my lack of knowledge, and consider the ways I could help them now that I did not know about then, I realize how much our field needs a clinical training curriculum.

Sometimes I encountered scary situations. I have spent many sleepless nights worrying about a baby I have just seen. This anxiety helps motivate me to stay in daily contact with families until the problem is resolved. I ask the parents to call me every evening and leave a message if I don't answer the phone.

My suggestions for new private practice LCs are as follows:

- Spend time observing other IBCLCs in private practice.

- Designate a space in your home for your home office.

- Learn about being a businessperson.

- Keep a list of professionals to whom you can refer families, such as doctors who will clip a frenulum, counselors who specialize in postpartum depression, and so on.

- Make a business card, but don't worry about creating a brochure.

- Have a colleague with whom you can discuss matters.

- Join ILCA, and become involved in the activities of your local affiliate. If there is no affiliate, start one!

- Network with local breastfeeding support groups.

- Hire an accountant.

- Find a way to keep records that works for you.

- Find a medical library where you can spend time on a regular basis.

One LC in my area dictates her consult into a tape recorder and has an office worker transcribe it for her doctor's report. Another LC in my area does not answer her phone; instead, she pays someone else to answer it and set up appointments. If the mother wants to talk to someone on the phone, she is given a breastfeeding support group leader's telephone number.

Two pieces of equipment that I am glad to have are a scale and a camera. I learned from Chele Marmet that every IBCLC needs a scale. Doing a pre- and post-feed weight has changed my recommendations on many occasions. For example, I thought one mother had an oversupply. She had a rapid milk ejection reflex (MER), but the scale told me the baby had taken only one ounce at the first breast. As a consequence, I changed my recommendation for her from "one breast per feeding" to "keep doing both breasts per feeding."

I am more of a "picture person" than a "word person." Early in my LC career I arranged for a professional medical photographer to teach our ILCA affiliate how to photograph mothers and babies. She made recommendations about the equipment we would need, and Chris and I bought the items she suggested. The camera has helped me to meet our profession's need for pictures that can be used to teach parents and health care professionals.

Sometimes I am frustrated that I cannot remember everyone I have seen, but I do remember many of the families I have photographed. Having women call back after giving birth to a subsequent baby is special. Being a detective—a problem solver—is rewarding. I feel that I learn from every family with which I work.

Some days I wonder, if I had known what I was getting into, would I have entered this field? I am glad I did not know, because I love what I do. Each day is different. I never know when the next call will come or what will happen.

I do not like some things about private practice:

- How do you make yourself available NOW?

- I have to do estimated income taxes for federal and state agencies. I have to pay my own Social Security taxes.

- I have to collect state sales tax and submit it on a quarterly basis.

- I have to keep detailed records of money transactions, expenses, income, and mileage.

- I had to obtain a license to conduct business in the city of Philadelphia.

- Writing the doctor's letter after the consult remains challenging for me, but I think I am getting better at it.

With the database I have set up, I can pull out all kinds of interesting information. For example, I have learned the following:

- Most of my referrals come from hospital lactation consultants. The hospital from which I receive the most referrals has just started its own outpatient lactation center. My numbers for this year have gone down as a result.

- I see about the same number of girl babies as boy babies. Over the past five years, I have seen 46.4 percent males and 53.5 percent females.

- The most frequent request for my lactation consultant services is for a baby who is not latching on, which was 39 percent of my business over the past five years.

- The second most frequent request relates to sore nipples, which is 28 percent.

- The third most frequent request involves a low milk supply or a baby with weight gain problems; it accounted for 18 percent of the babies I saw.

- In the past year, 44.5 percent of the babies I saw during their first week after birth and 16 percent during the second week after birth, so 60 percent of the babies I see during the first two weeks after they are born.

Currently my solo private practice is very part-time. It has been 16 years since I began, and I see an average of one family per week. I refer many calls to other IBCLCs. I work part-time for a city health department, so I have less time for private practice.

I enjoy the teaching I can do during a consultation. I like talking for the baby. It is my way of helping parents understand what the baby is saying. My township does not allow residents to operate businesses in their homes. I have a home business office, but I may not have people coming into my home, so all of my consults take place in the mothers' homes. I like seeing the mother's environment, her support system, her chairs, bed, and pillows. If the consult is not too complicated, I like to leave the mother in her bed with her baby at breast in the side-lying position. She is usually half asleep by then.

I think my rewards come from the strengths of the women I see and feeling that I am able to provide some assistance at a very challenging time in their lives.

DIANE WIESSINGER, MS, IBCLC

Cream rises. Without a little help, it may rise slowly. But the rise is inevitable, even if it isn't marked.

My academic background was in nature education and animal behavior; I never expected to become a La Leche League Leader. I went to a La Leche League meeting as a "thank you" for the phone help that got us through my toddler's nursing strike, and I just . . . kept going. Over a period of several years, I realized I was giving as much at meetings as I was getting and eventually became a La Leche League Leader. Training for leadership took me three years; it takes some people as little as a few months.

As a new Leader, I was convinced that most of the questions I was asked had answers, if I just looked in the right books or attended the right conferences. And so I acquired books and went to conferences. After a few years of this "dogged pursuit of knowledge," I realized two things: (1) I was beginning to know more than any other La Leche League Leaders I knew, and (2) knowledge has a price tag. The obvious next step was to become certified so that I could stop losing money. I was the first in my area to decide to become an IBCLC, and I prepared for it simply by seeing as many mothers as I could and buying and reading all of the basic books. Apparently it was a sound preparation; I did fine.

My plan from the outset was to make money in spite of myself—to give each mother every break I reasonably could. Our income was such that I could afford to do so. But I was stunned by the first "LC in Private Practice" session I attended at an ILCA conference. One of the speakers, a nationally known LC, said she made enough money to pay for her own clothes and conference costs. That was one of the most enlightening pieces of information I gained at that session. Another eye-opener was delivered by a woman who attended with a baby in arms. "Don't get into this field too soon," she said. "It'll suck you right in and take time away from your family that is rightfully theirs." Her comment reinforced my inclination to take things slowly.

I have let my business grow on its own, from the time my younger child was about 8 years old until now, when he has graduated from high school. At this point, I have been a certified LC for 11 years and a La Leche League Leader for 16. I have never advertised, beyond giving my fee schedule to doctors' offices and the local hospital and just doing my job the way I feel it should be done.

I operate from my home, which means I have no additional office expenses. It's a simple matter to slip in and out of work, because my supplies and literature are available all of the time. But the LC who warned against starting in too soon, because it can suck time away from family, must have operated a home office, too. This field is so fascinating that it's difficult to put it on a shelf after-hours, especially if the shelf is located at home.

We live in the country. Most mothers make some comment about the peacefulness of the setting, or the loveliness of the drive, or the quietness of the room. My living room has two antique pendulum clocks, and mothers may comment on the calm their ticking induces.

Our front door enters the living room, and the living room and dining room can be isolated from the rest of the house with sliding doors. The first thing I do when a client comes in is to slide the doors shut to "protect" her (rather than having them shut when she arrives). My credentials hang near the door, I have a bulletin board covered with baby pictures that mothers have sent me, and I may have my digital scale set up on the dining room table. Pump parts are hidden behind a chair and slings are lined up under the sofa; my quilted home visit bag fits under the piano bench; a sling with several dolls hangs over a chair; and a soft-sided bag with files and handouts is tucked off to the side. A pitcher of water sits on the table, with glasses for each of us. I've recently added a small sign saying, "Help yourself or ask for help any time," because mothers don't generally reach for it on their own and are always grateful when I think to offer it. Otherwise, the room looks like anyone else's living room. My computer and file cabinet are in a nearby room.

Because I don't see breastfeeding as a medical subspecialty, I try to convey the sense that it is a women's issue, not a medical issue. I wear no special clothing or name tag, although my IBLCE certificates hang in the front hall. Because I am a floor-sitter by nature, because I tend to strew papers and equipment about during a consult, and because I like to keep my body lower than the mother's (emphasizing that she is in charge and I am merely her helper), I explain that I'll be sitting on the floor and she's welcome to sit any-where she likes. Before I touch the baby, I excuse myself to wash my hands. I spend 30 seconds washing them (two rounds of "Frère Jacques" sung men-tally), and return to the living room still drying them on a paper towel—ca-sual evidence to her that they are clean. If I want to explore a baby's mouth or suck, I wear a non-latex glove or finger cot to avoid exposing the baby to latex.

My intake form has a release statement at the top, where I won't forget to have the mother sign it before we start:

> I understand that a consultation may include a visual and manual examination of my breasts and of my infant's mouth. I give permission for information from this and subse-quent consultations to be shared with my child's pediatrician, my own health care providers, my insurance company, and with other breastfeeding specialists as needed to further the understanding of breastfeeding generally or to improve my lactation consul-tant's knowledge base.

It is a very simple release form because of my setting and my clientele. In my practice, I feel a longer and more formal statement could actually invite prob-lems as much as protect against them.

The consult proceeds according to the baby's state: If the child comes in hungry, I save the rest of the form and the positioning information for later, providing the positioning tips as we go. Initially, I based my form on one from another LC. Over the years I have added and deleted items numerous times, gradually creating a form that suits my needs.

Initial consults usually last two hours. They seem to come to a natural end at that point; if they last 2 1/2 hours, I generally feel that I have pushed the mother beyond her tolerance. Anything less than two hours feels incomplete, and in most instances we simply can't finish in less time. Subsequent consults may last from a half hour (rarely less) to another two hours. Mothers also have the option of paying by the quarter hour, if we feel her questions can be an-swered with something less than a full initial consultation. If she ends up stay-ing more than 1 1/2 hours, it becomes less expensive for her to pay for a full consult.

Sometimes a baby nurses to satiety right away and can't be roused for ad-ditional practice. Sometimes the mother explains, apologetically though I sup-port her decision, that the baby was hungry before she came and she "just had to feed him." In such a case, he comes in asleep and shows no interest in eat-ing. In either case, we do what we can, and she comes back the next day without charge to finish what we had planned to do.

I have a lovely, quilted, box-shaped duffle bag for home visits, and use it during consultations in my living room as well. A pocket on the outside holds slippers, so that I can have "shoes" on in a client's home but not track any out-side dirt. Inside the duffle bag are two plastic shoe boxes, one containing things to do with nipples (shells, shields, Lansinoh™, dimple rings) and the other having to do with feeding (syringes, eye droppers, bottles and teats, tape). A cloth bag holds demonstration versions of bottles and bottle teats, SNS, shells and shields, a golf ball to demonstrate stomach size, and a three-prong electrical outlet adapter for pumps. Another cloth bag, differently col-ored, holds clean but not new nipple shields and a clean but not new SNS™ with new tubing. A small box holds an SNS put together from new spare parts. A small bag holds my positioning "props"—a plastic hamburger, helium-quality balloons, a lipstick, and a hand puppet with a wide mouth. Yet another bag holds a clean (but not new) pump kit. A new pump kit lies in the very bottom of the home visit bag.

I should explain what "clean but not new" means. One of my services is pump trials. For these trials, I reuse pump parts by washing them in hot, soapy water; rinsing them and leaving them in a bleach/water solution (about 10 percent household bleach) for several minutes; then autoclaving them in a standard kitchen pressure cooker for at least 20 minutes.

I am especially pleased with the pressure cooker. For far less than the cost of an autoclave, I can "cook" equipment at the same temperature and pressure as a hospital autoclave. (The temperature and pressure are stated in the owner's manual, which I checked before purchasing.) I place a vegetable strainer in the bottom so that parts do not come in contact with the water, which reduces but does not eliminate spotting. It is a home-style solution to a very real concern. Using the principle of informed consent, I describe my cleaning procedure to a mother before offering her the parts to experiment with; so far, no mother has expressed concern about my procedure.

Because any single step—the hot, soapy water or the bleach soak or the pressure cooking—should be adequate, I feel the triple-cleaning approach assures my clients that the parts they are using, while not new to them, are safe for this one-time use. I follow the same procedure for the "clean but not new" SNS and nipple shields, although I always insert new tubing. This way, for the cost of the tubing alone, a client can experiment with me. Will a nipple shield work for her? Does she feel she can manage an SNS? If the answer is yes, she buys new equipment to take home.

In addition to my home visit duffle bag, I rely heavily on a soft briefcase full of files with handouts and photocopied articles from journals and magazines. The files are Alternate Feeding, Breast, Culture/Family, Formula, Milk Supply, Nipples, Older/Solids/Wean/Work, Perinatal, Philosophy, Policy, Position/Latch-on, Pumping, Referrals, Special, Suck, Thrush, and Weight. I use both the duffle bag and the briefcase in my living-room consultations as well.

Every client who has a full initial consultation receives a client packet—a two-pocket folder with Linda Smith's "Rules for Helping Breastfeeding Mothers" on the front along with my name, phone, e-mail, and Web site address. The left inside pocket is labeled "Papers on this side are for future use or general interest" and contains a LLL meeting announcement, a discount coupon for our local LLL group, sheets on starting solids and on working, and other handouts not immediately necessary. The right inside pocket is labeled "Review these now. Insurance forms at back." Newborn and positioning information, and any sheets that will be of special importance to the mother's situation, are on that side. When I fill out her insurance forms at the end, I tuck them behind the other sheets. Attached to the outsides of the pockets are my business card and a sticker that says, "Milk supply depends on frequent and effective milk removal." To avoid copyright issues and save money, most of the handouts in the folder are written by me and copied on standardized-color paper (the sheet on weaning is always purple, the father's sheet is always ivory, and so on). I tell the mother or her partner to look over the sheets on both sides when they get home, and often suggest that the partner do the reading, pulling for the mother any handouts that seem especially important.

A great deal of thought and energy goes into the folders. Although I work with a highly literate population, I know mothers are often too stressed to make much use of them. On the other hand, I know that they have accurate information at their fingertips if they choose to make use of it; some sit right down and devour it all. It can only be reassuring for them to realize that their questions and uncertainties are so common that a handout has already been written about it.

Toward the end of a consultation, we make out a "cheat sheet" together—my version of a care plan. It is handwritten on triplicate paper. I write down anything of which she wants to remind herself, and anything of which I want to remind her. We review each phrase as it is written to make sure it is written the way she wants it. The top copy goes in the front of the right-side pocket, the second goes in my file, and the third may or may not be mailed with my report to her physician.

I use a Polaroid™ camera to record significant events for the mother—a nonlatching baby at breast for the first time, a new way of positioning the baby that doesn't cause pain. I also make up a colorful certificate for any mother returning a pump or finishing her involvement with me. The text reads: "This is to certify that ____ is a Pretty Terrific Kid* and is entitled to use the initials PTK, in recognition thereof (*and his mom is pretty terrific, too)." The certificate includes a line for the date at the bottom. It doesn't mention either me or breastfeeding, so whatever the outcome, I can leave the mother with a reminder that her baby is wonderful and she is, too. If the father has clearly been deeply involved—coming to consults or helping her pump, for instance—I may change the text on the computer to read ("and his mom and dad are pretty terrific, too"), or I may make a certificate for an older sibling. Basically, however, I think of it as a reward for *her* efforts.

My insurance packet includes a half-sheet of instructions, a pink referral slip to be signed by the appropriate health care provider, an HCFA-1500 form of which I keep a carbon copy, and a letter of explanation to the insurance company. It rarely works. For a while, I used both a lactation "superbill" and an HCFA form, but decided to drop the superbill after a conversation with an insurance agent who called with questions about a client's claim: "Let's see, now. I have this HCFA form in front of me, and this form I don't understand . . . ." Enough said. But with or without the superbill, the lactation services insurance coverage tangle desperately needs resolution.

I have a consultation notebook that has the intake sheet, copies of doctor reports and "cheat sheets," and looseleaf paper on which I write notes from phone calls and consultations, along with the makings for insurance packets. I tape insurance codes from the lactation superbill to the inside and a year-long calendar to the cover. When I no longer seem to be involved with a client, but her child is still of likely breastfeeding age, I take her papers out of the notebook, staple them together, and file them on a bookshelf, alphabetically by first name. (I am much more likely to be able to place a woman after several years by her first name than by her surname.) If I haven't heard from the mother in a number of months, I transfer her file to the basement, where I have a file cabinet of old insurance forms, old clients, archaic breast pumps, and old rental forms. I don't yet have a computerized system for keeping track of clients or pumps, but I use the Quicken™ software program that came with my computer to track my finances.

Soon after a mother leaves a consultation, I write the physician's report, using it as my notes from her visit. An exception is the mother who visits repeatedly. I continue to make notes, but mail a letter summarizing those notes only when something changes significantly or perhaps when nothing has changed for a long time. My doctor's reports include my letterhead, a strip at the top listing the baby's and mother's names; the baby's birth date and weight; dates of visits with baby's age and, usually, weight; reason for the initial consultation; and current recommendations. Below that is a report in narrative format, with key words or phrases in bold. With rare exceptions, the letter is one page long. I prefer a narrative style because I think it makes the letter a bit less "medicalized." At the same time, putting key points in bold allows the reader to absorb the gist of it without reading the entire report. I include any pertinent articles or handouts that I think the recipient would learn from, usually described (accurately) as information I shared with the mother. While this information may directly contradict the physician, I never let on that I know this fact. It's a gentle approach that may have changed a few opinions after repeated exposures.

I had very little feedback from area health professionals for the first decade or so of my unpaid and paid work with mothers. Sometimes I was intensely frustrated by the silence. "I can yell," I told my husband, "or I can whisper. It doesn't seem to make any difference, so I just don't know how to pitch my voice. It's like being deaf!" But years of maintaining a consistent level of professionalism, closer to a whisper than to a yell, have slowly paid off. I've come to think of the process as dropping pebbles into a deep well. Year after year, pebble by disappearing pebble, I have tried to be accurate, pleasant, deferential, and prompt—no incidents that would cause anyone, anywhere, to think ill of me. Rather suddenly, in the past several years, the pebbles have become visible at the surface. No one has anything negative to say about me, and mothers are quick to recognize this fact. Physicians and midwives from every office in town have referred mothers to me, although some are much more likely to do so than others. While physicians may not seek me out, they are inclined to say, "Oh, good," if a mother reports that she has begun working with me. More than one has said, "Well, that's not what I would have suggested, but if Diane says you should try it, then I think you should," or, "You might want to try this, but see what Diane thinks." When I ask a mother where she got my name, she is likely to say, "from everyone." Gaining this recognition and respect has required no effort on my part beyond doing my best for the mothers and babies.

Income is another story. Clients who have paid for a full initial consultant can subsequently call me free of charge. Most do not abuse the privilege, transferring their less specialized questions to La Leche League meetings and other nursing mothers, but I spend many free hours on the phone. My fee for a second consultation is far less than that for a first. If a mother needs to come repeatedly, I usually do not charge for some visits. For women whom I haven't seen, I charge by the quarter hour for phone help, after a free 10- to 15-minute conversation in which I either answer their question or determine that they need additional help. I rarely talk to, or meet with, or write a report about, fewer than two women in a day, but most days I receive no reimbursement for my time. On one unusual day, I dealt with nine women without any payment. It is the way I choose to operate, but there's clearly room for increased income.

My filing system began with my first La Leche League phone call: a mother of twins, one of whom was still hospitalized. "Why are you calling me?" I wondered. "What do you think I could possibly know?" But I set up three files in a kitchen drawer: Problem—Cesarean, Problem—Multiples, and Problem—

Pumping. Over the months and years, those files expanded to the following "problem" headings in two drawers of a four-drawer file cabinet:

- Adoption
- Allergies
- Baby's health
- Birth
- Biting
- Bottle/nipple confusion
- Breast
- Cleft
- Clothing
- Culture
- Depression
- Discipline
- Donating
- Down syndrome
- Drugs
- Engorgement
- Family
- Fertility
- Foreign language
- Fussy baby
- Getting started
- Grieving
- HIV
- Jaundice
- Kangaroo care
- Lactose intolerance
- Latch-on
- Legal rights
- Let-down
- Mastitis
- Milk supply
- Mothering skills (infant)
- Mothering skills (older child)
- Mother's health
- Mouth
- Multiples
- Nipples
- Nursing older baby
- Nursing strike
- Nutrition
- Oversupply
- Position
- Premature
- Pumping/hand expression
- Relactating
- Reluctant nurser
- Second child
- Separation
- Sleeping
- SNS
- Starting solids
- Stools
- Stress
- Sucking
- Thrush
- Weaning
- Weight gain
- Working

As a file grew too thick to be manageable, I would subdivide it. "Mouth" is now "Mouth" and "Cleft," and may be subdivided yet again to create a "Tongue-tie" file. If I were starting over, I would choose some word other than "problem" to precede each file name, but it does distinguish those working files from my "lactation consultant" files—IBLCE, ILCA, LC correspondence, conferences, LC insurance, handout masters, and so on—and my "administrative" files—pump company business, "thank you" notes from mothers, political issues, the local breastfeeding coalition, WIC, and so on.

I now try to have at least two copies of anything I rely on frequently; I may make 10 copies of something I hand out frequently. When I have only two copies of a paper left in a file, one goes in a "to be photocopied" bag for one of my periodic trips to the copy store.

A typical week will include perhaps two initial consultations, a few follow-up consultations, a pump rental or two, one or two equipment sales, and 20 to 30 phone calls with current and potential clients and others who simply need basic information. My net earnings have never exceeded 50 percent of my gross, even working out of my home, which makes an office away from home impractical without significant changes. Supplies (mostly pump-related and slings) and pump leases represent my greatest expenses by far—as much as 40 percent of my gross. Office expense (mostly copying, paper, and telephone) are my only other major expenses. Conference and travel costs generally amount to less than 10 percent of my gross, although I allot about $1000 for the ILCA conference every year. Pumps are my greatest source of income, with consultations second and speaking and writing third. Over time, the three categories have begun to equalize.

I use an "irritation pricing system." When I become irritated with how little I make for my time, I change something. At the start, I charged $5 for all follow-up visits, whether at my home or at the mother's, figuring that my heroes in the breastfeeding world could probably have fixed the problem in one visit and so it was not fair for me to charge for more. Then a "woman of means" asked me to come for four follow-up home visits some distance away at $5 each. After that, I changed my fee sheet. Some years later, a woman who lived a half hour away asked me to come for several follow-up home visits. I realized I much preferred to have women come to me, so I raised my home visit rate to 50 percent more than my "office" rate. Now, if a mother is willing to pay the extra money, I know she really needs to be at home and I go to her without irritation.

My inventory of 15 to 20 pumps is small enough that, with more than half of the pumps out on loan, I can fit it in my front hall closet. I have opted to stay with one pump company, and I stock all of the little bits and pieces a woman might need. To have those little items for pumps from more than one company would take up more space than I care to devote to inventory, and I would hate to make a pump available without having the spare parts for backup. Parts, files, a computer, and books take up one wall of our family room. Outdated materials are stored in the basement.

"Have a business phone with an answering machine," one LC advised, "and never answer it." That seemed like odd advice to me when I was starting out and trying to grow a business, but I remembered it and began doing the same thing myself a few years ago. An answering machine on a separate "business" line acts as a low-cost secretary. When the business phone rings, family members know it is not for them, and I can ignore it if I'm with a client or just want some unbroken time. I can always grab the phone partway through a mother's message, and I often do.

When I feel guilty about screening calls, I think of all the businesspeople whose secretaries allow them to work without interruption. My phone message always gives the name of at least one La Leche League Leader or IBCLC, so that no mother is ever left at a dead end, even for a few minutes.

In my small practice, I haven't had to be any more complex than that. If I want some time off, my message indicates that I'm not taking any new clients. I may continue to offer pumps, or I may send callers to another source for everything. Old clients continue to have access to me, but business slows just a bit while I catch my breath.

Although I remain an active La Leche League Leader, I have not experienced any difficulty in keeping my roles separate. I lead local meetings only a few times each year but am present for most of them, fielding questions as needed. The other Leaders and I work well together. My clients understand that I "wear a different hat" during meetings, and they recognize that the help I give freely to mothers at meetings is very different from the focused, lengthy sessions I offer as an LC. Occasionally I will arrange to meet with an existing client for free after an upcoming meeting, as a way of saving her some money, making it easy for me to meet with her in a limited, efficient way, and exposing her to La Leche League. My home number is available in a very limited way to LLL mothers—I'm listed as a resource for pumps and slings. All other LLL listings include only the other Leaders.

As noted earlier, I always have at least one La Leche League contact number on my phone message, and I have arranged for two of the Leaders to keep a pump and kit on hand. If I'm out of town, and the Leaders don't have the expertise they need to help a mother, they can at least help her protect her milk supply and feed the baby until I'm available. La Leche League offers a very different service from mine—free telephone help for simple questions, an accepting group of friends for a new mother just beginning to "get out," and a breastfeeding miniculture that helps ensure continued success after a client no longer needs me. Even if I weren't already a part of LLLI, I would cultivate friendships and connections with my local Leaders and encourage my clients to do the same.

A client who is having a really difficult time may be too uncertain to attend a La Leche League meeting, but may still benefit from the camaraderie of other new mothers. When I have two or more such clients, I may arrange a "Walking Wounded" gathering (a term I don't share with the mothers) at my house. I don't charge, and I don't offer much help. I just make simple snacks and water available and encourage them all to exchange stories, addresses, and phone numbers. If they seem unlikely to get together again on their own, we may meet at my house one or two more times. Some of the friendships and playgroups that have formed in this way have continued for several years.

One of my concerns is the frequency with which any of us—LCs or other breastfeeding helpers—may become a bottleneck in a mother's search for solutions. To help protect against my being part of the problem, my fee sheet includes the names of La Leche League Leaders, other LCs within an hour's travel time, doulas, massage and chiropractic therapists who are skilled with babies, and other pump sources. The bottom of the sheet includes the following statement: "There is always more help, if you want it—all the way to clinics in California!" I have had a mother ask about out-of-state options only once, but I feel better knowing that all clients are aware of the range of choices open to them.

My basic fees now approximate what the local market will bear. My small city is "centrally isolated" in a largely rural region of the state. Most of my clients are partners of low-income university graduate students or are students themselves. Most would feel forced to abandon breastfeeding if they had to pay too high a price to succeed. Insurance coverage remains unreliable for them. With only a few small changes I could "tighten things up"—charge for every non-client call that exceeds 10 minutes, charge a cleaning fee for pumps, charge the mother who comes for a weight check and stays to nurse and chat, charge a small fee for the books and videos that I now loan for free, eliminate my practice of charging 10 percent less than retail for equipment. Those small changes could significantly increase my income, but they are not in my nature.

Another LC in private practice in my town is no more assertive in her marketing or charging than I am. We aren't usually listed on each other's phone messages because we don't want the additional business. Like me, she has tended to take the business that comes her way without trying to increase it. We do agree to be on the other's phone line as backup during trips.

A few years ago, not long after she first started in private practice, the other LC and I went on a "retreat" together for a weekend, out of town. It was an extremely valuable exercise, and one that I'd recommend any time two or more of you are in competition. We wrote down all the issues we thought we should discuss and combined our lists. During the next 36 hours we worked our way through the combined list, checking items off as we completed them. Our points of discussion: teaching prenatal classes, pricing, fee schedules, renting pumps, advertising, expanding our roles/presence, forming a study group, fostering communication, comparing forms, using each other for a second opinion, doing joint consults, World Breastfeeding Week, what we hoped to gain from our loose partnership, what we hoped not to lose, dividing up the week to ensure time off, arranging for a central phone, the role of La Leche League in our practices, meeting regularly. It was an intense forging of both a business relationship and a friendship.

This kind of loose partnership between people who compete for business may be difficult to achieve, especially if your marketing efforts are at very different levels, but it is certainly worth attempting. At the very least, we learned a great deal about each other during the retreat and have cooperated extremely well ever since. Our arrangement hasn't led to a total partnership, but it has given me a top-notch backup, a second local brain to pick, and enormous moral support. I worked for years alone. Now that I have someone with whom to share my experiences, even if it's only occasionally, I'd sure hate to lose her. And what happens to the mothers we might have seen, if we had advertised more effectively? Those mothers who are persistent find us. Those who have persistent helpers find us. It seems to be the best we can do without losing the freedom we both have begun to crave.

I wish I could say that having a second PPLC in town has helped me keep breastfeeding issues from overwhelming my life. Our work is just too interesting to stay neatly confined in a regular workday, even when the load is shared. There is always another letter to write, e-mail to answer, phone call to make, and handout to revise. And the desk where most of this activity takes place is such an attractive nuisance! I may sit down to send out one e-mail while I wait for the water to boil and forget why I'm boiling it in the first place.

This job does not confine itself to working hours anyway. Mothers need pumps when they need them. They need to see you on weekends. My husband jokes about The Six O'Clock Call. Virtually every evening, sometime between 5:45 and 6:15, the business phone rings. Some callers who don't leave a message are probably telemarketers, but 6 P.M. is a typical new-mother meltdown time. The father is home from work and insists that the mother call for help, or he's there to take the baby so that she has her first chance to do so. Perhaps the mother has given it one more day and matters just aren't getting better. Or, if she's lucky, perhaps the grandmother has said, "I'll take care of supper. You get yourself some help." As an LC in private practice, your suppertime is someone else's crisis time. Which is more important tonight: the baby who hasn't eaten in eight hours or getting your lasagna to the table on time? Which will be more important tomorrow night, and the night after? Too many years of always putting someone else's baby first will wear you out, however, which explains why collaboration and limits are important.

Doing most of my consulting at home has meant that my children—already of school age when I began—could take care of themselves for the relatively short times that I spent with a client. I was still at home and able to step in if I was truly needed. This system has made it possible to fit my work in around meals, errands, and family time. The reality, however, has been that business issues have run neck and neck with family time: "We can go as soon as I finish this doctor's report." "Sorry I was late picking you up. A mother called." "I can't go that weekend. There's a conference." And always, of course, something seems to be more important than housework. A La Leche League Leader told me years ago, "My husband complains about the time I devote to League work. He doesn't understand that, if it weren't the League, it would be something else." We are women with passionate energy. If we don't direct it toward breastfeeding, it's a fair bet we still wouldn't direct it toward housework.

No, I don't make what you could call a living. I do make much more than enough to pay for my own clothes and cover all my costs, including conferences. I am my own boss, I take time off whenever I choose (although I often trail several clients along with me into my "time off," sometimes calling them from vacation spots at my own expense). My reputation is good and created itself without marketing efforts. I could earn significantly more than I do, if I were cut from a slightly different cloth, so I feel that my basic approach must be sound. I also like to think that, although I have indeed been sucked heart, mind, and soul into this fascinating field, I haven't shortchanged my family too badly in the process.

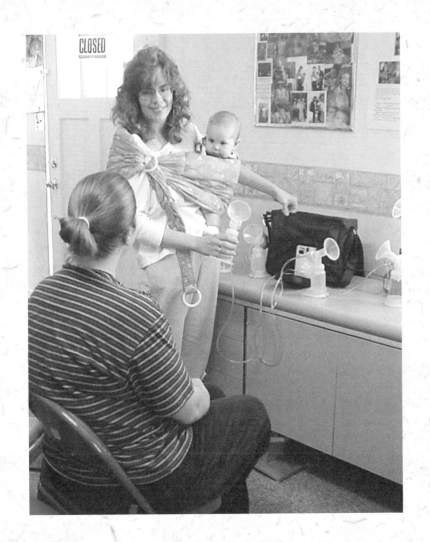

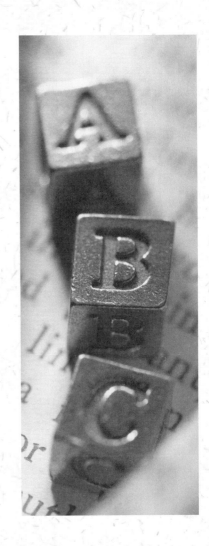

Business Skills

Operating a PPLC Business

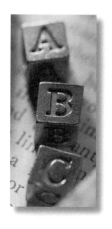

7 Overview of Business Skills

Linda J. Smith, BSE, FACCE, IBCLC

Do you have what it takes to be a successful private practice lactation consultant (PPLC)? In Part B, Business Skills, we explore the legal, financial, and administrative skills that you'll need to turn this work into a career.

In this book, we take the position that "success" means that your lactation consultant private practice is more than just a hobby—it is your livelihood. The key to achieving that success is having a business-like attitude and sound business skills. Success on the business side means you're happily making as much money as you want, the administrative details of your practice are manageable, and you comfortably comply with all laws, codes, and regulations of your community and your profession. Your clients are satisfied with the results of interacting with you, and they refer others to your practice.

The business side is the most challenging aspect of PPLC work for many of us. Most LCs entered this profession because we genuinely want to help mothers and babies and to use our skill as caregivers. Many of us practiced for years, even decades, as volunteers. In fact, the LC profession has grassroots origins: We learned from other mothers, then from other peers. Being in business is a whole different ballgame for many of us.

Furthermore, because of the long history of aggressive and unethical marketing of infant formula, and because of the poor breastfeeding advice often given by paid providers of health care, many of us are very suspicious and distrustful when "breastfeeding" and "money" are used in the same sentence! Some of this suspicion is justified. This skepticism makes starting a breastfeeding-related business even more challenging.

The chapters in Part B, which were written by successful PPLCs and a consultant to successful PPLCs, provide a framework for developing the business side of your practice. Debi Page Ferrarello discusses how to develop a carefully thought-out business plan as the first fundamental step. Elizabeth Brooks, a lawyer/LC, presents an overview of legal issues with which you must deal. Diane DiSandro analyzes crucial financial practices, including third-party reimbursement. Jane Bradshaw addresses the ins and outs of hiring staff. Dennis Smith provides sound philosophy and specific advice for PPLC business-oriented computer purchases. Debi Ferrarello's guide to marketing complements the new IBLCE/ILCA material being developed. Finally, Chapter 14 includes some sobering business pitfalls that could derail the best-intentioned LCs.

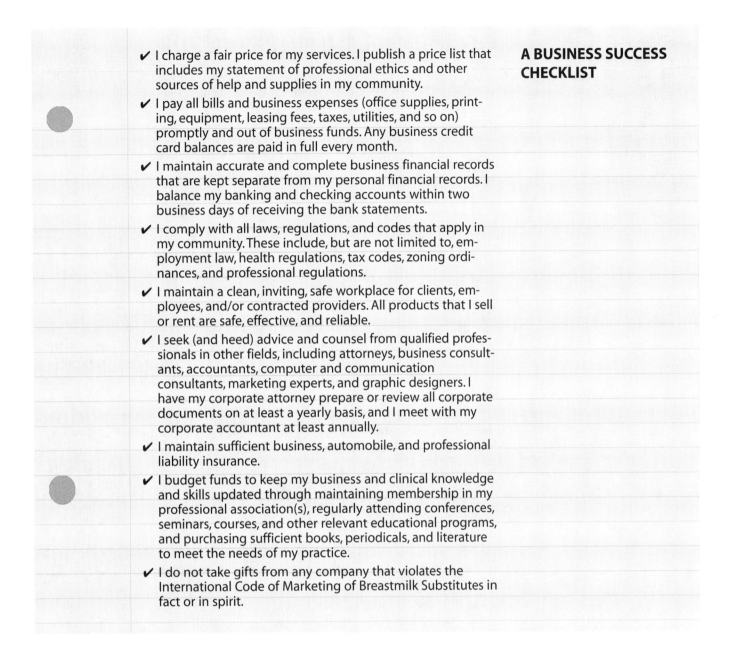

✔ I charge a fair price for my services. I publish a price list that includes my statement of professional ethics and other sources of help and supplies in my community.

✔ I pay all bills and business expenses (office supplies, printing, equipment, leasing fees, taxes, utilities, and so on) promptly and out of business funds. Any business credit card balances are paid in full every month.

✔ I maintain accurate and complete business financial records that are kept separate from my personal financial records. I balance my banking and checking accounts within two business days of receiving the bank statements.

✔ I comply with all laws, regulations, and codes that apply in my community. These include, but are not limited to, employment law, health regulations, tax codes, zoning ordinances, and professional regulations.

✔ I maintain a clean, inviting, safe workplace for clients, employees, and/or contracted providers. All products that I sell or rent are safe, effective, and reliable.

✔ I seek (and heed) advice and counsel from qualified professionals in other fields, including attorneys, business consultants, accountants, computer and communication consultants, marketing experts, and graphic designers. I have my corporate attorney prepare or review all corporate documents on at least a yearly basis, and I meet with my corporate accountant at least annually.

✔ I maintain sufficient business, automobile, and professional liability insurance.

✔ I budget funds to keep my business and clinical knowledge and skills updated through maintaining membership in my professional association(s), regularly attending conferences, seminars, courses, and other relevant educational programs, and purchasing sufficient books, periodicals, and literature to meet the needs of my practice.

✔ I do not take gifts from any company that violates the International Code of Marketing of Breastmilk Substitutes in fact or in spirit.

Karen Evon, IBCLC, and owner of Maternal Expressions, a storefront practice in Folsom, California, writes:

> Motivations vary for wanting to open a storefront business. Many dream of expanding a private lactation consultant practice to reach more mothers and babies. Some have previous retail experience in another setting and feel confident about what to do. Others view being their own boss and doing things their own way as exciting and liberating. However, the reality is that within the first five years 90 percent of new businesses will fail. New business owners will misallocate an estimated $10,000 to $40,000 before opening their doors!

The onus is on PPLCs to behave ethically and legally, while charging a fair amount for the services provided. If you don't want to deal with the business aspects of a private practice, you should either volunteer your time as a mother-support group leader or peer counselor, or pursue employment at a hospital, clinic, or medical office. The bottom line? Take care of business at least as well as you take care of mothers and babies.

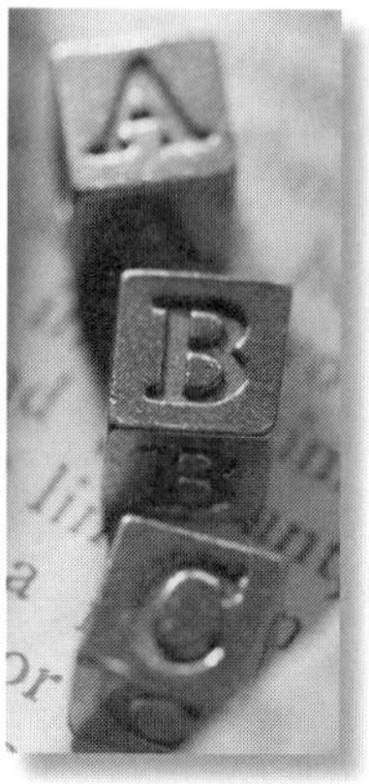

8 Creating a Business Plan

Debi Page Ferrarello, RN, BSN, MS, IBCLC

NEEDS ASSESSMENT

You've made the decision. You want to be a lactation consultant in private practice. Now you need to do a little research before you go any further. You need to learn how breastfeeding needs are currently being met in your community, who your potential referral sources are, and who your competition is. This time spent assessing the needs in your community represents an investment in your future.

You may already have some idea about how breastfeeding needs are being met in your community. Perhaps you have served as a volunteer counselor or you work in the birthing unit of your local hospital. However, now you will want to expand your outlook a bit. Call local pediatric practices and ask where they send mothers who experience breastfeeding difficulties. Do they have an LC "in-house"? Do their nurses or physicians try to manage breastfeeding issues themselves? Do they refer to a lactation consultant in private practice?

Check with the local nursing mother-support groups. Do they see unmet breastfeeding needs in your area? Ask where they refer mothers whose lactation issues fall outside the scope of the support group.

Explore the services offered by each hospital in the area. Does it have lactation consultants on staff? What services are available for patients after discharge?

Finally, remember to ask mothers themselves. You might consider conducting *focus groups* for mothers with young babies. You could invite mothers of infants to come to a comfortable location where you could ask them about their breastfeeding experiences, the help and support they received, their perception of their postpartum needs, and their level of receptiveness to the services you would like to offer. You will want to be considerate of their time, so be sure to provide for their comfort. Incentives, such as a free gift, are often needed to encourage busy people to participate in a focus group. You might find mothers to invite by posting a notice in a pediatrician's office, toy store, or consignment shop, by contacting a parenting support group, or by taking out an ad in a parenting newspaper. *Before you invest too much time, effort, and money into establishing a private practice, you want to determine that a community need exists for your services.*

Before you "hang out your shingle," you will want to take stock of *your* needs and the needs of your family. Starting your own business requires an enormous amount of time, energy, passion, and commitment. Is your whole family on-board with your dream?

One of your biggest considerations is your *time*. You can start a practice on either a part-time or full-time basis, but be clear that your LC practice is not a hobby. To do the job well requires attending professional conferences, reading professional journals, and networking with other professionals. You can be a breastfeeding enthusiast without being in private practice. However, establishing a private practice requires the commitment of a professional.

Think about your time. If you have small children at home, you may find part-time work better suited to your needs than full-time employment. Many successful lactation consultants in private practice started by working part-time. When the business is small, and so are the children, many LCs have been able to juggle both. They may do some initial immediate problem solving and appointment making by telephone, scheduling appointments for the evenings when their spouse comes home. Others trade child care with friends. Often, with everyone's support, a small practice remains flexible enough to fit the needs of a family.

As your business grows, you may find that a casual part-time arrangement no longer works well. As you simultaneously talk with prospective clients on the phone while racing to rescue your baby from your toddler's grasp, it dawns on you that you're not doing either job effectively. You can wear many hats, but not at the same time! It's time to set some boundaries on your time.

Whether you are planning to work full-time or part-time, it is a good idea to establish "work hours." During your work hours, you can see clients, do follow-up phone calls, read journals, and do promotional activities. During these work hours, dress for work, plan your agenda, and invest your time in your business.

Another consideration in assessing your needs is *income*. As with most new businesses, it takes some time for a lactation practice to generate income, and it is not likely to generate a large income ever! On the other hand, compared to other businesses, a lactation consultation practice can be started with very little expense. Whereas most businesses take an average of five years to operate in the black, your LC business may generate at least a small profit the very first year. Some lactation consultants work for an employer, such as a hospital, or in another field, gradually decreasing their employed hours as their private practice expands. However, there comes a time when the employed work actually interferes with the practice growth, as lack of availability for consultation takes its toll. I found that the surest way to guarantee that women would call for my services was to schedule myself for work elsewhere! At some point, it becomes necessary to "take the plunge" and pour all your professional energy into making your private practice become a success.

Doing home visits requires the least amount of capital outlay. You need a phone, a reliable car, and some portable tools of the trade, such as a good scale, paperwork, and other LC supplies. You will need some space in your home to store your supplies, a computer on which to write your health care provider reports, and a filing cabinet for your client charts. Many LCs find that doing home visits is an easy and cost-effective way to begin a private practice.

ASSESSING YOUR NEEDS

Clients appreciate being able to avoid packing up the diaper bag, figuring out the car seat, and leaving the comfort of home. LCs often learn a great deal about a client by visiting her home. Yet while home visits offer some advantages and require very little in terms of equipment and space, they do consume an enormous amount of time. Be sure to factor the time it takes to gather your supplies and travel to and from the client's home into your fees. Home visits may also involve some risk to the LC. Know something about the neighborhood before you head out, and carry a mobile phone in case you run into trouble or get lost.

Having mothers come to you greatly increases the number of clients you can see in a given period of time. Some LCs see clients in a room in their home, some in a separate home office, and others in an outside office.

If you're planning to see clients in your home, remember to keep your practice professional! Having a new mother sit on a Lego-laden chair, with the dog drooling on her feet, may not give you the aura of expertise and calm for which you are striving. Also, clients tend to see services rendered in a living room as more casual, and they may consider your time with them as similar to a social call. There is an emotional discrepancy between the nurturing relationship in a cozy living space and the very business-like bill for professional services rendered.

It is generally preferable to have a separate office space for your work. If the space is dedicated entirely to your business, discuss the potential tax advantages with your accountant. What is necessary in terms of workspace? Consider that many new mothers won't be traveling alone with their newborn. Most often her partner, and sometimes an assortment of friends and relatives, tag along. You will want to have enough furniture for everyone to sit down. Be sure to provide at least one piece of furniture that is comfortable for nursing a baby (or two!). A footstool is also helpful. You will want to have space for your computer, files, supplies, and an impressive array of texts and journals. Easy access to a clean bathroom and sink must be available, as you will want to wash your hands before touching the baby, and everyone will want to use the facilities.

A home office offers some other advantages. Aside from possible tax benefits, it usually gives you great flexibility in your hours, and you can't beat the commute. On the other hand, it may become difficult to separate your home life from your business world. Will your children respect your time "at work" if "at work" means "in the next room"? Will you be able to turn off the phone so as not to be distracted from your dinner party?

Some lactation consultants establish a practice in a separate facility, by renting or buying space. Some distinct advantages ensue from working out of an outside office. An aura of professionalism surrounds a practice in an office building. Clients expect professional service and expect to pay a fee for that service. It is easier to delineate working hours from time "off" when your workspace is separate from the rest of your life. Signage may attract more business, increasing your client base.

The office space comes with a considerable price, however. The income you generate must now cover rent and utilities, in addition to your supplies, communication system, insurance, salary, and benefits. You will need a space large enough for consultation, supplies, a waiting area, a restroom, and sink. You will need to furnish the area with the comfort of postpartum women and their families in mind. Thus you will need to increase your client base, increase your fees, or pursue some combination of the two to cover the additional costs. Yet, you will need to remain aware of your competitors' fees and services. Are they doing home visits for the price of your office consultation? How can you position yourself so attractively that clients are willing to come to you, pay your fees, and see the value? We will talk about that issue more when discussing the marketing plan (see Chapter 13), but these considerations need to be taken into account at the very beginning of your planning.

YOUR MISSION STATEMENT

Right now, before you go any further, contemplate what you are all about. Consider how your lactation consultant practice fits into who you are. Why do you feel compelled to create a path in unfamiliar territory, carving out a niche in your community? What service do you hope to provide? Why? By what principles will you establish your policies, develop your protocols, and grow your business?

Webster defines a mission both as a calling or vocation and as a specific task with which a person is charged.[1] Your mission statement defines your calling, clarifies your purpose, and gives you a framework on which to build. It represents a standard against which you can judge all of your practices and a lens through which you can view your purpose.

Mission statements may be broad enough to encompass your entire existence or specific to your work. I have found it helpful to first write my mission statement for life, and then to create my mission statement for my work to fit within the broader scope. For example, the mission statement that defines my life is as simple as "For the glory of God." Out of that very broad statement flows the mission statement for my work. At one time, that statement was "To provide technically excellent, lovingly compassionate, and respectful lactation consultation services." At the present time, a colleague and I have established a nonprofit corporation whose mission is "To provide expert clinical breastfeeding services to mothers and children, regardless of income, and to provide health care professionals with evidence-based breastfeeding information and supervised clinical opportunities."

Most companies have a mission statement. Take a few minutes to go on-line and seek them out for examples and inspiration. Out of the mission springs the vision. Out of the vision springs the practice. It is worth spending the time, at the outset, articulating your mission.

The resource list at the end of this chapter lists several recommended books. These materials can help you as you clarify your mission. In turn, having your mission clearly defined can help you as you develop your business plan.

YOUR BUSINESS PLAN

Your business plan tells you where you are going to go, how you are going to get there, and how you will know when you have arrived. Where your mission statement paints with broad strokes, your business plan is written with a fine-point pen.

A business plan has been called a "powerful declaration of your goals and intentions, a written summary of what you aim to accomplish and an overview of how you intend to organize your resources to attain those goals."[2]

If you plan to borrow money to start your practice, your business plan will need to be very detailed. You will need to demonstrate exactly how you will earn the money needed to repay the loan. If you do not plan to borrow money to open your business, your plan may be less detailed, but will still give you an edge as you seek to establish your niche in the marketplace. According to Janet Attard in *Business Know-How*, if you are risking "relatively little overhead and money, you can get by with a simple outline of ideas. You will make predictions of what it will cost you, who will buy your services and what they'll pay for them."[3] The business plan translates your professional vision and goals into business-speak. This endeavor will be tremendously helpful to you because, after all, your practice is a business. If you want to stay afloat financially, so that you can continue to meet the needs of mothers and babies in your community, you must develop some business skills and learn to speak the language. The plan will help you to spell out, step by step, how you will meet your professional goals.

What goes into a business plan? Its contents depend on how the business plan will be used. At least thinking through each area will prove invaluable to you as you establish your practice. In general, a business plan contains the following:

- Cover page
- Mission statement
- Table of contents
- Business description
- Risk assessment
- Assessment of competition
- Financial analysis
- Insurance information
- Operation procedures
- Marketing plan
- Executive summary
- Supporting documents

Let's look briefly at each component.

The **cover page** includes a title, such as "Business Plan for Laura's Lactation Center," your name, address, and the date. The **table of contents** lists each part of the plan, with page numbers. Put your **mission statement** on the very next page, so that it will set the tone for the rest of your plan.

The **business description** describes, in some detail, your practice. Include the history of your practice, what services you plan to offer, and to whom. The business description paints a portrait of your practice. Write about the physical location of your office, or describe your policy regarding home visits. Think of every aspect of your business. List products you will carry, if any, as well as the suppliers and the types of potential customers. List the wholesale and retail prices for each item.

The **risk assessment** demonstrates that you have given thought to the "what if"s: What if a new product makes breastfeeding obsolete? What if you become ill and unable to work? What if Breasts R Us opens next door? Identify potential problems and address them in this section.

The **assessment of competition** shows that you are going into practice with your eyes open. You are aware of similar services being offered in your community, yet still believe that you can find a niche in the market. What do you have that your competitor lacks? How will you communicate that special quality to the public? What special need will you address? Your assessment of competition will identify who the competitors are in your area, how they practice, whom they serve, how much they charge, and how you differ. Not all of your "competitors" will be IBCLCs. Some will be lay counselors, visiting nurses, triage nurses at the pediatric clinic, or mothers-in-law. Identifying your competition and learning all you can about them will help you as you develop your marketing plan.

Doing the **financial analysis** can be very tricky for lactation consultants. Not only is it not the forte of most of us, but we are treading where few have gone before. Only scanty information is available to help you determine the income potential of a lactation consultant in private practice.

The financial analysis lays out your fees, projected sales, funding sources, and projected income, as well as all of your start-up costs and ongoing expenses. Basically, the financial analysis presents a detailed budget for your practice.

Let's start with your initial costs. You will need stationery, charting forms, and a computer, as well as such tools of the trade as a digital electronic scale and alternative feeding devices. Some of these articles must be purchased; the option of leasing is feasible with other items. If you plan to sell products, what will your inventory costs be for the first year? Calculate the cost of your phone, postage, educational materials, and advertising. If you will make home visits, include related automobile and parking expenses. If you will rent or buy space, include those costs in your calculations. Doing this work ahead of time will give you some idea how much money you need to open your business and help you to see some of the costs that must be absorbed in your pricing.

The financial analysis section is also where you list your fees. Since lactation consultation is a service industry, thinking about your fees for services rendered is very important. If you plan to use a sliding fee scale to accommodate clients of different financial means, offer professional discounts, or accept coupons, you will want to spell that policy out here. LCs set fees in several ways, most of them very "unscientific." Some check out the prevailing rate for pediatrician visits and charge that amount for a consultation. Others go by "feel," as in "This amount feels about right." Still others ask competing LCs in the area what they charge and set their fees accordingly.

Another option is also possible. First, think about what a health care professional with your educational background and years of experience *should* earn annually. If you haven't a clue, do some research. Find out what physical therapists, occupational therapists, and speech therapists charge in your area. When a home health agency sends out a nurse specialist, such as an enterostomal therapist, what does it charge? Doing this research will put you in the ballpark. The amount charged for health care provider visits varies greatly from region to region.

Once you have decided what a salary for an IBCLC of your experience ought to be, you will need to determine the cost of your overhead. Overhead includes your rent, real estate taxes, and/or mortgage, if you have an office, as well as your car costs, phone expenses, and so on. Add the yearly cost of your overhead to the amount of your annual salary. Now divide that number by 50 weeks. (You're allowed to have a vacation; be nice to yourself.) This amount should equal your weekly income.

Next, determine how many *billable hours* would be reasonable for a full-time LC in private practice. The time you spend reading journals, delivering brochures, attending conferences, and promoting your business is not billable, but it is an essential part of a thriving practice. Would you spend half of your time actually seeing patients? A third? If you estimate that half of your working hours would be billable hours, and that a full week would be 40 hours, you will need to divide your weekly income figure by one-half. If you estimate that an excellent LC in private practice would spend only one-third of her hours with paying clients, use that divisor. The result is the hourly rate that you should charge your clients.

Take a deep breath. How does that figure look to you? Too high? Actually, it's probably too low. Some sources recommend adding 30 percent to your salary to cover benefits. And remember that self-employed people pay a very high rate of income tax, keeping only about half of every dollar that they bring in.

Still sound too high? Consider this: In my area, having a cartoon character like "Barney" come to a children's party for an hour costs $125 (!). Skills needed: a purple suit and a big hug! A plumber charges $70–80 per hour for labor. My mechanic charges $45 hourly. A haircut at the cheapest shop in town is $11 and takes about 15 minutes. That's $44 per hour plus tips. A sick visit with the nurse practitioner at the pediatric office costs $40 and takes 10 minutes.

Still sound too high? A recent edition of the *Philadelphia Inquirer* listed salary ranges for various industries. The salary range for "consulting and professional services" was $45,000 to $200,000, for "health care/medical devices" $50,000 to 120,000, and for "pharmaceuticals" $45,000 to $185,000.

Practice stating your fees out loud. Write them down. Tell friends and colleagues. Think of the monthly cost of the artificial stuff people feed babies.

Not everyone will value your services. A mother who has her acrylic tip fingernails filled each week may tell you that your fees are too high. She does not place the same value on your services that you do. I feel no need to adjust my fees when a mother does not value my services. Sometimes, however, paying my fees would truly be a hardship. I am *always* willing to work out a plan with a mother who really wants my expertise, but my billable income must allow me to do that.

I believe that setting fees too low harms our profession. Setting fees too low sets a precedent for third-party payers. In other words, why should an insurance company pay someone $75 if someone else will provide the service for $50? At too low a rate, the LC would be hard-pressed to pay for the continuing education needed to keep her skills sharp and the activities needed to promote her practice. *We need to establish fees that allow us to practice with excellence.*

Once you have reflected on your costs and your fees, you can begin to calculate a break-even analysis. This is the point at which your income and expenses balance. How many clients per week do you need to see to break even? To make that number more realistic (and more complicated), include your sales projections. You may calculate that you would need to do 15 consultations per week to break even, but only 10 if you rent five breast pumps and teach one prenatal breastfeeding class. Be prepared to adjust your numbers once you have been in practice for a few months.

Include any other funding you may have from another agency, foundation, or other source. If you are taking out a loan, include the loan payments in your financial analysis. Computerized accounting programs can help you to put all of this financial information into a usable format.

Insurance information is also included in the business plan. Spell out each type of insurance you carry, the policy number, cost of premiums, amount of coverage, and name and address of each insurance company. Include your malpractice insurance, liability insurance for a home or outside office, and car insurance if you do home visits. If you plan to have disability insurance to give you some income should you become unable to work, include that information as well.

Operation procedures include the policies and procedures specific to each aspect of your business. Start with the legal form of your practice. Specify what legal form you have chosen and why. Include relevant licenses, permits, and zoning ordinances.

List your qualifications for the job of running your practice. Consider all of the administrative tasks of running a business. How will you take care of accounting, billing, inventory, and bookkeeping? Spell out how often you will do each task, what reports you will generate, and on what time table. If you plan to hire someone or contract out some of this work, specify their credentials, qualifications, and hours.

Identify policies for insurance billing, returned checks, and deferred payments. Write procedures for client interactions, including telephone greeting and messages, conducting a consultation, and reporting to the primary health care provider. If another person will work with you, you will need to be more specific about your policies and procedures.

The **marketing plan** lays out how you plan to attract new clients and keep the ones you already have. It is vital to every practice, and creating one can be a lot of fun. We will discuss promoting and marketing LC services in depth later in Part B of this book.

The **executive summary** capsulizes what you are going to do and how. If you are seeking funding, put your most persuasive paragraph here explaining why your lactation practice is a good risk. If you are applying for a loan, you will need **supporting documents** such as your tax returns, the results of your needs assessments, and references.

Writing a business plan can seem like a daunting task. However, investing the time to consider all of the business aspects can help you to turn your practice into a viable business. Numerous resources are available that can help you with the process. There is software both on-line and in office supply stores that helps to organize and format the information. There are good books available in your local library, bookstore, and on-line that can guide you as you learn to speak the language of business and formulate your plan. In addition, the Small Business Association Web site provides a basic business plan at no cost to you.

Your business plan is not a static document. You will need to revise it periodically, especially when beginning your practice. Factors not yet known to you will likely affect both your income and your expenses. Plan on your business plan being flexible.

Setting goals for your business helps you crystalize where you want to go. Dream about what you would like your business to be. Set specific one-year, five-year, and ten-year goals to help you to realize those dreams. Your goals may relate to the number of clients you hope to see, sales income you hope to generate, services you would like to add, and areas of professional growth. Refer to your goals often. You may even want to keep them posted near your desk. They keep you focused on where you're going, and help you to recognize destinations when you reach them, which is very satisfying.

DON'T LET SUCCESS RUIN YOUR LIFE

How will you define success? You can measure your achievements by how they measure up to your goals. You can, and should, take stock monthly, quarterly, and yearly. You may need to revise your goals along the way, but always keep them in sight. When you meet goals, celebrate your accomplishment.

Think for a minute about what success means for the lactation consultant. The numbers and dollars matter—they enable you to stay in business. Our profession is so much more. Economist and author Paul Hawken has this perspective:

> But if you undertake a service role to a customer, your outcome will always be successful, because your role is to inform and care for the customer. Even if this means "no sale," you have performed your role and are therefore successful.[4]

When you care for and educate a client, you are successful. Success in your life, however, encompasses so much more than success in your practice. Success in your life means finding balance as you consider your time, talents, relationships, and gifts.

Having the phone ring constantly may seem like a dream come true at this point in your practice. If you practice with excellence and work diligently to market your services, the phone will indeed ring often. Without planning and clear priorities, the dream come true can turn into a nightmare. You can easily become so busy meeting the needs of others that the needs of your own family, friends, and self go wanting.

Now, before you go much further, is the time to sit down and reflect on your priorities. How will you set limits with your practice? How will you ensure that your stated priorities are really the priorities by which you live? Many LCs become addicted to heroism. It feels more satisfying to step into a crisis and act the role of the savior than it does to read a story to a toddler, enjoy dinner with your family, or take a walk with a friend. Helping others is truly virtuous and to be encouraged. But, all too often, lactation consultants in private practice lose the perspective needed to live fully balanced lives.

It is also tempting to turn money making into the goal. Quoting Paul Hawken once again, "We are speeding up our lives and working harder in a futile attempt to buy the time to slow down and enjoy it." Albert Einstein once said, "Try not to become a man of success, but rather try to become a man of value." There is wisdom in those words.

How, practically speaking, can you set limits in your practice? Start by adopting the mindset and the language of a professional. Lactation consultation is your job, and your vocation, but not your life. Use phrases like "My hours are . . ." and "I have an appointment available . . . ." Consider collaborating with others in private practice so that you can each have some time "off."

Is there someone whose practice you feel comfortable enough with that you can cover for each other?

This type of professional collaboration offers some significant advantages. If there is someone whose philosophy complements your own and whose practice you respect, you might consider sharing marketing costs. Being willing to refer to another consultant and accepting referrals from her can help both of you sharpen your skills as you discuss cases and share ideas, while meeting more needs in the community. Finally, you can each enjoy more time off, focusing freely on other aspects of your life. It is also good to think about how you feel about adding a partner to your practice, and, if so, how you will determine that it is time.

SUMMARY

Being a lactation consultant in private practice can be tremendously rewarding. Investing time at the outset of your venture can help you to chart a course for your business to succeed. By doing a needs assessment, you will establish that a community need for your services exists. Your mission statement will help you to see the big picture of your life, out of which flows your business endeavor and other aspects of your life. The business plan will spell out the business side of your practice—that is, how you will function day to day, who will perform administrative tasks and how often, and how you will operate in the black financially. Your marketing activities will be ongoing and designed to effectively attract new clients and nurture your existing relationships. Finally, keeping sight of your life priorities and mission can help you to keep your business in perspective and find balance in your life.

NOTES

1. *Webster's Ninth New Collegiate Dictionary*. Springfield, MA: Merriam-Webster, 1991.
2. Sohnen-Moe, C. M. *Business Mastery*, 3rd ed. Tuscon, AZ: Sohnen Moe Associates, 1997.
3. Attard, J. *Business Know-How*. Holbrook, MA: Adams Media, 2000.
4. Hawken, P. *The Ecology of Commerce*, New York, NY: HarperCollins, 1993.

Books

RESOURCES

Attard, J. *Business Know-How*. Holbrook, MA: Adams Media, 2000.

Beckwith, H. *Selling the Invisible*. New York, NY: Warner Books, 1997.

Blanchard, K., and Bowles, S. *Raving Fans*. New York, NY: William and Morrow, 1993.

Davidson, J. *Breathing Space: Living and Working at a Comfortable Pace in a Sped-up Society*. New York, NY: Master Media, 1991.

Edwards, S., and Douglas, L. C. *Getting Business to Come to You*. New York, NY: Putnam, 1991.

Holtz, H. *How to Succeed as an Independent Consultant*. New York, NY: John Wiley & Sons, 1988.

Jones, L. B. *The Path: Creating Your Mission Statement for Work and for Life*. New York, NY: Hyperion, 1996.

Korn, I., and Zanker, W. *Starting a Home-Based Business (Full or Part Time)*, New York, NY: Citadel Press, 1993.

Lasser, J. K. *How to Run a Small Business*, 7th ed. New York, NY: McGraw-Hill, 1994.

McKenzie, J. F., and Smeltzer, J. L. *Planning, Implementing, and Evaluating Health Promotion Programs*. Needham Heights, MA: Allyn and Bacon, 1997.

Pollan, S. M., and Levine, M. *The Field Guide to Starting a Business*. New York, NY: Simon & Schuster, 1990.

Riordan, J., and Auerbach, K. (eds). *Breastfeeding and Human Lactation*. Boston, MA: Jones and Bartlett, 1998.

Sohnen-Moe, C. M. *Business Mastery*, 3rd ed. Tuscon, AZ: Sohnen Moe Associates, 1997.

Williams, B. *In Business for Yourself*. Chelsea, MI: Scarborough House, 1991.

Web Sites

www.businessknowhow.com: General business information

www.SBA.gov/starting/indexbusplans.html: A free business plan outline from the Small Business Administration

www.Amazon.com: Browse for business books to suit your taste

Other

Medela, Inc., manufactures electric breast pumps for lease and purchase. If you have an account, your representative may be able to help you with a business plan and with insurance billing information.

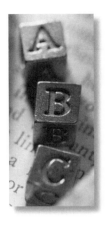

9 Legal Considerations

Elizabeth C. Brooks, JD, IBCLC

As a lactation consultant considering private practice, you confront the same legal issues facing any new small business owner. Your goals are probably quite simple: You want to set up your business properly, so it is easy to manage. You hope to avoid paying a lot of taxes. You want a simplified paperwork or recordkeeping system. You want to help mothers and babies happily breastfeed (although your cynical side is scared that someone will slap you with a silly lawsuit). You want to protect yourself, your personal assets (the house!), and the assets of your business.

Don't panic. This is not difficult legal territory. Hundreds of thousands of self-employed, small businesspeople have come before you, and they have all shared the same questions (and nervousness) about setting up shop. Your hometown has dozens of lawyers who can help you set up your business.

ACT LIKE YOU DO THIS FOR A LIVING

First, a bit of nonlegal advice. Ours is a young, growing profession. Every time you confer with a mother, you have an opportunity to market *the profession* of lactation consultation. As an IBCLC, you have an obligation to stay informed about lactation matters and to present yourself in a professional manner. What sort of impression do you leave about yourself (specifically) and lactation consultants (generally) if you scrawl your consult notes on Post-it notes attached to your grocery list? To do so creates a recordkeeping headache—and you'll risk losing (or foregoing) credibility in the eyes of the mothers you serve, and the other medical professionals with whom you are ethically required to interact. Even if your private practice will operate a mere 10 hours per week, you should *look* and *act* like the professional that your shingle claims you to be.

Promise yourself that you'll invest in yourself and in your business. You don't have to spend a lot of money, but spend what it takes to purchase the equipment and supplies necessary to do your job well. Use a sturdy bag or briefcase to carry your materials, not a filthy backpack. Use handouts that are clear and snappy (and proofread)—not crooked, faded copies. Order stationery, envelopes, and business cards that are attractive (and proofread) and reflect your style. Prepare (and proofread) your reports to health care providers promptly; send copies of everything to the mother. During your lactation consultation with a nursing mother, you will no doubt be leaning, squatting, and sitting. Wear comfortable, functional clothing that permits these movements, while allowing you to look polished. Slacks and a turtleneck go on just as easily as jeans and a T-shirt, but leave a better impression. Every time you come into contact with someone, you are telling a story about yourself and your chosen profession. Do it well.

HOW TO PICK A LAWYER (OR ACCOUNTANT)

Before you hire a lawyer, do your own research about opening a private practice. Buying this book was a great start! The more information you have, the better your lawyer (or accountant) will be able to serve you. Also, you'll save money in legal fees: Why pay an attorney to teach you basics that you can easily learn on your own? Lawyers, like lactation consultants, are professionals. They get paid for the time they spend giving you their expertise. The more you know before you sit down with your lawyer (or any other professional, for that matter), the more you will glean from the meeting. Once you have a better idea of the sorts of business and legal decisions you'll have to make, you can better evaluate who your lawyer should be.

Please Make This Easy for Me

Do you want to find a good lawyer? First, get a list of names and phone numbers of attorneys in your area who advise small businesses. Use the checklist on the following page to generate your list.

Once you have your list of names and numbers, call the attorneys' offices. Ask the following questions:

- Is the lawyer taking on new clients who want to establish and run a small business?

- What are the fees or rates for such legal consultation, and when must they be paid?

- Is there any material about the firm or the attorney that can be sent to you (or, does he or she have a Web site you might visit)? This information can give you an idea of how long the lawyer has been in practice, and whether this is the attorney's main area of practice.

- Is it possible to arrange an introductory meeting (at no cost to you) to meet the lawyer face-to-face? You aren't looking for your legal consultation here—you want to know if this lawyer is willing to take a few moments to market himself or herself to you, so you can decide whether to actually hire this person.

You'll be surprised at how many lawyers you can weed out with these telephone inquiries—and you might take a few notes for when you open your own private practice. Was the person who answered the phone courteous and informative? Did you get a live person, or did you leave a message on a voice messaging system? Was your call returned promptly? The questions you are asking are typical of any potential new client; if the attorney's office can't capably and impressively answer these "bread and butter openers," you might consider crossing that name off your list.

If you plan to meet the lawyer in person before hiring him or her, take stock of the office when you arrive. It doesn't have to be a fancy, but it should be run efficiently and effectively. Are there stacks of files and papers everywhere? Is the phone ringing off the hook? Does the staff (or the lawyer) look harried? You can judge a lot by these appearances. Again, you'd do well to make mental notes of what you would avoid (or duplicate) in your own private practice.

✔ Call some other IBCLCs in private practice in your area. Ask each for the name and number of her attorney, and whether she would recommend that lawyer.

✔ Think about the many mothers you see. One of them may be an attorney—or know someone who is. She may be thrilled to counsel *you*, for a change! Don't forget the barter system, either: You may find that you can "exchange" your professional services as a lactation consultant for her professional services as an attorney.[1] (The same holds true for other aspects of your business. Before they were breastfeeding, mothers were accountants, Web site designers, graphic design artists, bookkeepers, and so on. You may have several untapped resources right in your client index.)

✔ Ask small business owners you know (your hairdresser, your cleaning service, the local restaurateur) if they would recommend the attorney they used. If so, get that name and number.

✔ In the Yellow Pages, look under "Attorneys" and "Lawyers." There may be a separate entry for "Lawyer/Attorney Referrals." If specialties are listed, you want someone who handles "business/small business" law; that area may appear as "corporation, partnership and business law."

✔ Call your county or state bar association (the professional association for lawyers). Ask for its attorney referral service, and explain that you need a lawyer who can advise you as you establish and run your private practice. You can consider several attorneys, comparing their areas, locations, hours of office operation, and so on. Many attorneys who are listed under these referral programs have agreed to give you an initial consult for a reduced (or even waived) fee.

✔ If the local bar association doesn't operate a formal referral service, it may have "sections" (committees) for attorneys in the same practice area. Try to get in contact with the lawyer who chairs the Small Business or Commercial Section. That attorney is probably pretty good (after all, he or she is willing to do the important but unpaid work of running a substantive section of the bar association). The section may have its own attorney referral system, either formal or informal. There also may be a Women's, Young Lawyers', or Minority Lawyers' Section, if you would prefer to bring your business to an attorney fitting these descriptions.

✔ Find out whether your local chamber of commerce or a local "small business development center" has a list of attorneys willing to work with small businesses.

When you have narrowed your list of candidates, you are still entitled to know—before you hire anyone—how an attorney's experience and track record might be of value to you as an aspiring small business owner. You may have been able to tease out this information from the materials you received in the mail or from the attorney's Web site. Ask the attorney:

• *Are you licensed to practice law in this jurisdiction?* An attorney who has passed the bar exam somewhere—anywhere—is quite capable of doing legal research, advising you, and preparing legal papers and can charge you for such professional service. You need a lawyer licensed to practice in your local jurisdiction, however, if you must file papers in court. As you start up your business, your lawyer is not likely to be running into court. Rather, the attorney will be looking at state laws and regulations and preparing documents to send to government agencies. At some point down the road, if you must go to court on behalf of your business (perhaps to collect on unpaid breast pump rental fees), it would be nice to have a lawyer who has actually set foot in the courthouse.

- *What is your experience in the area of setting up a small business, and advising small business owners?*

- *In what other areas of law do you practice?* If your lawyer is a one-person shop offering representation on everything from personal injury cases to federal antitrust law, you might find your little company lost in the shuffle of bigger cases. Remember: A good general practitioner will be able to advise you in many legal areas—or to know where to look for answers.

- *Are paralegals, administrative assistants, or law students available to assist you in matters involving me and my company at lower rate?* Don't turn your nose up: A competent administrative assistant or paralegal is perfectly capable of preparing many of the documents you will need. Spend the more costly "attorney dollars" getting the legal advice only an attorney can provide!

- *How will you keep me informed of progress on matters involving me and my company?* Will you always have to initiate contact with your lawyer? Or does the attorney have some way to keep you "in the loop"? Bear in mind that many attorneys will not use e-mail for communicating confidential client information, as there is no guarantee of privacy.

- *What is a reasonable estimate of the total bill for your services, including fees and expenses?*

Now that you know how to get a good lawyer, here are some other homework assignments.

JOIN THE INTERNATIONAL LACTATION CONSULTANT ASSOCIATION AND YOUR ILCA LOCAL AFFILIATE

If you want to open a private practice, the best place to start is with other lactation consultants, whether they are hospital-based or work in private practice. *Join or start a local ILCA affiliate group.* It will be a fabulous resource for you. You can discuss cases and evidence-based practice with other, more experienced IBCLCs. You can ask questions in a relaxed, information-sharing atmosphere. As you become better known to your colleagues, you may find that they refer business to you. Attend the meetings and read the newsletters, because this sort of learning and chatting is what networking is all about. Your confidence, both as an IBCLC and as a businessperson, will increase as you spend time with people interested in the same line of work. You might also consider joining your local chamber of commerce or Rotary organization. These organizations include your neighbors who currently run small businesses. Their members will have plenty to share about starting a business in your community.

Professional Liability Insurance

If you plan to open a private practice, you should obtain a professional liability (malpractice) policy as an "allied health care professional—lactation consultant." It is quite affordable: One large Chicago-based firm charges $150 per year for a self-employed lactation consultant working with mothers for 20 hours per week. If you practice full-time, 20 hours is a realistic figure for the amount of time you will spend in face-to-face consultations with mothers (versus work on other aspects of your business, such as paperwork and bill-paying). Even if your state does not require allied health care professionals to carry malpractice insurance, you should do so anyway. While the risk of a lawsuit against an IBCLC is low, the fact remains that we are a litigious society. Nurses and doctors are sued all the time. As more IBCLCs enter the work force, more will find themselves drawn into lawsuits. Even unfounded lawsuits require a formal response. Professional liability insurance is designed to give you the help you need (a lawyer to represent you) if your professional integrity has been questioned.

You can select "occurrence form" insurance, which covers you for any incidents that arise while your policy remains in effect (even if you don't carry it now). A "claims made" policy must currently be in effect when the claim is made. Whichever kind you select, it should cover you for errors of negligence as well as malpractice. You would also be wise to ensure that your policy covers battery (the civil tort of "unwanted touching"). An IBCLC, by the very nature of her work, often touches a mother's breast or a baby's mouth. If your policy has an exclusion for battery claims, you may be left out in the cold! See Appendix B for some sources of malpractice insurance.

Many IBCLCs wear several hats: They work part-time at a hospital or pediatric practice, and part-time in private practice. You may have additional insurance coverage under your employer's "blanket" malpractice policy for work you do at that office. Look carefully at the fine print. When your roles blur, you may find yourself dropped through a loophole where the insurer can deny coverage. For example, suppose that you counsel a mother at the pediatric practice where you are the in-house lactation consultant three days a week. You advise her to rent a hospital-grade breast pump as part of your care plan to increase her milk supply, and leave her with a list of local breast pump rental stations (including your own). The mother comes to your home office the next day (when you are in private practice mode) to simply rent a pump. Are you seeing her as a private practice IBCLC—or is she still "seeing you" as an extension of the care she sought from her pediatrician?

General Liability Insurance

You'll want to be covered for negligence resulting in injury to others while you are on their premises (i.e., making a home visit), and while they are on yours (i.e., coming to your house to rent a pump).

Homeowner's Insurance

What does your homeowner's policy currently cover? If you anticipate having people come to your house as customers—not as guests—your homeowner's policy may *not* cover for accidents (someone who slips and falls or crunches your garage door while parking, for example). Because so many businesses operate out of homes these days, your homeowner's insurance agent may be able to set you up with a **business-in-the-home rider** to cover against such losses.

Business Insurance

Just like your home, your business should be insured against loss. Imagine a fire destroying all of your files, supplies, and computer equipment. You've not only lost the actual objects, but your ability to do business (and keep earning income) will no doubt be interrupted. Insurance is available to cover these possibilities.

Car Insurance

If you plan to use your car in your business (to travel to see mothers or to deliver breast pumps), be sure your policy protects for such business use of the car. Also, keep track of those miles: They are a legitimate tax deduction.

Breast Pump Insurance

If you rent breast pumps to mothers, be sure this equipment is insured, either under your business policy or through the (very affordable) insurance offered by the large breast pump companies. These pumps are worth hundreds of dollars. If you have one in your car trunk and get rear-ended, you'll be glad you have insurance to pay for its loss.

Medical and Disability Insurance

Now that you are opening your own business, you may be leaving a job that offered you several benefits, including health care insurance, worker's compensation, and personal disability insurance. These sorts of safeguards against loss of income due to injury or illness will be vitally important to you now that you are self-employed.

BUSINESS LICENSE AND ZONING CONSIDERATIONS

Now is the time to take a trip to town hall. Find out what your local government officials (city, township, or county) require in the way of a business license for a self-employed, small businessperson. Usually you will pay a small fee, perhaps annually, to have a "license to do business" in your municipality.[2]

Zoning considerations may apply as well. Does your town restrict the kinds of signage you can have at your front door? Will there be foot and car traffic to and from your home? Does the town allow you to have a business in your home at all? In some areas, strict zoning codes govern the type of business activity you can conduct from home.

If you plan to see clients within an office setting, you may need to obtain a building safety permit and/or a certificate of occupancy (which shows your location has been inspected and found to be safe for you and your clients). Check with your local fire department.

D id you ever think of yourself as a retailer? You may well be. The interactions you have with a mother may create more than one legal relationship between the two of you. If you sell her a breastfeeding product (a pillow, a book, a bra), you take on a *commercial* role in addition to your IBCLC role. You are the seller; the mother is the buyer. In the eyes of the law, you are just like Sears Roebuck and Company. Have you thought about how you'll handle commercial transactions such as returning products, taking checks or credit cards, or offering discounts?

Check with your state department of revenue. Often, the fees you earn as a lactation consultant are considered a "service," which is *not* subject to sales and use tax. Once you start offering equipment to mothers—whether you're selling it or renting it—you will probably come under an obligation to collect (and remit) sales taxes for the state. Thus, if the mother buys a nipple shield from you, you have to collect the appropriate sales tax from her. Several times each year, you will send in the tax you've collected to the state revenue department. Some local authorities (the city or county) impose a sales tax on top of what the state charges.

You will need to obtain a sales tax license from your state. This process is usually fairly simple. Your state wants you to start and maintain a successful business within its borders: Take advantage of the state's inherent desire to assist you in doing so.

SALES TAXES AND TRANSACTION PRIVILEGES

D o you know how to run a small business? Does "cash or accrual method of accounting" mean anything to you? You don't need to learn it all right now, but you need to have some idea of what you are planning to get yourself into.

You might be pleasantly surprised at how eager people are to help an aspiring small businessperson. Some obvious places to look for information are the library, town hall or municipal government offices, your local chamber of commerce, and any big book store. Connect with associations of executives such as SCORE (Service Corps of Retired Executives), a nonprofit organization of retired executives eager to share their experience with new business owners. Check the local community college or any adult education program (whether accredited or not) for classes about opening a small business, using computer software, or keeping track of business records.

The Internet

The Internet is teeming with information—almost too much. Be savvy as you surf. Consider and evaluate the source of your information, just as you evaluate written resources. A ".com" is a *com*merce entity. A Web site with this address extension is a business venture. Even if you don't have to pay money to use the site, someone has. Are the facts you're seeing slanted to endorse one particular viewpoint (the advertiser's)? A ".gov" site is run by a government agency. Stop cringing: State and federal bureaucracies these days are easy to access, fun, flashy—even hip. To see how, just pull up www.irs.gov, the site of the venerable Internal Revenue Service (IRS). An ".org" is a nonprofit entity; an ".edu" is an educational institution.

BASIC RESEARCH ON BECOMING SELF-EMPLOYED OR STARTING A SMALL BUSINESS

Often you can accomplish more than one goal by venturing onto the Internet. For example, many materials available from the IRS about business taxes also include how-tos (complete with examples) about setting up your business or keeping your records. For some reason, people become paralyzed with fear when they must deal with taxes and the IRS. While the paying of taxes may not be fun, the tax folks are generally quite helpful. They'd rather help you set it up right at the front end than tangle with giving penalties at the back end.

Not hooked up to the Web yet? *Do it.* If you haven't purchased a computer or Internet access yet, you can often test-drive the Internet using computers at the public library. You will have a wealth of information at your fingertips— not only about business and taxes, but also on breastfeeding management and advocacy. It is a standard of practice in other professions to be proficient in computer-based research. Shouldn't IBCLCs have a similar high standard?[3]

Gathering Federal Tax and Small Business Information on the Internet

The IRS has a very consumer-friendly site. Look what 20 seconds in front of a computer offer you! Visit www.IRC.gov on the Internet. The IRS home page is "The Digital Daily," updated each day. Click "Tax Info for Business," and you reach a page chock-full of tantalizing offerings for businesses of all sizes. You'll no doubt be drawn to the "Small Business and Self Employed Community" heading. Click once, and you access another page that just can't wait to help you. Want your free, single copy of the "2001 Small Business Resource Guide, CD-ROM 2001"? This disk represents a collaborative effort between the IRS and the Small Business Administration (SBA) "intended to be a one-stop source of easy access to federal tax and other regulatory information important to small business entrepreneurs. The CD contains business tax forms, instructions, and publications needed by small business owners. In addition, the CD provides an abundance of other helpful information, such as how to prepare a business plan, finding financing for your business, and much more."[4] How's *that* for a party favor?

Prowl around the IRS site some more. It allows you to download publications or forms in Adobe Acrobat® (PDF) format. With PDF format, you can view the document on your computer screen just as it was printed by the government. You can type directly onto the form and then print it out; the printout will look just like the official IRS version. If you prefer, you can use "text only" to quickly read through the information (because Adobe downloading can take longer). If your computer isn't currently equipped with Adobe Acrobat, the site provides easy instructions as to how you can immediately add it to your computer (for free). Also, almost all tax forms can now be filed electronically.

Head back and click the "New Business" button when you reach the "Small Business and Self Employed Community" page. You can pull up several options with timely advice. Look at how succinctly the "Before you Begin" page lays out the sorts of regulations you need to think about when starting up a small business:

- Business licenses (which come from the local authorities)
- Certificate of occupancy (to use office space outside your home; local)
- Business organization (the legal structure of your business; a state authority function)

- Registering a business name (a county or state role)
- Protecting your ideas (through patent, trademark, and copyright protections afforded by federal authorities)
- Business (and professional liability) insurance (local)
- Sales and use tax numbers (issued by the state)
- Employer responsibilities, if you have people working for you, including unemployment insurance, worker's compensation, minimum wage, and health and safety requirements

In short, the IRS Web site allows you to download every form, instruction sheet, pamphlet, and publication the IRS has to offer—which is a lot. Be sure to peruse IRS Publication 583: Starting a Business and Keeping Records, which "provides basic federal tax information for people who are starting a business. It also provides information on keeping records and illustrates a record keeping system." What more could you ask?

Another resource for the aspiring entrepreneur (that's you) is the Web site of the Small Business Administration www.sba.gov. Again, the agency is just itching to help the new businessperson. Click a button on the SBA home page for "Starting Your Business." From here, you can access dozens of helpful pages, with enticing names like "Your First Steps," "Startup Kit," "Do Your Research," and "Training." You can even add your electronic business card to this Web site when you're up and running! (Go to "Business Card," type "lactation consultant" at the "search all fields" option, and see what pops up.)

The SBA also provides great opportunities for you to learn, either on the Web or through free (or low-cost) classes near your home. Go to the SBA home page and click "SBA Classroom" to find out what the department has to offer on-line or at a nearby SBA office. Try clicking the "Outside Resources" button, which takes you to a page that is described as the SBA's "3,779 Outside Resources and Great Business Hotlinks." You might look into SCORE as well. These mentors-in-waiting offer free counseling (even on-line) and free or low-cost workshops for the new entrepreneur. Try "Women in Business" to see if any links look interesting to you.

Gathering State Tax and Small Business Information on the Internet

Several states have created easy-to-use Web sites, enabling you to quickly learn what is required to start a business within their borders. The federal IRS and SBA Web sites have links to several states' Web pages, another easy way to access these sites. Why do you care? Because businesses in the United States are created and conducted according to state law, even if you must also pay federal taxes or obey federal laws. When you form your business entity, it is done under the rules, regulations, and authority of your state government.

Let's use my state of Pennsylvania as an example. I start at www.state.pa.us, the home page for the Commonwealth of Pennsylvania. When I click the "Business in PA" option, I reach a page with several tempting entries, such as "Start a Business," "Business Taxes," and "Maintain a Business." By clicking and surfing a bit, I can reach every department within my state government that has a stake in seeing that I successfully start my new business venture. After all, I represent precisely the sort of revenue-generating commerce every state likes to attract. My state officials want to make it easy for me to figure out which forms must be filled out and where to send them.

Your community-level government officials may not be "wired" yet, so you'll want to call or visit your local officials for information. Many municipalities, however, have very sophisticated Web pages; indeed, the Internet may be the only source for some information (which local commissions could not otherwise afford to print on paper).

What Does Your Research Reveal?

Probably your first decision is: What form should my new business take? When you boil it all down, there are just three basic forms of business ownership: sole proprietorships, partnerships, and corporations. Some states have created business forms that are unique within their borders; they are designed to make it easier for the small entrepreneur to start a business, without putting any personal assets on the line. Select your business form carefully. It affects everything from how you report and pay taxes to how you keep business and financial records.

Sole Proprietorship

A sole proprietorship is an unincorporated business owned by one person. The person *is* the business.[5] In this simplest form of business ownership, the sole proprietor has maximum freedom to make business decisions and minimal legal restrictions. As the owner, you receive all the profits that are earned, and it is easy to discontinue the business if you so choose. All income and expenses are reported on your individual tax return (in schedules attached to your federal 1040 form).

The primary disadvantage of a sole proprietorship is that business liabilities are also personal liabilities—meaning that the owner can be held personally responsible for all debts of the business. In other words, creditors may tie up your personal assets (your furniture or house!) to settle debts, even though you didn't use them in the business. Sole proprietors have limited ability to raise capital; funds are restricted to whatever the owner can personally secure (the furniture and house again). This constraint could hamper your ability to operate the business effectively during the early low-profit periods or to expand later on.

Partnership

A partnership is a relationship between two or more persons, who join to create an unincorporated business, each offering their money, skill, labor, and so on, and each expecting to share in the profits and losses.[6] The advantages are that a partnership is easy to organize, and it offers greater financial strength than a sole proprietorship. It combines the managerial skill, judgment, and expertise of the partners. The entity attains a legal status apart from the partners themselves, while each partner has a personal interest (stake) in the business. A partnership doesn't pay income tax; rather, the profits or losses "pass through" to each partner, who report them using schedules on their own federal 1040 tax returns.

Partnerships do have some drawbacks. Each partner has unlimited liability for the losses caused by each partner (meaning one bad apple can cause the whole lot to pay damages). There is also shared authority and decision making. Choose your partners very carefully! An IBCLC who has wonderful rapport with mothers may still make a lousy *business partner*.

Some Recent Improvements on Partnerships

Many states have laws permitting creation of a special business entity called a limited liability company (LLC), a limited liability partnership (LLP), or an S corporation. Here, the owners/partners are *not* personally liable for the business's debts and liabilities, except to the extent of their investment in the company. Voilà—your furniture and house are protected! Ask your Secretary of State's Office, or possibly the Department of Commerce, whether such an entity is recognized by your state, and how you would go about registering yours.

Why did some states make this change? Very simply, it is an incentive for you to start a business. The self-employed or small businessperson enjoys the protections afforded to a corporation: If the business fails or you get sued, your furniture and house are safe. Better still, you retain the paperwork and tax-paying simplicity of a partnership. The income and expenses are divided among the shareholders—who may be just one person—who then report them on their individual tax returns.[7]

Thus, you'll keep the tax and recordkeeping advantages of a partnership, but you retain the managerial aspects as well. If you work with another person, can you happily arrive at joint business decisions? While increased paperwork responsibilities come at the front end (to establish and register the entity with the federal and state agencies), it is a "one-shot" deal.

Corporation

A corporation is a business entity with an identity separate from its owners, the shareholders (or stockholders). Corporations are formed when shareholders give money or property in exchange for capital stock.[8] The shareholders own the corporation, although its day-to-day operations may be handled by managers and a board of directors. Some corporations have their stock publicly traded on Wall Street; others are privately held (meaning the shares may be owned by a small group or by one family).

Why form a corporation? The business has a perpetual "life"; it exists in spite of (rather than because of) the personalities of its owners. Stockholders have limited liability (the furniture and house again), and ownership is easy to transfer (through the sale of stock). It is also easier to raise capital, and corporations are readily adapted to small and large businesses.

The disadvantages? A corporation is subject to "double taxation." That is, the business is taxed at both the corporate level (taxes are paid when the corporation pays out dividends) and the shareholder level (income taxes are paid on the dividends received). Organizing and registering a corporation under your state's laws can be complex and cumbersome. Corporations are subject to extensive state and federal controls.

Identification Numbers

You Have a Personal Number

To process tax returns, federal and state tax agencies use a special taxpayer number to identify who you are. Most of us in the United States use our Social Security number (SSN), issued by the Social Security Administration. Its format is 000-00-0000. If you operate as a sole proprietorship or partnership, you'll probably report your earnings using your SSN.

As a lactation consultant in private practice, you may have to supply your number to other people or entities that have their own reporting responsibilities to the government. How so? Imagine that a colleague you met while attending your local ILCA affiliate group meeting has asked you to fill in for her at a breastfeeding talk she is giving to pregnant mothers. She'll pay you the $75 she would have earned that night. That IBCLC will need to know *your* SSN, because she must explain (in her own business records) why she is paying you $75 out of her business checkbook.

Your Business May Have a Number

Another taxpayer identification number is issued by the Internal Revenue Service. The employer identification number (EIN) is formatted as 00-0000000.[9] The IRS uses the EIN to figure out who must file certain kinds of business tax returns. EINs are used by employers, corporations, *sole proprietors, partnerships, certain individuals,* and a few others. Even if you work all by yourself, and you report your earnings by attaching a schedule to your tax forms, you may still need an EIN (if you formed your business as an LLC, LLP, or S corporation).

Obtaining an EIN is very easy.[10] Some things to remember: You should have only one EIN as a sole proprietor, even if you operate more than one sole proprietorship. If you change your business into a partnership or corporation, get a new EIN, as each separate partnership and corporation must have its own EIN.

You May Need to Get Some Numbers

You may need to *get* numbers from others with whom you deal. Remember that talk you did for your friend? Now you want to go out of town, and she's going to cover for you. That $75 you paid her needs to be accounted for in your business records. You'll need to know your colleague's "payee identification number," which is either her SSN or her EIN.[11]

IF YOU WORK ALONE, ARE YOU AN EMPLOYER?

Step back just a bit. It is perfectly legal, ethical, and desirable to use deductions (and other means) to *reduce* the amount of tax you must pay. This statement is true for an individual taxpayer, and it is a business concern. But you *do* have to pay the legitimate taxes owed by your business.[12] The tax folks decide how much you owe by looking at how you set up and run your business. In this area, the business of lactation consulting can create some headaches.

Employer for Tax Purposes

If you don't have any employees, you're not an employer, right? The answer to that question is sometimes complex: It depends. A person who does work for you may be classified as a common-law employee, a statutory employee, or an independent contractor. These designations concern the self-employed lactation consultant, for it is the classification of the person that determines which tax forms you must file (and which taxes you must pay).[13]

Employee or Independent Contractor?

Generally, you must withhold and pay a whole bunch of taxes (income, Social Security, and Medicare) on income (wages) you pay to an employee. You can't get around the issue just by giving different labels to the people who do work for you. The IRS will look at all the circumstances.

A *common-law employee* is anyone who performs services for you, where you control *what* will be done and *how* it will be done. You're considered an employer when you have the *right* to control the details of how the services are performed, even where the person has freedom of action.[14]

Want an example? You and another IBCLC are very compatible. She has worked as a hospital IBCLC, but is interested in branching into private practice (like you). You are feeling overwhelmed with the number of calls you get from mothers needing consults. The two of you come up with a great idea: Your friend will join you on several home visits over the next few months. You can show her how you do your charting, write letters to doctors, and handle follow-up with mothers. She can learn the ropes of private practice, all with your expert guidance. You will, of course, pay your friend for the time she gives to help ease your workload. You'll also get consent from all the mothers first.

Nifty idea, right? Absolutely. Under this scenario, however, someone receives money from you, does consults under your careful tutelage, and prepares paperwork under your guidance. The IRS is very likely to consider her your *employee*—even though the arrangement is short-term, and even though the two of you have no plan to enter into an employer–employee relationship.

You do not have to withhold or pay taxes on money you give to *independent contractors*. Independent contractors are usually self-employed people—lawyers, building contractors, plumbers, seamstresses, and IBCLCs—who offer services to the public, for a fee. It is tempting to avoid the employer's tax payments by simply explaining that any money you've paid to an outsider is going to an "independent contractor."

The IRS is wise to this tactic. It will carefully consider the "degree of control and independence" you exert over the person paid in this manner. The general rule is that "an individual is an independent contractor if you, the payer, have the right to control or direct only the result of the work and not the means and methods of accomplishing the result."[15] If the IRS decides the payee is an employee, you'll have to pay the taxes.

The IRS generally examines three areas:

- *Behavioral control.* Does the business have a right to direct and control how the worker does the task? An employee is generally given instructions as to when, where, and how to work, what tools to use, and what procedures to follow. An independent contractor will do the job on her own, as she sees fit. Training? Employees get training from the business: They go on company time, and the company pays the tuition. An independent contractor is responsible for her own training, on her own time and dime.

- *Financial control.* How much control does the company exert over the business aspects of the payee's job? An independent contractor usually has unreimbursed expenses; an employee is repaid by the boss for out-of-pocket expenses. An independent contractor often has made a significant investment in the facilities and materials used to provide her services. The independent contractor incurs ongoing costs—whether or not she is working right now. She is also free to make her services available to anyone willing to pay for them. Lastly, independent contractors are often paid a flat fee (not a wage) and may make a profit or a loss.

- *Type of relationship.* The IRS will look at the entire situation to see what kind of relationship the two parties envisioned. A written contract can describe the relationship the parties intended to create (including one that says you are doing work as an independent contractor). If a worker receives such benefits as insurance, vacation, and sick pay, she is probably an employee. Hiring someone for an indefinite period also tilts you toward employee.

YOU'VE CHOSEN A BUSINESS ENTITY; WHAT ELSE SHOULD YOU CONSIDER?

The IRS has created a very helpful booklet to help you narrow your concerns as you contemplate opening a private practice.[16] You will have to pay taxes on the money generated by your lactation consultation business. The federal and state governments set their own rules as to what sorts of tax a business is responsible for, but they often echo each other. The taxes you must pay (and when) also depend on what business form you decide to take. While we are putting the cart a bit before the horse, here are some basics to guide you.

Four types of business taxes exist:

- Income taxes
- Self-employment taxes (Social Security and Medicare tax for individuals who work for themselves)
- Employment taxes (paying the government the income tax you have withheld from employees)
- Excise taxes (on products and industries not related to breastfeeding)

Income Taxes

All businesses (except partnerships) must file an annual income tax return. Partnerships report their annual income on an information form. Many LCs simply report this income on IRS Form 1040, attaching Schedule C: Profit or Loss from Business (Sole Proprietorship). You may even use the simpler Schedule C-EZ if you operated only one business as a sole proprietorship, without a net loss.

Note that income tax is "pay as you go." Back in the good old days, when you had a "regular job," your employer withheld income taxes for you from your paycheck. As a small business, you will pay the amount of income tax that is due when you file your tax forms in April, *unless* you are required to pay "estimated tax." That requirement means you must pay your income taxes up front, if you expect your lactation consultant in private practice business to be so successful that you will owe more than $1000 in taxes on your business income this year.[17]

Self-Employment Taxes

The self-employment taxes consist of Social Security and Medicare tax for self-employed people. You must pay it if the net earnings in your private practice exceeded $400 this year. Again, you may find that your annual 1040 form is all that you need. You would attach a Schedule SE: Self Employment Tax.[18]

Employment Taxes

Recall the earlier discussion of employee versus independent contractor. If you do, in fact, have employees whom you pay, you will need to file forms to report (1) Social Security and Medicare taxes, (2) federal income tax withholding, and (3) federal unemployment tax. You can see why a self-employed businessperson would be eager to avoid this complicated bookkeeping. One reminder: You don't have to withhold taxes on money you pay to an independent contractor, but you still have to report those payments on a simple information form.[19]

Excise Taxes

Thankfully, a lactation consultant can probably ignore excise taxes. They are paid on the manufacture or sale of certain products (such as alcohol, tobacco, and firearms).

Simple, short information forms are required when you make or receive payments in your business, apart from wages to an employee. For example, suppose you paid $600 or more for services to your company by people who aren't employees—such as the lawyer and accountant you hired to prepare your tax forms, or the graphic artist who designed your company logo. You will report the payments made on IRS Form 1099-MISC, Miscellaneous Income. The IRS gets a copy, and so does the person you paid. The government compares your information return with the tax forms filed by the person who got your money to make sure that person or company reported it.

The same drill occurs if you received money from another IBCLC when, for example, you did a talk for her.[20] She'll file an IRS Form 1099-MISC, and give you a copy. You, of course, will admit you received this income when you prepare your annual income tax return.

WHAT CAN YOU DEDUCT? THE INFORMATION ON INFORMATION FORMS

You Can Dream

Imagine you have a lactation consultation with a young heiress. She is so thrilled when she and her babies learn to breastfeed happily that she gives you a bonus—a very big bonus. Let's hope we are all, one day, forced to file IRS Form 8300: Report of Cash Payments Over $10,000 Received in a Trade or Business.

Let the rest of this section serve as a mere primer on the sorts of deductions you can legitimately take from the taxes your company will pay.

Business Expenses

You can deduct business expenses on your income tax return, as these are the costs of running your business.[21] To be deductible, the expense must be (1) *ordinary*—common and accepted in your profession, like stationery, office supplies, breast pads, and newborn feeding cups and (2) *necessary*—helpful and appropriate for your profession, like use of a car.

Business Bad Debt

Sometimes a mother won't pay you for your consultation or her breast pump rental. You can deduct this "business bad debt" (where you were unable to collect money owed) as an expense on your business tax return. These unpaid-for goods and services are usually shown in your business books as "accounts (or notes) receivable."

Business Start-Up Costs

The money you spend to research whether you should go into business is considered a "capital expense." These "capital expenses" might include advertising, market surveys, training, and even the cost of this book. You can recover your start-up costs by "amortizing." That means you deduct a little chunk of the total start-up costs over several years.

Lots of office equipment lasts for more than a year (such as the computer, the fax, and the desk and chair). These expenses are usually "depreciated," which means you deduct a portion of these expenses over several tax years. Just to make you crazy, the IRS will let you deduct the amount of certain depreciable property (such as a computer) in the year you purchase it.[22]

Car (and Truck) Expenses

You can deduct the cost of operating and maintaining the car you use in your business, even if you drive the same car for personal use. You can deduct the actual expenses (i.e., gas, insurance, tolls, parking, depreciation), so long as you divide your expenses between business and personal use. It is easier to use the "standard mileage rate." Just keep track of the miles you drive for business purposes (using a little notebook you can buy at any stationery supply store). Each year the IRS announces the rate (for 2001, it was 34.5 cents per mile). Multiply the number of business miles by the standard milage rate to calculate your deduction. Note that you can still deduct parking and tolls even if you use the standard mileage rate.[23]

Depreciation

If property you acquire to use in your business is expected to last more than one year (e.g., a desk, chair, file cabinet, storage shelves for pumps), you can't deduct the entire cost of the items in the year of purchase.[24] Instead, you must spread the cost over several years, deducting just one chunk at a time (on the Schedule C or C-EZ with your 1040 form). Some "listed property" is subject to extra recordkeeping rules for depreciation. You care about this factor because it includes computers and cell phones.[25]

Insurance

Remember that professional liability insurance you bought? Deduct the cost! If you bought health insurance for you and your family as a small businessperson, you may be able to deduct as much as 60 percent of that expense as well.[26] If you purchased credit insurance (on loss from bad business debt), that may be deducted. An employer may deduct a whole host of other insurances, such as worker's compensation insurance and contributions to state unemployment insurance funds.

Interest

Some of the rules are quite technical, but you are entitled to deduct the interest you paid on money borrowed for business purposes.[27]

Legal and Professional Fees

You can deduct fees you pay to a lawyer or accountant who advises you about your small business. You can also deduct fees paid to have your business tax forms prepared for you.

Travel, Meals, and Entertainment

These costs are the ordinary and necessary expenses of traveling away from home for your business (for example, to attend a lactation conference to earn the CERPs you need as an IBCLC). They include (1) transportation costs (i.e., your plane fare), (2) taxi/limo/car rental costs, (3) baggage and shipping costs (to get materials there), (4) lodging for overnight stays, (5) laundry/cleaning while you are there, (6) business phone calls and faxes, (7) tips, (8) meals (though usually you can claim only 50 percent of your meal costs), and (9) entertainment expenses for a client or customer (again, usually at a 50 percent rate). These sorts of deductions have been abused in the past, so the IRS looks rather carefully at any deductions in this area. If you keep your receipts, you can show they were legitimate deductions.[28]

Other Business Expenses

Other business expenses likely to affect a lactation consultant in private practice include (1) advertising, (2) donations to business/professional organizations (e.g., ILCA), (3) educational expenses (seminars and training manuals), (4) licenses and regulatory fees, (5) subscriptions to trade or professional publications, and (6) supplies and materials.[29]

Business Use of Your Home

Lactation consultants in private practice will want to carefully study the rules governing business use of their home. Even if you do not have an office in your home where you see mothers for lactation consults, you no doubt use a portion of your home to store files and business records, to make phone calls and schedule appointments, and to pay business bills. If you can meet the IRS's carefully crafted definition of the "business use of your home," you can deduct all the expenses associated with using that part of your house. Let's explore this possibility in some detail.[30]

Very specific requirements must be met if you plan to deduct expenses related to the business use of your home. Your use of the business part of your home must be *exclusive* and *regular*. That means the area you use (i.e., the spare bedroom you converted into an office) can be used *only for your business*.[31] It won't count if your children regularly come into your "office" to play video games. Also, the space must be used in your business on a *continuing* basis. You cannot use the space only occasionally—even if it isn't used for anything else at the idle times.

In addition, the business part of your home must be either *your principal place of business, a meeting place for you and your customers,* or *a sepa-*

rate structure apart from the house. Once again, the IRS has spelled out exactly what this requirement means. The *principal place of business* is that part of your home used to exclusively and regularly conduct the administrative or management activities of your business. Even if you go elsewhere to do your work (i.e., home visits), you qualify if you use your home office to do such work as (1) billing, (2) keeping books and records, (3) ordering supplies, (4) setting up appointments, and (5) writing and forwarding reports. The business part of your home may be a *meeting place for you and your customers.* For example, you may have clients who come into your home during the normal course of business (i.e., to rent a breast pump), even if you also go elsewhere to work (i.e., make home visits). Lastly, you may have a *separate structure* (apart from your house) used in connection with your business, such as a studio or converted free-standing garage. If so, this business use of the home can be deducted.[32]

How Much of a Deduction Can You Take?

You can deduct *in full* those expenses related only to running the business, but not the house (e.g., advertising, business taxes, supplies). "Direct expenses," spent only on the business part of your home (e.g., painting the office), are also generally deductible in full. Other expenses can't be broken out so neatly. You must divvy up some expenses involved in running your house between personal and business uses. To do so, you multiply by your "business percentage" to see how much you can deduct for those "indirect expenses" that are spent to run the entire house (such as homeowner's insurance, rent, repairs, depreciation on your home, and utilities[33]).

You can claim deductions for the business use of your home only if you use Schedule A of IRS Form 1040: Itemized Deductions. Being self-employed, you'll show business income and expenses on Schedule C (IRS Form 1040), Profit or Loss from Business. You'll figure out your business expenses on IRS Form 8829, Expenses for the Business Use of Your Home, and transfer the deductible numbers over to line 30 on Schedule C.

One note of caution: Don't "double deduct" your real estate taxes and mortgage interest. Recall that some deductions on your 1040 form are yours no matter how you earn a living (i.e., mortgage interest and real estate taxes). If you use part of your home for your business, multiply by your "business percentage" to know how much of the deduction is claimed by you the *person* (on Schedule A) and how much is claimed by you the *business* (on Schedule C).

KEEPING TRACK OF THIS PAPERWORK IN A PRIVATE PRACTICE

As a Businessperson

You have an obligation and duty, as a small businessperson, to keep accurate records of your business venture. Good records will help you monitor the progress of your business, prepare your tax returns and financial statements, identify the source for money received, keep track of deductible expenses, and support your tax returns.

Business and tax law don't prescribe any special sort of recordkeeping. Any system employed should make sense for your work as a lactation consultant, and many computer-based programs can track both your clients and your business records. Select your accounting method wisely,[34] so your accounting system can make it easier to track your business income and expenditures.

Supporting documents (e.g., purchase receipts, invoices, deposit slips, paid bills, canceled checks) contain all the information that is to be recorded in your books. Supporting documents show your gross receipts (income you receive in business), your purchases, and your expenses. They substantiate your tax claims. It helps to keep them organized: try using an expanding file folder, divided by month and year. Simply drop your receipts into the appropriate pocket. You will also need supporting documents to figure out the depreciation on your assets (such as office furniture).

How long should you keep your business records? "As long as they may be needed for the administration of any provision of the Internal Revenue Code."[35] Translation: Most business records should be kept for a maximum of seven years but you'd be wise to keep *forever* the paperwork or records used to create and support your tax returns.

As a Lactation Consultant

Quite apart from your duty to keep good business records, you also have a duty to keep accurate files reflecting the actual work you do as a lactation consultant: client files, phone logs, letters to physicians, sales and rental receipts for breastfeeding supplies.

If you are in private practice, working alone every day, it is very easy to slide into recordkeeping techniques that make perfect sense to you—but that might confuse anyone looking over your shoulder. This is precisely what you should assume happens whenever you commit pen to paper. While your clients are entitled to confidentiality (which means you don't talk to anyone about her case without the mother's permission), that excuse doesn't mean your paperwork is free from examination. Will you be able, even years from now, to examine a file about one of your mothers and reconstruct your consultation and follow-up? Will the abbreviations and forms you use be clear to an outside reader? To an outside reader who is not a lactation consultant? Strive for files that are accurate yet concise, legible, free of personal opinion, and written at the same time as the events you describe. Keep them as long as required by your local jurisdiction, which usually specifies "until the child reaches the age of majority"—often 18 years or more.

ARE YOU READY?

Don't panic! You can do this! Almost all of us have the inherent desire to perform our responsibilities well. You are not likely to get into trouble if you give thoughtful preparation to the creation of your private practice. You've already tackled the most difficult part: You've earned your IBCLC credential by spending thousands of hours assisting breastfeeding mothers and babies. If you can apply even half that much vigor to the planning of your small business, you should be up and running in no time.

SUMMARY

You do have serious legal considerations as you establish your private lactation consultant practice. Fortunately, this is easy legal territory. Plenty of help is available as you decide when, and in what form, your private practice will open. Do some research—on your own, at the start—about opening a small business. Use the Internet, join your professional association, get out and talk to other IBCLCs. Consider carefully the various forms a small business can take: Once you've decided, it triggers several other ongoing responsibilities (such as when, how, and whether you pay taxes). Then, find an attorney who is experienced in establishing and representing small businesses and one-person shops in your community. Protect yourself (and your family) by purchasing professional liability insurance and other insurances for business losses. Learn—from the start—what files and papers you must generate, not only about your consultations, but also about your business. Your private practice is a business: It brings a myriad of legally enforceable responsibilities as money flows into, and out of, your enterprise.

NOTES

1. You must report these barter exchanges on your income tax return. See IRS Form 1099-B (and its separate instructions): Proceeds from Broker and Barter Exchange Transactions.

2. Lactation consultants generally are not required to have an *occupational license* (from the state) to work as an IBCLC (the way an RN needs a license to work as a nurse, or a hairdresser needs a license to cut your hair). An occupational license is different from a business license; the latter you *will* need.

3. In the meantime, humans are available to help you. Call (800) 829-3676 to order IRS Publication 454: Your Business Tax Kit (an assortment of forms and publications to help taxpayers operating a business). From your fax machine, dial (703) 368-9694 and follow the prompts to receive IRS publications. Dial (800) TAX-FORM to get IRS Publication 910: Guide to Free Tax Services. Call (800) 829-1040 for 24-hour tax assistance; (800) 829-4477 offers recorded tax information and automated refund information; (800) 827-5722 (during the day) is the Small Business Answer Desk at the Small Business Administration.

4. You can also obtain your single, free copy by calling (800) 829-3676 and asking for IRS Publication 3207.

5. IRS Publication 334: Tax Guide for Small Business (For Individuals Who Use Schedule C or C-EZ).

6. IRS Publication 541: Partnerships.

7. See IRS Form 1120S (and its separate instructions): U.S. Income Tax Return for an S Corporation; IRS Form 2553 (and its separate instructions): Election by a Small Business Corporation; and IRS Form 8832 (with attached instructions): Entity Classification Election.

8. IRS Publication 542: Corporations.

9. IRS Publication 1635: Understanding your EIN.

10. Fill out IRS Form SS-4, Application for Employer Identification Number (which you can download from the IRS Web site). For immediate gratification, apply for your EIN by phone. Once you have filled in your SS-4, you call the Tele-TIN number noted on the SS-4, and it can be assigned *immediately*.

11. When you have every-once-in-a-while business payments such as this one, you may have to report them on certain "Information Forms" with the IRS. See IRS Form 1099-MISC (and its separate instructions): Miscellaneous Income.

12. Procrastination and delay are still permitted by the government, as long as you plan for it. Visit the IRS Web site's Forms and Publications page, and view any of the 65 different forms for postponing your filing (and even paying) of federal taxes.

13. IRS Publication 15: Circular E, Employer's Tax Guide, and IRS Publication 15-A: Employer's Supplemental Tax Guide. To help you figure it out, look at IRS Form SS-8 (with attached instructions): Determination of Employee Work Status for Purposes of Federal Employment Taxes and Income Tax Withholding.

14. The same deal goes for *statutory employees*. This issue is less likely to be a concern for the self-employed IBCLC. Those who are considered, by law (statute), to be "employees" are a driver distributing beverages or foods or dry cleaning, a full-time insurance agent, someone doing piecework for you at his or her home, or a full-time traveling salesperson soliciting orders on your behalf.

15. IRS Publication 15-A at 3.

16. IRS Publication 583: Starting a Business and Keeping Records.

17. Use IRS Form 1040-ES: Estimated Tax for Individuals, to figure out and pay the tax. For more, see IRS Publication 505: Tax Withholding and Estimated Tax.

    One handy tip if you are employed elsewhere (in addition to your private practice): You may be able to avoid estimated tax payments on your small business if you have your other employer withhold more taxes from that paycheck. See IRS Form W-4V (with attached instructions): Voluntary Withholding Request.

18. IRS Publication 533: Self-Employment Tax.

19. IRS Form (and separate instructions) 1099-MISC: Miscellaneous Income.

20. IRS General Instructions for Forms 1099, 1098, 5498 and W-2G.

21. IRS Publication 535: Business Expenses, and IRS Publication 334: Tax Guide for Small Business.

22. For more on this "section 179 deduction," see IRS Publication 946: How to Depreciate Property.

23. IRS Publication 463: Travel, Entertainment, Gift and Car Expenses.

24. IRS Form 4562 (and its separate instructions): Depreciation and Amortization (Including Information on Listed Property).

25. This "listed property" also includes some items you probably don't have to worry about ("property generally used for recreation or amusement," unless that includes toys you buy to amuse the toddlers whose mothers you are seeing).

26. See Chapter 7, "Insurance," in IRS Publication 535: Business Expenses.

27. See Chapter 5, "Interest," in IRS Publication 535: Business Expenses.

28. IRS Publication 463: Travel, Entertainment, Gift and Car Expenses.

29. See Chapter 13, "Other Expenses," in IRS Publication 535: Business Expenses.

30. IRS Form 8829 (and its separate instructions): Expenses for Business Use of Your Home, and IRS Publication 587: Business Use of Your Home (Including Use by Day-Care Providers).

31. A lactation consultant may be able to avoid the "exclusive use" test if she uses a part of her home to store inventory or product samples, such as the breast pumps or other breast-feeding supplies you store on a shelf in your house. Ask your accountant or lawyer to look into this point for you. See IRS Publication 587, p. 3.

32. Assume you meet the definition for "business use of your home." You still need to figure out how much of your home is actually used for business (divide the business square-foot area by the total area of the house, or divide the number of business rooms by the total number of rooms) to get your "business percentage." See IRS Publication 587.

33. The first phone line into your house is *not* deductible, although a second line installed for business use only can be deducted, as can long-distance charges on any line, when the call involves business.

34. Usually you will summarize your business activity in your "books." Journals (which you can get at any stationery supply store) are where you record each business transaction shown on your supporting documents (i.e., receipts), and ledgers contain the totals from all of your journals.

35. IRS Publication 583: Starting a Business and Keeping Records, p. 14.

Books and Articles

Bornmann, P. Chapter 31: A legal primer for lactation consultants. In Walker, M., ed. *Core Curriculum for Lactation Consultant Practice*. Sudbury MA: Jones and Bartlett, 2001.

Bornmann, P. *Legal Considerations and the Lactation Consultant*. La Leche League International Lactation Consultant Series, Unit 3. Wayne, NJ: Avery Publishing Group, 1986.

Pennsylvania Bar Institute. *Counseling Small Businesses, vols. I and II*, PBI No. 2001-2766, 2000.

Pennsylvania Bar Institute. *LLCs and LLPs in Pennsylvania*, PBI No. 1999-2382, 1999.

Riordan, J., and Auerbach, K. *Breastfeeding and Human Lactation*, 2nd ed. Sudbury, MA: Jones and Bartlett, 1999, pp. 709–744.

Sohnen-Moe, C. *Business Mastery*, 3rd ed. Tucson, AZ: Sohnen-Moe Associates, 1997, pp. 67–97.

Wilson-Clay, B. Lactation consultants: Are we a profession yet? *Current Issues in Clinical Lactation* 2000, 57–63.

IRS Forms and Publications

IRS Form SS-4, Application for Employer Identification Number (Rev. 2-98)

IRS Pub. 15, Circular E, Employer's Tax Guide

IRS Pub. 15-A, Employer's Supplemental Tax Guide

IRS Pub. 334, Tax Guide for Small Business (for individuals who use Schedule C or C-EZ)

IRS Pub. 505, Tax Withholding and Estimated Tax

IRS Pub. 535, Business Expenses

IRS Pub. 583, Starting a Business and Keeping Records

IRS Pub. 587, Business Use of Your Home

IRS Pub. 1066, Small Business Tax Workshop Workbook (Rev. 4-99)

IRS Form 1040-ES, Estimated Tax for Individuals

RESOURCES

IRS Form 1120S, U.S. Income Tax Return for an S Corporation, and Instructions for Form 1120S

IRS Pub. 1976, Independent Contractor or Employee?

IRS Form 2553, Election by a Small Business Corporation (to be an S corporation)

IRS Form 8829, Expenses for the Business Use of Your Home

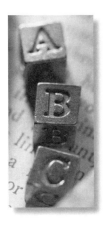

10 Financial Considerations

Diane DiSandro, BA, IBCLC

Finances... no one wants to talk about them. In fact, the financial aspect of running a private lactation consulting practice is something that sends most lactation consultants running screaming into the night. The truth is that if you choose to work as a lactation consultant in a private practice setting, the financial aspect of your practice must work as well.

Keep your ears open at any gathering of private practice lactation consultants. You will hear many people claim that one just cannot make a living as a private practice lactation consultant. You will hear complaints from lactation consultants who barely make enough money to cover their expenses or to pay for attending the conferences necessary to keep up their credentials. Certainly this struggle must happen in other professions as well, but because many lactation consultants come from a volunteer counseling background, we seem to better accept or at least resign ourselves to not making a living at our chosen career. Physicians must be equally committed to their profession, and equally committed to helping and healing their patients. Nevertheless, few physicians are unable to make a living by practicing medicine.

To establish a thriving private lactation consulting practice, you must first and foremost make a conscious decision to go into business for yourself. As discussed earlier in this book, ask yourself the hard questions: Is opening a business really for you? Are you organized enough to run a business? Are you self-motivated enough to work on your business when you do not have to answer to anyone else? Do you have the discipline to "go to work" when you do not feel like it, or when distractions arise? Most importantly, do you want to own your own business?

Once you make the decision to go into business for yourself, *then* you can decide to make that business anything you want it to be, and you can be successful. You can choose to make your business helping mothers to breastfeed their babies, but you must realize that you are now a business owner. One reason that many private practices fail is that the lactation consultant never decided to "go into business" for herself.

If you really do not like the idea of running a business or feel that you cannot deal with the financial aspects of business ownership, be honest with yourself. If mostly you just want to be a lactation consultant, find someone to hire you. You can help mothers in a hospital setting, in a physician's office, in a WIC clinic, or even working for another lactation consultant's private practice.

FINANCIAL FORECASTING AND PLANNING

One of the most important aspects of owning a profitable business is ongoing financial forecasting and financial planning. If done correctly, your accounting will do more than just tell you how much money you are making and how much you will owe in taxes. It will help you see the trends in your business.

Your overall business plan definitely needs to include a financial section. Do you have enough capital to start your business? Do you have enough reserves to live on until your new business starts producing? How much money do you need to earn to make your practice financially worthwhile? Refer back to Chapter 8 for more information on how to determine in what setting to start your practice and if you have enough capital to get under way.

If you lack adequate capital in the form of savings, you will need to find it. Maybe you can make do by just leveraging initial costs on a credit card, but be aware that the interest rates can swamp you if you do not make enough to pay off your debts in a timely fashion. Perhaps you could borrow capital from family members, but here again there are risks. What if your business fails? How will borrowing money affect your relationship with that family member? Are you willing to accept these risks?

You could take out a bank loan, although it is difficult to find a banker who is willing to take a risk on a small business. The Small Business Administration can help by working with banks to secure a loan for you that you might have been unable to secure on your own. It is usually easier to obtain a home equity loan (as long as you are a homeowner, of course). Once again, there are risks involved. You will be risking your home on the bet that your private practice will thrive.

Financial forecasting becomes even more important once you actually open your practice. As stated earlier, forecasting will help you see the trends in your business. Which months are busier? During what time of the month do you see the most mothers? Are you busier near holidays? Or are impending holidays slower (and therefore generating less income) for your business?

This knowledge will help you keep your business financially healthy. If you know in advance that August tends to be a slow month, then you will want more cash in your reserves by the end of July to help you make payments during the "quiet" times. If April crushes you with income tax payments, sales tax payments, and estimated tax payments for the first quarter of the current year, then you can plan in the months prior to April so that you will have the funds needed to meet your obligations.

At the end of every month, and again at the end of the year, you should put together an **income statement** (see Figure 10.1) to review the profitability of your practice. An income statement summarizes your practice's profit or loss during a given time period, such as a month, a quarter (three months), or a year. It is quite easy to construct if you use your computer to do your accounting. Otherwise, you can set up a spreadsheet listing all of your direct sources of income (e.g., consultations, sales, breastfeeding classes, pump rentals, fees garnered by speaking engagements). Subtract from that total amount the direct costs of those activities, such as the cost of goods sold and the cost of the pumps you carry. This calculation will yield your **gross profit**. Subtract from your gross profit the other expenses of running your business, such as salaries, postage, advertising, telephone, printing costs, insurance, con-

Income Statement, January 2002
For
Baby Yours Lactation Consultants

INCOME		$4800.00
Consults	$2500.00	
Sales	$750.00	
Pump rentals	$1250.00	
Breastfeeding classes	$300.00	
Speaking engagements	$0.00	
COST OF GOODS SOLD		$410.00
COST OF PUMPS LEASED		$420.00
GROSS PROFIT		$3970.00
OPERATING EXPENSES		
Advertising	$50.00	
Car: Parking and tolls	$12.50	
Office expenses	$78.00	
Telephone/Internet service provider	$170.00	
Postage	$28.00	
Office salaries	$425.00	
Depreciation on office equipment	$54.00	
Other expenses	$6.00	
TOTAL EXPENSES		$823.50
NET INCOME BEFORE TAXES		$3146.50
NET INCOME		$2139.62

tinuing education, travel, and supplies. This result tells you your profit before taxes. Finally, subtract the amount you pay in taxes. Now you know how much money your business is making.

Having a financial plan for your practice is important if you want to run your business, rather than have your business run you. Many private practitioners feel out of control in their business lives. They work and work, but do not have a sense of getting anywhere. They always work in "panic" mode, running from emergency to emergency with no sense of what they need to do to run their businesses effectively.

Once you know the sources of your income and your major expenditures, you can assertively grow your business and direct it in the way that you want it to go. Does consulting bring in 40 percent of your money but sap 90 percent of your time and energy? You may want to rethink how you approach that issue. Do pump rentals bring in 40 percent of your money but take up only 15 percent of your time? That could be an area in which you choose to market for growth. Perhaps retail sales account for 25 percent of your income, but tie up most of your money in inventory. Or maybe you just really hate tracking inventory and purchasing items and collecting money owed to you. You can choose to close down that aspect of your business. If any aspect consumes significantly more time or mental energy than it is worth, you should take another look at whether that particular aspect belongs in your practice. Without keeping good financial records, you will not be able to discern these issues.

BOOKKEEPING AND ACCOUNTING

Accounting does not need to be a scary prospect. As with anything else, once you understand some of the basic principles and realize what they can do for you, accounting will not be intimidating. Simply put, accounting is just counting your money. It means keeping track of how much money you make, and keeping track of how much money you spend on your business. Of course, making money is not the main reason most of us become lactation consultants, but if our practices are not financially stable we will not be able to afford to continue helping the new mothers and babies as we wish. We need to make money for our practices to be successful. For this reason, the time spent on bookkeeping and accounting can be among the most enjoyable hours of the day. It is a time when you can feel good about the work you have done and the success of your practice. And if you have spent an entire day working without getting paid, it is the time you face yourself and ask why.

As a private practitioner, you will want to take an active role in your bookkeeping. It is, after all, your business! Even if you plan to hire an accountant, you need to understand the basic finances of your business. The best way to do so is to remain actively involved in your accounting. You need to have an understanding not only of your income, but also of your business expenses. Otherwise, you will find yourself working and working, putting money in the bank, only to find out with surprise that there really is no money in the bank. You may want to consider doing your own bookkeeping in the beginning, especially if you are a sole proprietor. If you start small, it is not tremendously difficult to learn, and it will save you from having to hire a bookkeeper. You learn quickly in a small business that every time you hire someone else to do a task for you, you must pay him or her a portion of your hard-earned money. If you wait until you no longer have the time to do your own bookkeeping, you will probably be earning enough money to pay someone else to do the job for you.

When starting a business, many people make the mistake of setting it up based on other, more established businesses. They set up the office with all the technology and support services that they may one day need, only to find that they do not have the money required to support their establishment. In the early days of your practice, you can probably get along with very little. When you find yourself running out too often to the copy shop, then perhaps buying a copy machine is warranted. When the day comes that you do not have time to do consultations because you spend all day on the phone, then it may make sense to hire someone to answer your phone for you. In the beginning, however, you can save a great deal of money by doing most of these tasks yourself.

You can keep your books by many different methods. You can do it the old-fashioned way in a ledger, but these days probably your most important business expenditure will be a computer (see also Chapter 12). It does not have to be the newest, biggest, and best computer around, but you do want it current enough and with adequate memory to support the basic software applications that you will need. One application in which you will probably want to invest is a small business accounting package, such as QuickBooks® or Peachtree® Accounting. These programs make it incredibly easy to do your own bookkeeping, and they generate income statements, produce profit and loss reports, and run reports comparing this year's activity to last year's.

Even if you work with a bookkeeper or accountant, you must still be able to understand your monthly income statements so as to know how much your business is worth, how much money you are making, how much you owe others, what your inventory needs are, and what your cash-flow situation is. You will want to monitor your income and expenses on at least a monthly, quarterly, and yearly basis so that you can make the best decisions for the health of your business.

It is crucial to keep meticulous records of your business finances, especially when dealing with your tax liabilities. You can deduct your business expenses from your taxes, but only to the extent that you know what they are and can prove that you spent that money on your business. Because you do not want to pay more in taxes than you really owe, you need to keep receipts in an organized fashion. If you are self-employed in the United States, you must file Schedule C with your federal income tax return. An easy way to organize your receipts is to make file folders corresponding to categories on Schedule C: COGS (cost of goods sold), office supplies, advertising, equipment rental/lease, travel, wages paid, legal/professional fees, supplies, insurance, and so on. This process forces you to file the receipt by tax category and makes it virtually painless to do your taxes at the end of the year.

The most important thing about accounting is simply that you *do it*. To be effective, you must keep records of your expenses and income on a regular basis. It is impossible to remember at the end of the week (or month, or year) all of the minor expenditures you made. If you have a business meeting over a quick breakfast, you can write that expense off. So what if it is only $3.50? And who cares about the $0.75 you put in the parking meter? Why should you pay taxes on that money needlessly? It is amazing how quickly those little expenses add up! Nevertheless, if you cannot remember when or exactly how much you spent, you cannot use it as a deduction.

Before you start, you must make some important accounting decisions about your business. If you are working with an accountant, it would be good to discuss these options with her or him. You need to decide on your business year and on your accounting method.

For most home businesses, the business year will correspond to the calendar year, January 1 through December 31. If you are a sole proprietor, you will pay income taxes based on the calendar year anyhow, so it simplifies matters if your business year matches it.

The other option is to establish a separate fiscal year for your business. A fiscal year can start at the beginning of any month of the year and end with the last day of the month prior—for example, July 1 through June 30. This decision does not have anything to do with when you actually start up your practice; you can open your practice in September and still use the calendar year as your business year if you so choose.

When deciding on an accounting method, you must choose between the cash basis and the accrual basis methods of accounting. The cash method is easy and works the way most of us are accustomed to dealing with our finances. It works well for most home-based businesses. Basically, money is income when we receive it, and expenses are recorded when we actually make the payment.

Accrual basis is a method of bookkeeping in which you regard income or expenses as occurring at the time you ship a product, render a service, or receive a purchase. Under this method, the time when you enter a transaction and the time when you actually pay or receive cash may be two separate events. If you have a lot of inventory, you must use the accrual method of accounting. Your monthly balance statements will list receivables (money owed to you but not yet received) and accounts payable (money you owe others but have not yet paid) as assets and liabilities.

Once you have reached those decisions, you simply begin your record-keeping. Put succinctly, you need to keep track of all money received and all money spent in your practice. You record all of these transactions either in your computer software package, in a spreadsheet, or in a revenue and expense journal. Each item is assigned to the appropriate account; for example, your business stationery is assigned to the "office supplies" account. This task should be performed as the transactions occur, but at least on a weekly basis. Once again, if you set up your computer or journal accounts to correspond to the categories on the IRS Schedule C, it will greatly simplify your tax preparations at the end of the year.

Save your receipts, copies of bills you sent to clients, check stubs, deposit slips, a petty cash journal, and other paper records as proof of your activities. Also, keep a mileage spreadsheet as a log for the business use of your car, along with a mileage reading from the first and last days of your business year to help determine the percentage of business use of your vehicle for tax purposes. Keep a phone log, especially if you use your home phone for your business in the beginning.

When you start your practice, and periodically as time goes by, you will incur expenses for items that will be in service for a long period of time and that will contribute to the operation of your practice. These **fixed assets** include such items as your computer, office furniture, vehicles, and buildings. Because of their long-term value, fixed assets are treated differently than are other business expenses. Typically, fixed assets are not written off of your taxes at once. Instead, you deduct the purchase price of an item over its useful life, not just the year in which you make the purchase. This process is known as **depreciation**. You need a listing of items that you will depreciate over time.

If you rent breast pumps, you will need records of which pumps you have, to whom they are rented, income received from them, and money you paid to either buy or lease them. If you sell items, keep track of the cost of the items (cost of goods sold), the price for which you sold them, and your inventory. You may also need to keep track of taxable revenue to pay sales taxes based on your state and city's regulations.

If you travel to a conference, keep track of your expenses, from registration down to tipping the bellman. Keep meals and entertainment costs separate from airfare, hotel, and registration expenses.

On a monthly basis, add up your income and expenses and create an income statement as discussed in the "Financial Forecasting and Planning" section. You need to balance your checkbook, review statements to make sure that you are current with any vendors with which you do business, and send out statements to any of your customers who owe you money. This effort keeps you in touch with the financial health of your practice, and it helps you plan for the future. You may wish to update your cash-flow statement at the same time.

If you use computer software to maintain your books, these end-of-month activities will take only a few minutes of your time. One of the joys of computerized accounting is that you need enter a transaction only once. The computer keeps track of each item and makes it available for profit and loss statements, income statements, and yearly or monthly comparison reports. It keeps track of which items are taxable so that at the end of the month or quarter (whenever you must file your sales tax with your state), you simply print a report of the amount owed. If a vendor continues to bill you for an invoice that you have already paid, it is easy to search and find the documentation you need to prove you made the payment. You can quickly identify all of your clients who owe you money and send them monthly statements with the click of your mouse. If you enter bills to be paid when they come in the mail, your computer will remind you when they are due, even if it is not for 90 days!

M ake sure that you have a billing system that works for you. You deserve to be paid for the work that you do, but if you forget who owes you money, you may never receive it. Decide early what your payment terms will be for your clients, and let them know from the beginning. You may want to receive payment in full at the time of the consultation. If the consultation ends and your client discovers that she does not have her checkbook with her, you need to stay on top of the issue until you receive payment. Ideally, she will go home and send you a check immediately. Many times, however, that is not the case.

Getting paid promptly is always better than having to bill for your services later, and you are more apt to be paid when the client is standing right in front of you. Make it easy for your clients to pay you. Do you accept cash, checks, credit cards, and debit cards? Consider setting up a merchant account with your bank so that you can accept credit cards or debit (ATM) cards. A fee is involved each time you process a credit card payment, but these payments do not bounce as checks can, and you receive your money promptly. Your clients will also appreciate your efforts to accommodate them. Some computer accounting packages offer services so that you can process credit card payments through your computer rather than having to buy or lease a terminal. You can also e-mail invoices to your customers and accept electronic payments.

Studies show that bills that are more than 90 days past due are significantly less likely to ever be paid. It is your job to make sure that all of your clients pay their bills promptly. A timely phone call to your overdue client often results in a remittance of payment. Of course, phone calls can also consume a lot of your time. Why should you spend your time trying to collect overdue debts for time already spent rather than using it to see more mothers and babies? It is usually more efficient to send billing reminders on a monthly basis to all clients who owe you money. With a computer, you can sort your overdue clients in an accounts receivables aging report. This report will reveal how many days overdue a given bill has become. You may wish to make phone calls to those clients who are more than 90 days past due. You can use red ink to stamp bills with "Second Notice" or "Final Notice." You can also choose to charge a monthly finance charge to help cover the costs incurred by repeated billing. For ongoing clients (e.g., breast pump rentals), you may want to send out monthly statements showing them exactly where their account stands. Professional-looking bills and statements make your debtors take you more seriously.

If your practice includes numerous overdue accounts, consider hiring a collections agency to help you settle some of your larger debts. Such an agency generally charges a percentage of the money collected, but if you feel that the client absolutely will not pay you, a percentage of the money owed is better than nothing! Sometimes just the threat of being sent to such an agency may prompt a client to settle her account with you. But be careful. Harassment charges can be brought against you if you threaten such an action and it can be proven that you do not have a relationship with an agency and were just trying to "scare" the client into paying you. Of course, referring a client's account to a collections agency will create a great deal of ill will and is not something you want to do except as a last resort.

PICKING AND USING A CPA

Picking the right Certified Public Accountant (CPA) is critical for your business as well as for your peace of mind. He or she must be someone you trust and someone with whom you feel comfortable. You should share the same basic philosophy about your business and the handling of your financial affairs. Running a small business, especially a home-based business, entails many unique considerations. You want to look for someone who is well versed in small business accounting.

Ask around for recommendations. You could check with your local chamber of commerce or Small Business Administration. If you are on-line, check out www.cpadirectory.com. Ask other self-employed people in your community. Consider hiring someone who is also self-employed and works out of his or her home. You can be certain that this entrepreneur knows the ins and outs of home business accounting!

You must decide what your accounting needs will be. Are you looking for a bookkeeper to do all of your accounting? Do you plan to do most of your own accounting on your computer, and need a CPA only at tax time? Make sure he or she is also a qualified tax preparer so that you do not need to hire a separate tax consultant.

Make appointments to interview several CPAs. Ask about their qualifications. Find out how much they charge and what services they offer. Ask for references from others in private practices, especially others in your setting. How often will the CPA meet with you? Does this schedule fit your needs? How does the accountant like to work with small business owners? Will the CPA give you a break on prices if you keep your books in a computerized accounting package? Many accountants charge significantly less if you can just hand them a computer disk or printout of the "books" from your computer program. It is tallied, organized (if you make it so), and clear; it takes the accountant much less work, so the savings can be passed back to you.

If you work in a home office, make certain that your accountant is fluent in home office tax preparation. In March 1997, *Consumer's Report* published an article on tax preparation. CU researchers submitted income tax information from a home office to a private CPA, a tax attorney, an income tax preparation company, and an accounting firm and also did the return using income tax return software. The private CPA was the only one who filed the return correctly. Writing off part of your home is rather tricky, and the tax laws change frequently. No matter who prepares your income tax return, once you sign it as being correct, you are liable; make sure that it is done right.

Hiring an accountant whose financial philosophies are similar to your own will let you sleep at night. Some accountants will find every last loophole to give you more write-offs on your taxes, even if it means stretching the truth a bit. Be aware that if the IRS audits you, you as the business owner bear the ultimate responsibility. With a conservative CPA, you may pay a little more in taxes, but you will not have to worry if you are audited.

CAPITAL AND OPERATING EXPENSES

How much money will you need to start and run your business? **Capital** is the money used for starting up your practice or for making a large change for the growth of your business. **Operating expenses** are the standard expenses you encounter on a regular basis for the maintenance of your practice.

Your capital needs will depend heavily on the type of practice you wish to open. You should take the time to write down the particulars of your practice the way you would like it to be. Where will you practice? Converting a room in your home into an office will probably be less expensive than buying or leasing a commercial property. Do you plan to hire employees who will need office space in which to work? Do you have access to items you need for your office? File cabinets, computer, fax machine, desk, copy machine—list the things you have and the things you will need. Try to be sensible about what you need to get started and which items can wait until your practice is on its feet. Do not forget the "little things," such as clipboards, forms, file folders, and practice supplies (e.g., gloves or finger cots, supplies for cup feeding or finger feeding). Do you need more professional clothes than you usually wear? You will want a separate phone line for your business even if it is located in your home. At some point, you will want a second phone number to be dedicated to fax and/or computer use, but could wait for a while. Do you have a two-line phone?

In addition, you need to consider your normal operating expenses. If you have employees you must pay them, whether or not you make money. If you do not work in a home office, you must make rent or mortgage payments. There are phone bills, utility bills, office supplies to be purchased, postage, professional liability insurance, insurance for the business use of your home, or similar liability insurance to protect you if someone is injured in your office. There are conferences to attend to maintain your credentials, subscriptions (e.g., *Journal of Human Lactation*), and dues. There is car upkeep and gas if you do mostly home consultations. There will be child care expenses if you have young children. If you rent breast pumps or sell items, you will have pump lease payments to make and the costs for replacing your sales inventory as needed.

Try to come up with a realistic idea of how much money you will need to stay in business, then plan how you will make that sum. If you need to borrow capital to get started, that can be done (remembering to factor in your loan payments as part of your operating expenses). If you find that your expected operating expenses far exceed the amount of money you think your practice will realize, then you must adjust your expectations. Find where you can increase income and where you can cut expenses.

You need to be in control of your practice, and yet be able to achieve those goals that are important to you. I started my practice on a shoestring, doing mostly home consultations when my children were young. At that time, I could not guarantee that my home would be clean enough on a moment's notice, or quiet enough to conduct consultations the way I wanted. As my children reached school age and my practice grew, I found that I did not have time to see all the mothers who wanted my help because I spent so much of my time driving. At that point I dedicated part of my home as an office. I spent the money to upgrade the furniture and to make my office into a space in which I was proud to see my clients.

As time passed and I grew busier, I realized that I had outgrown my home office. To continue my practice at the rate it was growing, I needed a "real" office, with a receptionist, waiting room, and at least two consulting rooms. "Good news!" you might think. But it was not good news to me. I like the fact that I sometimes have quiet weeks when I can work on projects (like an outline for a conference session) or just catch up on my paperwork. I like the freedom of working alone. And I was worried that if I had rent to pay and a payroll to meet, then I would have to stay busy! When I had a quiet week, instead of enjoying the change of pace, I would worry about meeting my expenses. If a mother might have benefited from a quick bit of phone advice, I would have to make an appointment to see her to ensure that I had enough income to support my business.

I was stressed and unhappy about the way these thoughts were coming, and the direction in which my business appeared to be heading. So I made my decision. I decided to slow down, step back, and maintain my home-based office. I traded the awesome, high-profile practice for my own awesome, comfortable setup. Sometimes I have to refer clients to another lactation consultant because I do not have enough time to see everyone who calls me. But I am happy with my business, and you cannot put a price tag on that satisfaction. I can practice the way *I* choose, giving my clients the individual, unrushed attention that they need, and my stress level is lower because I am doing things the way I want them to be done.

TAXES AND LICENSES, INCLUDING SALES TAX

Make sure you know the laws pertaining to your local community before you set up your business. Talk to your accountant or attorney about any licenses you may need to set up your practice in the area you have chosen. Some localities put no restrictions on where you may set up a business, whereas others are quite strict. Some areas will not allow a commercial enterprise to exist on property zoned for residential use.

And then there are taxes. When setting up your books, make sure that you remember to put aside enough money to cover the taxes that you will owe. Myriad taxes apply to the self-employed person. You will pay federal income tax, state income tax, and possibly local income tax. Depending on how much money you make, you may have to submit quarterly estimated tax payments to all three revenue departments. If you have employees, you must withhold and file payroll taxes. Depending on your locality, there may be a business tax, a school tax, an occupational privilege tax, or per capita taxes. Find out what rules apply in your area. Not knowing is not considered an acceptable excuse for not paying the appropriate taxes. A self-employed person has to pay Social Security tax when filing federal income taxes each April 15. You must be disciplined enough to set aside this money weekly or monthly, or not enough will be left to pay your taxes when they are due. The IRS is not a very forgiving agency in that way!

If you sell products or rent breast pumps or other equipment, you may have to collect sales tax for your state or municipality. Contact your state's Department of Revenue to find out whether you need to collect this tax, what the sales tax rate is in your area, which items are taxable, and how to apply for a sales tax license.

If you use computer accounting software, you can designate each item as either taxable or nontaxable. Your computer will then keep track of the amount of sales tax owed each period. You may have to remit your sales tax yearly, semiannually, quarterly, or monthly, depending on how much you usually owe. You can generate a *Sales Tax Report* on the computer showing all income for the past tax period so that you will know the amount of sales you made, how much of that was taxable sales, and how much sales tax you actually collected. You can just choose to have the software "pay sales tax," and it will calculate and print the check to the proper agency if you have taken the time to set up your information correctly. Otherwise, you will need to keep a journal, entering each sale made and tallying how much sales tax was collected. Be sure to look at the amount collected periodically so that you will have enough money to cover the payment to your state when it is due. Very stiff penalties are assessed for late remittances. Many states will now allow you to file your business tax returns and payments electronically; check your state's Web site to see how to register to e-file your sales tax or payroll taxes.

EQUIPMENT LEASING AND PURCHASING; VENDOR PAYMENT SCHEDULES

Much of the equipment that you will need for your practice (e.g., baby scales, computers, office machinery) can be either leased or purchased. Talk to your accountant about which options are better for your practice. This decision largely depends on how you set up your practice and how much initial capital you have. If you open a home office, you may be able to use the furniture that you already own. If you open a free-standing office, you will need to furnish it: the workstations for your employees, your own office space, a filing system, furniture for a waiting room. A busy office with a staff and many people working in it will have different needs than a one-person office. You will need a different type of phone system, space and furnishings for each employee to do his or her job, a heavier-duty copy machine, more computer workstations, and sturdier office furniture than does a lactation consultant who sees just one person at a time and then does her own recordkeeping when the consultation ends.

PUMP RENTAL STATIONS; GETTING PUMPS BACK

Many lactation consultants find it convenient to open a breast pump rental business as part of their practice. Good-quality, clean pumps are then available when you need them for your clients. You know they are in good working condition, and you can show the mother how to use her pump properly. The client appreciates not having to seek out a pump, and the lactation consultant can make a bit of additional income.

Contact a breast pump company (e.g., Medela, Inc. or Hollister, Inc.) to get information on setting up a rental station. Find out the company's prices to purchase or lease the pumps. Ask the suggested retail price for which you would rent the pumps. Ask about the payment terms. Does the firm expect payment from you in 30 days, 60 days, or 90 days? Does it offer a price discount based on the number of pumps you lease? Does it offer cheaper rates if paid in advance instead of monthly? Must you lease a minimum number of pumps to open an account? What kind of marketing tools does the company have to help you establish your business? How many competing rental stations does it have currently operating in your area?

Once you decide to open a rental station, you need to get the word out. Contact your local doctors, community breastfeeding support groups, hospital maternity units, and neonatal intensive care units to let them know that you have breast pumps available for mothers who need them. See Chapter 13 for more ideas on how to market your new rental station.

The breast pump company will supply you with books of rental agreements at no charge. Look over the agreement you will have the customer sign and make sure that it satisfies your needs. If not, you may want to design your own.

If you are starting with only a few breast pumps, you can probably keep track of them visually and by knowing which rental agreements are active. When you add more pumps to your station, however, you will need to find a more comprehensive manner of keeping track of your equipment. You can build a file card system, where you have a card for each pump. List the pump's serial number and the date that you put it into service. Make columns for the renter's name, phone number, the date on which the pump was rented, monies due, or anything you want to see at a glance. Get dividers for your card file box and make labels for "in" (not rented), "short-term," each month of the year, and "out of service." When you rent a pump, take the card from "in" and fill in the necessary information, and then file it behind the month when the pump is due back. Each month you can quickly find which rentals are up for renewal so that you can contact or bill the customer.

As your rental business grows, it will become increasingly difficult to keep track of your breast pumps manually. Few computer programs are available to help you perform this task (see also Chapter 12). One such program is an add-on to InfoNation's TLC (The Lactation Consultant) software. This software package allows you to chart consultations that you perform, with an added module that lets you track breast pump rentals and inventory. It is rather expensive for a private practitioner, but it does make your recordkeeping much easier. You can find more information about this software at www.infonat.com. Another program you might look at is Pump Track, sold by Barbara Wilson-Clay. For more information on this software, see her Web site, www.lactnews.com. Alternatively, you might find someone who can write a program to fit your business. My husband developed a computer program tailored to the way I run my rental business. You can also network and talk to others who have large rental businesses to find out how they operate.

Stay aware of your overdue rental items. As with any type of billing, the longer the bill goes unpaid, and the more the rental charges add up, the less likely you are to receive your money or to even get the pump back! Both of the major breast pump companies offer loss and damage insurance on the breast pumps that you lease from them. I strongly urge to you spend the money to carry this waiver. If even one of your pumps is not returned, it can cost you several hundred dollars. If you do purchase the loss and damage waiver, make sure you know how it works. What specific information do you need to have the company accept the claim? Generally, you will need a rental agreement properly and completely filled out, signed, and dated by the renter. Medela requires that you have either a driver's license number or Social Security number for the renter; Hollister requires both numbers. You will need the customer's street address, even if she uses a P.O. box number for the mail. The more information you have about the customer, the easier it will be to collect on a defaulted rental, whether through the pump company or through a collections agency.

Contact your renters before their rental periods expire. Let them know how to return the item or renew the rental. Bill promptly if money is overdue. Check return addresses on envelopes to make sure the mother has not moved and forgotten to tell you. Consider including a clause in your rental agreement that deals with overdue payments. My rental agreement gives me the right to charge all overdue amounts at a very high daily rental rate. I seldom exercise this right, but it gives me the ability if someone is overdue by a few months to write to that person, quoting the applicable paragraph of the contract, and giving her the option of paying me in full within a certain time frame (e.g., two weeks) or having the overdue period sent to a collections agency at the higher rate. If a delinquent renter has the option of paying $150 today or having an agency hound them for $450 in two weeks, you will frequently see that payment in the mail in a few days!

COMPENSATION

Being compensated for our work seems to be a big stumbling block for many lactation consultants, especially if the LC comes to the field from a background as a volunteer La Leche League Leader or nursing mothers counselor. However, as a lactation consultant you are a health care professional. You deserve to be paid for your work, just as any other health care professional would be.

The major obstacle you must overcome is your own mindset. You are a professional. You have skills that allow you to help other people. Other people are willing to come to you for your expertise. Would you go to consult with a professional without expecting to pay them? Find a phrase that works for you and practice saying it aloud. "I would be glad to set up an appointment to meet with you. My fee is $_____." Be firm. If the mother really just has "a few questions" but does not feel she needs to make an appointment, refer her to one of your local community's volunteer breastfeeding support groups. It is good to get new mothers hooked into this type of support network, and it frees up your time for seeing paying clients. Of course, if a mother truly does not have the means to pay you, you may choose to see her for a very small fee. Frequently, however, we project that the finances are more difficult than they really are. If you can save a new mother from buying artificial baby milk for even a week or two, that move has probably covered the cost of your consultation.

Third-Party Reimbursement

Third-party reimbursement occurs when someone else pays you for the consultation on behalf of the client, usually an insurance company. Some insurance companies contract with lactation consultants to see the people whom they insure and then pay the LCs directly. Other companies reimburse the mother for her consultation if she submits a claim form and a copy of your bill. Some insurance companies cover lactation consultations, but only if they are referred to a visiting nurse agency. It is a benefit for your clients if you are well versed in which companies cover your services and how they cover it.

Accepting third-party reimbursements directly (instead of having the client pay you and seek reimbursement from their insurers) can be very time-consuming. After you have authorization to conduct the consultation, you must file a claim for your services, then you must follow up on that claim. Frequently, the company says it has no record of receiving the claim. Even if the firm receives it, several weeks or months may pass before you receive your payment. Because of this delay and because few insurance companies in the United States cover our services directly, many lactation consultants choose to receive payment at the time of the consultation, giving the mother a receipt that she can submit to her insurance company on her own.

Getting prompt, accurate, and sufficient reimbursement for lactation care and services is an ongoing struggle at the grassroots level (that's us). The good news is that several recent U.S. policy documents (see the Forward) call for appropriate reimbursement for breastfeeding care and services. Keep billing, keep writing, and keep calling third-party payers. Eventually more insurance companies will figure out that paying for lactation consultant services is good for their financial bottom line.

Calculating Pay and Compensation

How do you decide what is fair when setting your fees? If other lactation consultants work in your area, find out what they charge so that you are at least in the same range that mothers expect to pay. If you are new to the profession, you should not expect to charge the same fees as someone who has operated an established practice for several years. This price checking and setting process has legal implications—consult with your attorney before comparing prices with others in your area.

Another way to set fees is to gauge roughly what a mother would pay for a trip to the pediatrician's office. Of course, the doctor would spend only several minutes with the baby, while you will probably spend an hour or two, but the fee structure seems to work for many lactation consultants.

Some consultants charge an hourly fee, whereas others charge a set fee for an initial consultation and perhaps a different fee for follow-up visits, if necessary. If you will do home visits, bear in mind that your travel time is also time out of your day when you cannot see another client. Either figure that time into your fees or set a separate travel charge (either a flat charge, an hourly charge, or a per-mile charge). Be aware of your operating expenses, and make sure that your fee will generate enough income to keep your business solvent.

How will you pay yourself? Some private practitioners draw a paycheck weekly, biweekly, or monthly. This policy would make sense mainly if you have a partner in your practice. Sole proprietors often just draw money from the business when they need it, leaving the rest of the money in the business. In this case, you would set up an expense account in your bookkeeping system called "Owner Draw," using it to keep track of money that you have taken out for personal use. Either way, you must make sure that you do not draw out money that needs to be allocated for paying taxes or running the business.

Types of Work

You may do several types of lactation consulting, and your fees may vary depending on your activity. You may do home consultations at the client's home or office consultations in your office. You may offer phone consultations, although you need to be very careful with them. A mother may call you for insufficient milk supply because her baby is nursing 12 times per day but not gaining weight. When you see her, you might discover her nipples have been bleeding for two weeks and she is limiting the baby to five minutes per feeding because she cannot stand the pain, or the baby may have ankyloglossia. You would be unable to "see" these problems over the phone. If the mother wishes to consult with you about a medication that has been prescribed for her or about milk storage guidelines in preparation for returning to work, however, these things can often be handled over the phone.

Some lactation consultants set a lower rate for phone consultations. I choose to keep my fee the same because I do not want the mother choosing a phone call based on price when a face-to-face consultation makes the presenting issue clearer and usually takes less time to identify a problem. It is more difficult to get paid when you consult over the phone, too. Consider taking a credit card number, and then send the mother a receipt after you process the charge. You may want to consider phone follow-up after a consultation for no fee, up to a certain point. Make sure you allow for that extra time when you set your consulting fees.

Some private practice lactation consultants contract out to do consultations for a visiting nurse agency. Some provide consulting services to employees of companies who are on maternity leave. You should have a contract drawn up detailing what is expected of you, what you expect of the company or agency, and your reimbursement and terms.

Related Sources of Income

If you are just starting your private practice from scratch, it is helpful to have other related sources of revenues to provide some steady income until your name becomes established and you have enough consultation work to keep you busy. It takes a while for your local doctors to get to know and trust you and your work. Depending on that factor and the amount of marketing you devote to your practice, it can be weeks or months before you receive enough referrals to begin consulting on a regular basis. Nevertheless, there are always expenses involved with starting a business, and you will want to have some money coming in to help you meet your financial obligations initially, and even when you are established, to get you through "quiet" weeks or times of the year.

Educational Services

An obvious and productive way for a lactation consultant to make some extra money is by teaching breastfeeding classes. Not only do you make money, but this step helps establish you as the breastfeeding "expert" in your community. Decide how and what you want to teach. Will you teach one class or a series of classes? Are they for mothers or couples? What do you want to teach? What will you charge? Where will you hold the classes? (See Chapter 19 for more on educational services.)

You can teach basic breastfeeding management classes, focus on just getting started, or teach mothers what they will need to do if they will be returning to work and want to continue breastfeeding their babies. You could run a series of classes that takes mothers and their babies through some of the changes over the first year. You will want to develop a good outline and handouts for your class participants, but classes can be taught with very little expense.

Where will you teach your classes, and how will you find participants? You can teach them in your home office or storefront if it includes an area suitable for a class. You can call your local hospital to see if it offers breastfeeding classes. If not, you can ask if the hospital has a room that you can use for teaching. Check with local obstetricians and pediatricians. They may allow use of their offices when they are not having office hours if you give preferential registration to their patients. It looks good for their practices to offer breastfeeding classes, and they can hand out class registration flyers to their patients for you.

Once a local physician recognizes you as a breastfeeding expert, you can earn extra money by offering in-service programs for the doctor's staff on breastfeeding. Teach them how to triage breastfeeding problems over the phone, how to handle routine breastfeeding questions, and, of course, how and when to refer a patient to a lactation consultant for help. You can also talk to your local hospitals about providing in-service programs for their nursing staff.

If teaching and speaking are your passion, work up some talks that you can give at conferences. You can contact La Leche League about speaking at their area conferences or health professionals seminars. Many lactation conferences take place around the country, as well as the annual ILCA conference. Consider writing articles or books if that is something you enjoy.

Retail Sales and Equipment Rentals

Equipment rental and sales are often part of a PPLC's business. Some of your clients may need a breast pump, and it is more convenient for them to get it from you. Also, you might as well make the money as opposed to sending the client elsewhere. You will be able to show her how to use it, and you can be sure it works properly. Medela and Hollister both have hospital-grade electric breast pumps that you can either buy or lease, and then rent to mothers who need them. As described earlier, you can contact these companies for more information on how to establish an account with them. Both companies will do marketing for you as an "added bonus," giving out your name and phone number to people who contact the company for information on finding a breast pump, either over the phone or on their Web sites. Be sure to discuss and read the fine print on any leasing agreement regarding the minimum number of pumps you can lease, shipping policies, insurance on leased equipment, stolen or lost pumps, and invoicing policies.

If you decide to rent breast pumps, you will need to have pump kits available for your rental clients. If you have a retail account with the pump company, it also has other items that you may wish to sell. Breast pumps for purchase, breast shells, books, nipple shields, supplemental feeding options, spare parts for your breast pumps, and breast pads are all items you might choose to carry for resale. Other items that many lactation consultants offer include nursing bras, nursing pillows, baby slings, breast milk storage systems, infant massage supplies, videotapes, and maternity or nursing wear.

Some lactation consultants feel uncomfortable combining retail/rental business with their consulting practice. They feel that a conflict of interest arises when the same person both recommends a certain product and profits from the sale. Others feel that they can delineate the differences and feel no ethical conflict in handling both business aspects. There is a very fine line here, and a practicing lactation consultant must be careful if she decides to open her practice to other income-producing pursuits. A client should never feel that you sold her a pump or other product that she did not need, or that you pressured her to buy or rent something that she did not want. One dissatisfied client can do a world of damage to your reputation. If you feel uncomfortable providing these products to your clients, don't. Others will sense your discomfort. The potential financial gain is not worth the risk.

The Downside of Retail Sales

If you decide to open a retail side to your business, it opens up an entirely different aspect to your finances. You will have to collect state and/or local sales taxes, and file the periodic returns. You will have to keep track of your inventory, do your ordering, and pay for the products whether you sell them or not. A substantial amount of money can be tied up in inventory. Most companies insist that you purchase in whole-case quantities or that you meet a minimum order amount. If you rent breast pumps, you will probably be able to sell the personal kits needed by each user. But what if you decide to carry baby slings, set up an account, order several, and then find out that they do not seem to sell well in your office? The money you invested in these items may remain tied up for several months or more. You probably want to start small, and then expand your inventory as you see a real need, and as your financial situation allows.

Think through the decision carefully before you take on a new item. I decided years ago to expand and carry a line of nursing bras. The line I chose comes in 38 different sizes, both soft cup and underwire, and both seamless and regular for both soft cup and underwire. If I choose to carry all varieties, that would be 4 styles of 38 sizes. I would have to stock 152 items just to have one of each to show a given customer! Also, it is not practical to decide not to stock a certain size. Of course, most of my clients do wear nursing bras, but they are primarily not coming to see me to buy a bra. You can imagine the mental gymnastics one must go through in deciding which items to carry. Make sure that you are not tying up more money in inventory than you think you can support.

Keep detailed records on your product inventory. You will need a designated space to store the items you carry, and you will want to know how many of each item you have on hand at any given time. Once or twice per year, you should go through and physically count each item to make certain that the number you have matches the number that your records show. If you carry only a few things, you can probably set up your inventory in a columnar pad or spreadsheet, with a column for each item. When you sell something, put the date and customer's name on a line and subtract that item from your inventory. Once you get beyond a certain point, however, it becomes difficult to keep your records manually. Again, using a computer greatly simplifies this task. If retail is an option you expect to use for extra income, make sure to shop for an accounting software package that has the capability to track inventory.

Setting up your inventory records can take a lot of time, but once it is done it becomes a great time-saver. It will probably make sense to take an entire day with no appointments to set up your inventory records. If you get only half of them entered, and then are interrupted, and then sell a few items, your inventory records will be out of balance before you even get started! Initially, you will need a complete count of your entire inventory. Next, set up each piece as a separate item; that is, establish an item name or number for each piece. You will need to know the vendor from which you purchase it, a description of the item to show on purchase orders, either the same or a different description to show on sales receipts or invoices, your cost when you purchase the item, and the price you plan to charge customers for the item. In addition, you should know whether you need to collect sales tax on the article. Identify which account to charge your purchases against (probably Cost of Goods Sold) and which account to credit when you make a sale (probably Sales). You will need to enter exactly how many items you have on hand today. Depending on your program, you may pick a reorder quantity so that your computer can remind you when you are low and need to place a new order. The computer will keep track of what is currently on order, what has been received, and when payment is due for each shipment.

When your vendors raise their prices, remember to go into your records and change the purchase price, and possibly your retail price as well. Once your records are set up, maintaining them takes very little time—but must be done regularly.

SUMMARY

You can really do this! You succeeded in acquiring your clinical knowledge and skills, and you can also acquire financial knowledge and skill—and attitudes. Deciding to go into business for yourself by opening a private lactation consulting practice represents a major change in your life. It can be a time of great excitement, and one of the best opportunities you have ever given yourself. You will need to make sure that the business aspects of your practice run well, so that you can go forward confidently to help families. Spend the time necessary in the beginning to set up your accounting system and to make sure that you understand it. It should work effortlessly for you, whether you do your own bookkeeping or hire someone to do it for you.

Make sure that you have adequate financial resources to open your practice, and set your fees realistically to cover your ongoing operating expenses. Stay vigilant with your financial forecasting so that you will not be surprised when tax time rolls around. Open your eyes to the many ways you can choose to practice. Find or create a niche in your community by providing the services that people need in an environment that they will enjoy. And then relax and take pride in being the owner of a business that you love.

RESOURCES

Adams, Bob. *Adams Streetwise Small Business Start-Up.* Holbrook, MA: Adams Media, 1996.

Savage, Jack. *The Everything Home-Based Business Book.* Holbrook, MA: Adams Media, 2000.

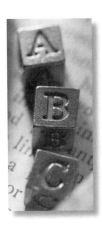

11 Hiring and Managing Staff

Jane Bradshaw, RN, BSN, IBCLC

The purpose of this chapter is to help the lactation consultant in private practice consider making the leap into hiring help. Recognizing and examining available resources and ways to take advantage of them will be discussed. Learning to think creatively and to see one's resources may take a real change of attitude. As most lactation consultants are trained as clinicians, not businesspeople, solving business problems—including getting help when needed—is often a major stumbling block to the success of a practice. The practitioner's own negative predetermined ideas and mindset can be the biggest obstacle. Nevertheless, innovative, practical, low-cost, high-benefit solutions are available and can be explored.

Are you feeling alone, overwhelmed, burned out, or tied down to your practice? Do you feel as if you can't leave town or even take a full day off because a mother might need a breast pump or a consultation? Do you feel as if you are shortchanging your family and pretty soon they will be shopping for a new wife and mother? Do you feel swallowed up by the enormity of details necessary to keep the practice running but are discouraged by the small amount of money you are making? The joy of the job, helping mothers and babies, may be starting to wane and you feel headed toward burnout. If you are feeling this way, look into getting some help.

When I talk to lactation consultants in private practice, many report that they cannot afford to hire anyone to help. Their practices are too small; they are barely making ends meet. Besides, there is no one in the area to help and the idea of becoming an employer and having to withhold and pay payroll taxes is too mind-boggling to even consider.

I once felt that way. For the first eight years of my practice, I complained to my colleagues, when I attended conferences, how I envied those who had someone to work with, another LC. I felt isolated and professionally lonely. There was no other lactation consultant within 50 miles with whom I could discuss cases, no one else to even answer the phone. If I spent the day away with my family, I came home to calls from women with engorged breasts, sore nipples, and babies who were refusing to breastfeed. Some mothers had given up breastfeeding entirely. I would lose clients, mostly to formula feeding, but also lose out on sales and rentals, the income that was vital to my practice. Losing a client affects every practice, whether it is small or extremely busy. Being unavailable for any amount of time hurts your reputation and may decrease your future referrals.

DO YOU NEED HELP?

What was my revelation in handling this problem? Getting help! In my case I had to learn to stop waiting for what I considered the perfect help, another lactation consultant wanting to join me in private practice, and realize that plenty of help was available, just not what I had expected. I learned that many of my duties did not have to be performed by an IBCLC and that the help and relief a good secretary gave me was amazing. Having clerical help reduced my stress and freed up my time to pay attention to the duties and responsibilities only the lactation consultant or business owner could and should be doing. Also, the employees I have hired have been so enthusiastic and knowledgeable about breastfeeding that they have relieved a lot of my feelings of isolation. After hiring my first person, I've never looked back. It has made such a difference in my life and has had the amazing result of increasing my business. Thanks to my employees, my stress has been reduced and I now take whole days and weekends off with my family. I can pay more attention to marketing my practice, as I am not tied down by the many business details that I used to shoulder alone. I still don't have anyone who can do consultations on a regular basis if I am away, but pumps can be rented, the classes can continue, and products provided when mothers need them. Thankfully, a good breast pump can usually preserve and protect the mother's milk supply and the baby can be fed until I return to work on the breastfeeding problem. My employees are all enthusiastic breastfeeding supporters who encourage the mothers not to give up and instruct them on correct use of the pump without overstepping their responsibilities. They are also trained regarding how and where to refer the mother if she needs immediate help and I am not available.

MY EXPERIENCE

Fortunately I had quite a bit of experience with employees from working with my husband in his busy veterinary practice. I had worked in his practice since 1981, often with one of my babies in the front carrier or toddling around at my feet while I waited on customers, made appointments, cleaned exam room tables, counted out pills, and mopped the floor. We actually child-proofed the veterinary hospital to the amazement of one of his visiting colleagues, who thought a child-proof latch was a security system for the restricted drugs! My husband's clients did not realize I was breastfeeding the baby while I answered many of their telephone calls. If the baby went to sleep in the carrier, I put her down in a port-a-crib in surgery, as it was a dark, quiet room, where she was out of the mainstream of activities. This experience has served me well, as I now hire mothers who bring their babies to work with them.

Along the way, I learned to order supplies, interview, hire and fire employees, and handle a payroll. Having contact with accountants and lawyers taught both my husband and myself a lot. Before we had a computer, I learned to sit down with the state and federal tax withholding booklets and pay as many as 17 employees, including 2 to 3 other associate veterinarians. This effort usually took two to three hours. The accountant talked us through the process of payroll the first few times, then it became just a routine task that took the time cards, withholding booklets, calculator, and accurate records. Paying the withholding taxes every month was also an exercise that took some practice and a few calls to the accountant that first year, but now is routine. With the wonderful, affordable accounting software that is now available, this process can be simplified greatly.

As a lactation consultant with a small practice of my own, I was convinced I could not afford to hire someone. I could not pay them for 40 hours of work per week. I could not pay professional wages, not even secretarial wages. No one else was certified in my area, either. The situation changed, however, when a dear friend returned to school to earn her bachelors degree and needed a "work study" program. She needed a part-time job to help her buy her books and give her some money for school. We decided I could be her work study program. She would work for me for the minimum wage, the same amount she would have been paid at the college. As I could give her better and more flexible hours that fit her class schedule, she would prefer working for me.

Initially my friend worked for me three days per week, from 11 A.M. to 2 P.M., answering the phone, renting rent pumps, weighing babies, and helping me with office paperwork, such as sending out monthly bills for rentals. Prior to her arrival, I had an answering machine with a message for parents to leave their name and number and I would call them back. Now that I had a live person to answer the phone, I changed my message to say "Our office hours are Monday, Wednesday, and Friday, 11 A.M. to 2 P.M. You may come to the office to rent or return pumps, or weigh your baby at that time. Services at all other times are by appointment. Please leave a message with your complete phone number and your call will be returned as soon as possible."

The results were amazing. My business grew by about 30 percent during the next year. This growth more than covered what I paid my assistant. I actually saw a difference in the first month. Having someone available to answer the phone—a real person—even for those limited hours increased my business. What I learned was that many people wouldn't leave a message but would call somewhere else hoping to talk to a real person, or often just wouldn't call back and would wean their baby to formula. I was still as available as I had always been and would call back mothers who needed lactation information. My employee, a former La Leche League Leader, had wonderful communication skills. She had breastfed her four children, including her twins, and enjoyed her work with me as much as I enjoyed her being there. We were a great team. Hiring her was my start in getting the help I needed.

FINDING AND HIRING HELP

If you are hoping for another IBCLC, your first worry may be that you cannot afford to pay her. Don't let your negative thoughts about what a potential employee may and may not accept stop you from investigating a relationship with someone with whom you would like to work. Not investigating your possibilities is probably your greatest barrier to getting help.

Another lactation consultant who is already employed in private practice or a hospital or clinic setting may be willing to work with you on a part-time basis. Because of her other income, she may be willing to take less pay or work for a commission. What other people are working in the area of lactation in your area? Be sure to include volunteer breastfeeding support group leaders. Often trained breastfeeding counselors from volunteer groups have served as a great source of employees for the LC with a small practice. These Leaders may not be certified IBCLCs, but they are often interested in working toward certification and may be well on the way to having the prerequisites. Is there an ILCA affiliate group in your area?

What if no other certified, experienced person is available and you are desperate for help? Look at your clients you have served. All except two of my receptionists have come from my client base. Whenever a mother praises you for the help you have given her, write that compliment down and give the mother a call when you need help. She may know someone or may be interested herself. Most of my employees actually came to me, asking whether I had any job openings and whether they could do anything for me without leaving their babies.

Take another good look at your referral sources. Ideally, you should have been asking your clients how they learned about you and your services. Pull out those records and make a list of the sources of your referrals. Call the people who have referred to you, including other clients and professionals, and let them know you are looking for help. Networking and word of mouth can be your best sources of potential employees. You can advertise your need for help by making a flyer that you mail to your clients, putting a note in with your pump rental bills, or putting a sign up on your office or on the outside of your home visit bag. Call the local La Leche League Leaders and tell them of the unfilled position. Call any interested people and invite them over for a cup of tea to discuss the possibility.

In addition, you can put a help-wanted ad in the newspaper. Expect a flood of people who send résumés and are curious about the job, but few who have a thorough understanding of breastfeeding, which is needed by a really good employee for our specialized type of work. However, if you have tried everything else, a newspaper ad may help you reach that perfect person who is not part of your network of contacts. Someone who has just moved into your area or has just began thinking of entering the work force may see your ad and respond. Be cautious about putting your phone number in the ad, however, unless you are prepared to spend a lot of time filtering out the people who are just curious and really have no basic knowledge of lactation. You can have people respond to you by phone or mail, or the newspaper can give you a P.O. box number or another anonymous way to receive résumés if you do not want to divulge your identity in the ad. Even if you do not include your personal contact information, some people will figure out who you are and call you. Be sure to include something in an ad that lets people know what you do and what you want in an employee. Consider using a statement such as the following: "Part-time secretary/receptionist for lactation consultant. Must be supportive of breastfeeding. Personal experience with breastfeeding preferred. Send résumé to . . . ."

After hiring people for my practice for almost 10 years, I have used a newspaper ad only once and did not find the employee I needed that way. I have usually found the best people through my clients or word of mouth. Many people ignored the requirements stated in the newspaper ad and sent me a résumé with no information about their understanding of or experience with breastfeeding. You can spend time doing brief phone interviews with everyone who responds in such a way but that résumé might be best filed away (probably in the trash). Anyone who cannot respond to a basic request in the ad about the type of person needed for a position does not represent a good candidate to work for you and is just responding to every help-wanted ad in the paper with the same résumé.

There is a work force consisting of women with the experience and attitudes you need who want to supplement their family's income but don't want to sacrifice the time with their children. They are just waiting for an invitation from you. They don't want to go into a high-stress, 40-hour-per-week job that demands all of their energy and time, but what you have to offer might fit their lifestyle perfectly. To find these people, tell everyone you know that you are looking for help and for the right person you would work out a flexible work arrangement that benefits both of you. When I say "tell everyone," that is what I mean. Don't hold back because you feel a particular person could not possibly know someone with the qualities you need. Tell your elderly neighbor, your pastor, the school bus driver, the postal carrier, and the principal at the school. It may surprise you that the most unlikely person will refer the perfect employee to you.

Who are potential employees for reception/office work?

- Your clients
- Breastfeeding support group leaders or attendees
- Aspiring lactation consultants
- Mothers with babies or small children
- Women with school-age children who are willing to work
- Older women with high school–age or adult children
- Neighbors and friends

Many things a lactation consultant/business owner does can be delegated to a trained, knowledgeable person. I currently have nine employees and use some volunteers every month. Five are part-time receptionists who cover the 40 hours per week my office is open; they bring their babies to work with them. The other employees are instructors for the various classes offered by my practice.

What kind of workers may be helpful in your practice?

- Another IBCLC: Of course, but when no one certified is available you can use the "Grow your own IBCLC" philosophy and hire someone working toward certification and help her along her way.
- Receptionist/secretary:
  —In-office: has regular hours, ranging from a couple of hours per week to full-time.
  —Out of office: someone who answers your phone on a regular or as needed basis, delivers pumps as needed, and so on. With "Call Forwarding," calls can go directly to her house or she can check your answering machine/voice mail at specific intervals.
- Pump delivery person: female or male. One IBCLC employed her teenage son to deliver pumps on his vacations from school. She was always careful to ask the mother if it was all right if her son delivered the pump and was never turned down. He would even set up the pump and give basic instructions on how to use it.
- Breastfeeding class instructor
- Childbirth instructor
- Massage therapist
- Exercise instructor
- CPR instructor
- Volunteers

You may also hire people who are usually paid as independent contractors, not employees, on a per-job or per-hours basis:

- Insurance billing clerk
- Bookkeeper
- Accountant/CPA
- Lawyer
- Web site designer
- Graphic artist
- Business advisor/computer expert
- Cleaning service

WHAT CAN AN EMPLOYEE DO FOR YOU?

For many small business owners, it is difficult to delegate responsibility. You may think there is not much someone else can do for you, but once you start delegating, training, and learning to trust your employee, you will see more and more she can do:

- Answer the phone and take messages
- Give basic information about your practice and what you offer
- Sell products—including understanding and showing the product to its best advantage and helping the client choose the right product for her needs, such as the bra that fits correctly, or the best pump for her needs
- Rent equipment, pumps, scales, and rechargeable power packs
- Give instructions on the correct assembly, use, and cleaning of pumps and other rental equipment
- Check and troubleshoot rental equipment for proper functioning; this duty includes being able to do basic troubleshooting over the phone when a mother calls to say, "My pump won't suck today"
- Send out bills for rental equipment and outstanding accounts
- Register people for classes
- Prepare materials and set up for classes
- Schedule and set up for consultations
- Do paperwork for insurance billing
- Make the bank deposit
- Maintain your inventory of products and place orders
- Shop for office supplies
- Weigh babies (and reassure mothers or schedule consults)
- Maintain client records
- File
- Clean
- Help you with marketing your practice
- Be an advocate for you and what you do

A mazingly enough, you may not have to pay a lot of money to begin your career as an employer. You can start gradually and increase the hours for the employee as your practice becomes busier and as you can afford to expand. Many people are willing to work for minimum wage if the job fits their lifestyle, such as working from home or being able to work just a few hours at a time and bring a baby to work. Bartering your services with another person is also a possibility. This approach would probably work best for a specific need that you have, such as someone developing a Web site for you, performing some legal work, or doing your taxes. Bartering is perfectly legal but must be recorded properly for IRS purposes. (The correct way to handle this issue legally is described in Chapter 9.)

A lactation consultant could work for you on commission. I currently pay 60 percent of the consult fee and 10 percent of the price of any items sold when another IBCLC fills in for me. This payment includes the time spent doing the doctor's reports and insurance paperwork that goes along with the consult. If you hire an LC to cover for time you want to be off, it represents money you would not have received if the employee was not working for you. The mother may not have needed or wanted your services by the time you returned from your weekend or vacation. Giving the LC a percentage is a small price to pay to keep your practice open and your reputation intact as being reliable and responsive to your clients. Other employees can also be paid a commission for each class taught, item rented or sold, or delivery made. A person could be paid a set amount just to check your answering machine for a day (for instance, $5 to $10) for up to an hour of her time. Then she could be paid an hourly rate for time she works over an hour if needed. One very busy LC who does home visits most of the day hires women, who are mothers at home, to call and check her answering machine every two hours during the day. She pays them $15 for every 10 phone calls they make or answer.

You can hire someone to work just a few hours every week, or you can look for someone who is flexible to work for you on an "as needed" basis. Some people would relish such a part-time job. Remember—you can begin gradually. It seems daunting to consider hiring someone to work 40 hours per week at a big salary, plus benefits, but this step is not necessary. Having someone send out bills, file, price merchandise, and answer the phone three or four hours per week might just be your ticket to a happier professional life.

You can usually find out what lactation consultants are paid in hospitals as well as the pay scales for other professionals such as physical therapists, occupational therapists, dietitians, and nurses. Do you have to pay your lactation consultant associate/employee the same rates? You and the employee must work out this issue. Currently there are not many job openings for lactation consultants. For the opportunity to work in her chosen profession, she may choose to accept what you can afford to pay her. If your practice has potential, the LC may be willing to join you and help promote your practice in return for greater rewards later.

I have found wonderful people who are willing to work with me for what I have to offer. They see the benefits of flexible hours that fit into their home life situation, and they may be able to bring their baby to work. Working for other businesses would demand much more of them than they are willing to give at this time. Don't overlook the value of providing a less experienced person with

HOW CAN YOU AFFORD HELP?

training that will make her more marketable in the future. Just be honest about what you can offer as pay from the start so no misconceptions arise. Some people will immediately decide they are not willing to work for that amount; others will look more favorably at the potential and benefits of the job.

A PROFESSIONAL LACTATION CONSULTANT

What should you consider when another lactation consultant is available to join you in your practice?

- Do you need someone to take your calls when you are off for a weekend or vacation, or are you so busy you need help on a more regular basis?

- What will your working relationship be? Does the LC just want to work for you or buy into your practice as a partner? Someone may start on a part-time basis and later seek to become a partner in the business.

- Assuming you want someone to help you part-time initially, how do you pay her? On commission for the work she does? Hourly? Salary? As an independent contractor?

- What is the LC's professional experience? Hospital? Private practice? Clinic? Doctor's office? Lay support group?

- How competent is she and what are her skills?

As stated elsewhere in this book, not every lactation consultant is prepared for private practice. It is a completely different experience working as an independent consultant without the safety net of the hospital or doctor's office behind you. Lactation skills are necessary but not enough to function independently. Take the time to get to know each other well before making a commitment, and then give yourself and the lactation consultant a probation time (three months or longer) during which both of you can determine whether this working relationship is to your benefit and hers. Learn each other's knowledge, experience, philosophy, and what you each want from the relationship. Come to agreements on the way you will handle different types of problems, when and how you will do follow-up, how doctor's reports will be done, and many other small details of practice. Write care plans that both can use for common problems. (One good resource for clinical policies is *The Lactation Consultant's Clinical Practice Manual* published by BFLRC; see Appendix B.) *Do* consultations together until you learn enough about each other, then get together and discuss your cases frequently so you continue to support each other and "sing the same song" to your clients and their doctors.

VOLUNTEERS

If you are firmly convinced you cannot afford to pay any help, start by using some volunteer labor. "Who would want to volunteer to help me?" you may ask. Surprisingly, many people are happy to donate a few hours of their time to help a worthy cause that they believe in . . . *you!* Most of my volunteers have been mothers whom I have helped. Some are so grateful to be able to breast-feed their baby, they would happily do a few things to free your time up so that you can provide your services to other mothers needing your expertise.

What could a volunteer do for you?

- Fold, address, and mail promotional materials for your practice, such as brochures and newsletters

- Help clean your office, sweep the walk, vacuum and dust, tidy up, and get the mail

- Answer the phone while you are with a client in a consult. Be sure to instruct and role-play exactly what should and should not be said. Only an experienced person should give out information—even your pump rental rates. You may want a volunteer to simply take messages that you return later.

- Address mailings

- Take packages to the post office or other delivery service for shipping

- Shop for you and deliver the items (e.g., office supplies, stamps) to you. You can give the volunteer a signed check made out to the particular store or post office, and the person can fill in the amount and bring you the receipts. Alternatively, or you can pay the volunteer back if she uses her own money.

- Deliver your brochures, newsletters, or other information to the local doctors' or midwives' offices

- Put up posters about your services at designated spots around town

- Help you run a mother's support group; bring refreshments, hostess, and mentor new mothers

- Come to your classes to talk about breastfeeding, childbirth, infant massage, working and breastfeeding, or some other topic for the benefit of new or expectant parents. This idea works especially well if the volunteer has attended your classes and is enthusiastic about the class's benefits.

One tip for dealing with volunteers: Always feed them! For the price of a basket of muffins, fruit, juices, and some tea, you can have several mothers working happily away for a couple of hours ensuring that your brochures are folded and mailed. The mothers usually end up having a great time, and the experience turns into a mini-breastfeeding support group meeting. If you have a newsletter, put in a section that thanks your volunteers publicly. A "thank you" get-together is a lot of fun. Provide food and maybe a small gift, a plant, or a box of tea to thank the volunteers for their time and efforts. Look for other ways to let the volunteer know you appreciate her. If a person helps you on a regular basis, you can offer to be a reference for future job applications. You may want to keep a folder on each volunteer with the hours that she helped you and the tasks performed that you can refer to if needed. Thus you can give a volunteer something really positive in return for helping you. Many wonderful people are happy to help you just to assist other mothers.

Once you get started using some volunteers, you may find that more people are willing to help you than you realized. One person might suggest or enlist another who would be willing to help you for a few hours. Another great benefit is that you may find a wonderful employee from your collection of volunteers. When people visit your office to help with some routine task such as folding and mailing out your brochures, you may discover a gem of a person who is smart, well-spoken, and willing to do more for you on a regular basis. She might be that wonderful first employee your practice needs.

THE JOB APPLICATION AND REFERENCES

Do require potential employees to fill out a job application, which should include all the basics, such as name and address, education, previous work experience, dates, reasons for leaving, and so on. Basic job applications are available at most office supply stores.

Next, ask the applicant to produce a résumé including her knowledge and experience, personal or professional, that makes her a good person to work with you. Completing this homework assignment will tell you a lot about a potential employee. I have learned this exercise is important. My rule is that if someone can't seem to get around to writing a simple résumé and bringing it to me, I won't interview or hire her. A résumé doesn't have to be long or involved, but if it's messy, has misspellings, contains poor grammar, or is scanty and incomplete, you can expect the same type of work from this candidate on your important paperwork. My best employees have had no problem whipping up a good résumé.

Look at the potential employee's work experience and discuss any former jobs with her. Discuss her skills and experience. Why did she leave previous jobs? Many good reasons exist for leaving or changing jobs, but if she was dissatisfied with all of her jobs, the applicant probably will not be happy working for you either. Look for dependability.

Require references and check them. If your applicant gives references who are all close friends, ask for more helpful references who can give work-related evaluations. It is not an insult to a potential employee to take this step. It is much easier to screen employees thoroughly before making the decision to hire than to be frustrated and seek a way to end an unhappy relationship later. When you call a work-related reference, ask what duties the employee performed, how well she preformed her duties, if any problems arose, and, most importantly, if the reference would ever hire her back. Many people hesitate to give much information in a reference, especially bad information, but will generally answer direct questions when asked.

SKILLS AND REQUIREMENTS FOR A CLERICAL POSITION

- Willingness to learn—absolutely the most important quality
- Good basic understanding of breastfeeding, especially breastfeeding of her own children
- Positive attitude about breastfeeding, childbirth, and all that you do
- Typing and basic computer skills
- High school diploma—for most positions
- Good verbal skills, including pleasant telephone voice, good articulation, and correct grammar
- Politeness
- Clean, neat appearance
- Good listening skills
- Good customer service skills
- Good spelling
- Accurate math skills to complete needed transactions, such as rental agreements and sales receipts

Many people bring résumés when looking for a job that include a lot of business experience, office work, and computer skills. After hiring and trying to work with a couple of these people, I've concluded that willingness to learn, trainability, and an understanding of breastfeeding are more important than business skills. If a person is fairly intelligent, I can teach her how to use my computer program competently and calculate rental forms in just a few weeks. If she really doesn't understand breastfeeding, however, I cannot give her that specialized knowledge in any amount of time.

Watch out for the "eager beaver" who is out to save the world and get everyone to breastfeed. Although you may agree with her philosophy, if she begins giving breastfeeding advice the minute anyone calls, she may create a problem. With some good training from you, she may turn out to be your best employee. If she cannot follow your guidelines, continues to give lactation advice, or disobeys your rules despite you educating her about her responsibilities, however, do not hesitate to end her employment.

DUTIES AND TRAINING

Spell out the employee's duties in detail. Start now by writing down all the things you do in your practice, and exactly how to do them. This effort will put you on your way to making your own policy and procedure manual. Next, look at those items carefully and divide the list into things you must do yourself and those tasks you can delegate. Now look at the list of things only you can do and be honest. Couldn't an employee handle some of those things? About the only tasks a lactation consultant who owns her own practice cannot delegate to a non-lactation consultant are doing consults, counseling mothers, keeping the checkbook, doing taxes, and handling payroll.

Note that the employee always does things with supervision. Training your employees in how each task is performed will prevent problems later. Take the time to write out exactly what she needs to do for each task in your practice.

For example, train your employee to answer the telephone correctly. Be specific. Write scripts for each type of call you receive. This strategy is recommended and used with receptionists in many other businesses, both retail and professional. A common business dictum is that "Your phone is the gateway to your practice," and the skill of your receptionist can be the deciding factor in whether the caller becomes a paying client. Practice with you being the caller and your employee responding to each type of phone call until she performs well and understands how she can answer the phone in a warm, positive way, encourage the mother to take advantage of your services, increase your business, yet not give lactation advice.

- The price checker: "How much do you charge to rent pumps?"

    Poor answer: "Our rental rates are . . . ." This answer gives only facts, and the price checker will probably choose the cheapest rental station in town and not realize all that you have to offer.

    Better answer: "Our rental rates include a free 15-minute 'pump consult,' in which our trained staff teaches you how to correctly assemble, operate, and clean your pump, free hospital delivery if needed, and telephone support on use of the pump. Our board-certified lactation consultant is available to give you more help with breastfeeding and pumping if needed. We also provide prescription forms your doctor may sign to help you with insurance reimbursement if the pump or consultation is medically indicated, and we carry all the spare parts you might need. Our rates are . . . ."

- The curious person: "What do you offer?"

  Poor answer: "We have breast pumps, classes, and books, and our lactaton consultant is available to help with breastfeeding problems." This answer may be accurate but too limited and is not warm and inviting.

  Better answer: "I'm so glad you called. We have wonderful classes for expectant couples, classes for after the baby comes, excellent books, fun support groups for mothers and babies, the best breast pumps that really work, plus we help to select the right one for your situation. Our board-certified lactation consultant can assist if you or your baby has any problem breastfeeding, and her services are often covered by health insurance. Mothers who use our services have a much easier time breastfeeding because we provide the support and information needed. May I get your name and address so I can send you our newsletter and some information? Also please tell me how you heard about our practice." A pleasant, warm, inviting tone welcomes people into your practice.

- The upset tearful mom who needs help right away: "My breasts are so sore and my baby is starving. What do I do?"

  Poor answer: "Have you tried lanolin on your nipples? That helped me a lot." This answer gives lactation advice and is a totally inappropriate response from someone in your office who is not trained as a lactation consultant and covered by liability insurance.

  Better answer: "We can help you! Our board-certified lactation consultant helps mothers with this type of problem all the time. She is out of the office right now on a home visit, and I am the receptionist. Let me get your name and number and some more information about your situation, and she will call you back in one to two hours." This is a very warm, encouraging response. The mother can begin to look forward to a solution to her problem.

- The person who wants help but doesn't want to pay: "I can't afford one of those expensive pumps or a consultation."

  Poor answer: "I'm sorry the consult fee and pump are too expensive for you." *Never* apologize for your fees and be sure your staff doesn't either.

  Better answer: "Our clients tell us frequently that we saved their families hundreds of dollars in formula costs and doctor's bills, as breastfed babies are so much healthier. We recommend and sell only breast pumps that are comfortable and efficient. If the baby can be kept on breast milk, it saves families much more than the cost of the pump." This answer emphasizes the value of the product and service over the price. The receptionist should never be apologetic about your fees and should show the potential client the value of your products and services. Your staff needs to believe in the value of your services. More importantly, they need to be able to put that value into words that the client will understand and appreciate.

Use the lists of everything you do to train your employee. Focus on one or two tasks each day until she learns the ropes. One day you might focus on rental forms, including renting and cleaning pumps. On another day, you might target using the scales, including weighing babies, recording weights, and cleaning and calibrating the scales. On yet another day, you might work on understanding your consultations, scheduling, setting up your consult room or home visit bag, making up necessary charting forms, filing insurance forms, and so on. Gradually, as the days go by, you should see more skills being checked off. Ask your employee to read all the literature and watch any videos about the products you sell. Role-play the common problems mothers have with their breast pumps and explain how to troubleshoot them. Training takes time and effort, but the result is a happier, better-prepared employee who is a benefit to you and your practice and becomes a real teammate.

Another great source of business information is other professionals and business owners in your area. Consider the following local resources:

- Veterinarian
- Dentist
- Doctor
- Lawyer
- Physical therapist
- Insurance agent
- Real estate agent
- Chiropractor
- Retail store owner
- Any other small to medium-sized business owner who has a staff that must deal with the public

All of these practices and businesses have their own professional associations and publications. Often their professions are older and more developed than the lactation consultant field, and they have more than one journal to which they subscribe, each dealing with a different aspect of the practice. Even retail stores have access to magazines and organizations related to their type of business. I have spent quite a bit of time reading one of my husband's journals, *Veterinary Economics*, which deals with practice and business management issues for his profession. I have picked up many good ideas that can translate to the business side of my LC practice.

Recently, my husband attended a big conference and came back with a computer program to train his office staff. The interactive program on CD-ROM teaches good client communication skills on the phone and in person at the reception desk, gives a pretest and post-test, and shows the learner typical client situations and different ways to handle them. Although the examples in this program are veterinary related, my staff trained by using the program, too. "Substitute 'mother and baby' for 'client with puppy,'" I told them before they started, "and when in the example the caller complains, 'My cat has fleas,' you substitute in your mind, 'My nipples are sore and I don't have enough milk.'" We all laughed and had a good time, but the exercise also opened up a great discussion on how we greet and speak to our clients. We learned that what we say, in person and on the phone, is powerful, shaping the client's impression of our practice. It is everybody's responsibility to turn the client into a satisfied customer, and those "price checker" phone calls are the most important calls of all. Our response can make the difference in whether that person will use our practice or go elsewhere to spend his or her dollar.

What can you look for from these other local resources?

- Samples of job applications
- Interviewing and hiring experience and advice
- Employee training information, such as the CD program mentioned earlier or information in other formats
- Examples of policy and procedure manuals

- Marketing tips

- Professional journals about practice management, business, and employees

- Experience and advice about dealing with employees and situations that may arise

- Information about different business files or computer programs, although many professionals now use very specialized programs sold only for their type of practice

How you approach these people and your personal relationship will probably determine their willingness to share with you. By approaching people who are not in competition with you, you are more likely to glean valuable information for your practice. Do *not* ask another lactation consultant who works in your area for this type of information, unless you plan to work together in some cooperative way that benefits both of you. That would be tantamount to asking her to train her competition. In a busy office situation, you may want to speak to the office manager with the permission of the owner. Generally, if you ask for something simple that is not time-consuming, such as what type of job application the business uses or whether you might borrow some of its old practice management publications, your resource will be happy to help you.

POLICY AND PROCEDURES

It is vitally important, to protect yourself legally, that the employee understands his or her role and your role. What the employee can and cannot say or do is best spelled out before employment begins, repeated during the probation/training period, and reemphasized whenever necessary thereafter.

Having a policy and procedures manual is of great benefit as soon as your practice expands to include even one employee. All of your employees should be required to read and understand this document. Creating it may sound like a huge undertaking, but you begin by writing down what you do a little at a time. Keep this information on your computer in a file, and print it out each time you make additions or changes; alternatively, get a three-ring binder and start writing with a separate page for each topic.

Reading your "manual" should be part of each employee's orientation and training and it can save you a lot of headaches as an employer in the future. One of the most difficult things any employer has to do some day is to correct or even fire an employee. Having the behavior you expect and your rules written down—even the most obvious things you may think don't have to be said—will be of huge benefit in these situations and can actually prevent many problems. You need policies about the most obvious reasons for dismissal, including lying, theft, drunkenness, drug use, habitual lateness, or unexcused absences. Also include a section on breaching confidentiality and note specifically what that means. Your employees need to know and understand that the intimate information a client reveals when coming to your office must be kept in strictest confidence, without fail. No information about your clients can ever be discussed or revealed outside your office. Even the fact that a client used your services is confidential. Your reputation will suffer greatly if personal information about any of your clients leaks outside your office. "What you learn here, remains here" should be your business's motto.

Topics in your policy and procedures manual might include the following:

- Vision statement for your practice: State in a few sentences or paragraphs your philosophy, goals, and beliefs for your practice.
- Client/customer relations policy: Politeness, consideration, appearance of your office, meeting the client's needs, and so on.
- Employee policies and expected behavior:
  - Job descriptions for every position in your office, including yours.
  - Conditions for employment.
  - Orientation, training, and probation period.
  - Pay period.
  - Benefits.
  - Personal appearance and cleanliness. If receptionists will touch babies, emphasize hand washing to protect everyone. Also, you may want to include a policy about piercing and tattoos. Many businesses that involve staff interacting with the public have rules for employees who enhance and protect their professional image such as "no visible tattoos, no facial piercing, no more than one (two, three, and so on) piercing(s) per ear." Of course you decide what is acceptable to you and your clientele. Your staff represents you to the public.
  - Attendance, tardiness, and illness. This problem will drive you crazy if you run into a person who is chronically late. It is best to set limits of how many occurrences are acceptable during a time period from the beginning. For example, you could decide "more than three occurrences within three months without a doctor's excuse or arranging for someone else to cover the shift can be reason for dismissal." You can always be more lenient, but excessive absences and tardiness can disrupt your practice. This written policy will give you the power to talk to the employee and take action if necessary.
  - Smoking. I recommend a "smoke-free" office for the health of your clients and their babies. It is also legal not to hire a smoker, even if she agrees not to smoke at your office. My experience has been that smokers are sick more often, can smell badly, which may be disagreeable to a mother who brings a baby to your office, and take every break you will give them to go outside to smoke.
  - Telephone usage (personal use versus abuse guidelines).
  - Bringing babies or children to work.
  - Disciplinary measures.
  - Reasons for dismissal.
  - Confidentiality.
- Procedures for every activity in your office:
  - General office duties: answering the phone, filing and recordkeeping, mail and deliveries.
  - Sales and rentals: exact procedure for each type of transaction, instruction manuals on each item you sell, business information from your credit card company about procedures and spotting credit card fraud.
  - Delivery of rental items (e.g., pumps, scales, battery packs).

— Making appointments and preparing for consultations.

— Registration and preparing for classes—have a detailed list of everything that needs to be done.

— Housekeeping.

This manual will become very useful when you have turnover in your staff. It makes training new people easier if you have a lot of the information they need written out.

The employee needs to know the consequences of not functioning within his or her job description. The biggest problems I have experienced are tardiness and absenteeism with a few employees, and overeagerness to counsel the mothers. If a mother calls with a counseling question and the receptionist knows the answer, she must be able to hold back on giving the answer and take the message to pass on to the lactation consultant. Giving the employee guidelines and role-playing on how to handle those calls can prove extremely helpful. She can reassure the mother that her question will be answered and that many others have called with this same problem or question. You can designate certain information that your receptionist can give out from printed materials you supply, such as guidelines on the correct storage of expressed mother's milk, correct assembly and use of a breast pump, and your rates for services, rentals, and classes. She should always identify herself promptly early in the phone call, stating her position as your receptionist, as many people start talking the minute the phone is answered and assume that they are speaking to the lactation consultant. The source of all information should be identified to the caller and a record of the call made for the lactation consultant to review.

Consider a policy stating that only the IBCLC, who has professional liability insurance, gives breastfeeding advice, because many questions seem simple at first, but often turn into a much larger problem. If your eager employee wants to do more, you can mentor her by encouraging her to learn more, take educational courses, and work toward becoming a lactation consultant. Explain clearly to employees that your policies and procedures are meant to protect all of you from possible lawsuits.

PAYING YOUR EMPLOYEES

What do you need as an employer to begin to pay someone beside yourself? You will need to set up accounts with the state and federal government so that you can report properly and pay withholding taxes for your employees. You will use your Social Security number or apply for an employer identification number (EIN) and a state tax ID number depending on what type of business you have (sole proprietor, partnership, or corporation). You will receive tax booklets and payment coupons that you send with each payment of the taxes withheld from the employee's check. Federal withholding is paid to an authorized depository, usually your local bank, and the state withholding is mailed to your state's department of taxation. You can find the contact numbers in your phone book for both your state and federal departments of taxation. Ask for the forms and information you need as a new employer to get set up and pay your employees.

You may also need to report your new hires to your state's department of taxation, along with the employee's Social Security number. Each new employee needs to fill out a W-4 form indicating how many deductions you should take from her paycheck.

Lastly, an I-9 form from the Immigration and Naturalization Service needs to be filled out and signed by both you and the employee. This form can be downloaded from the INS site (see the resource list at the end of this chapter). All U.S. employers are responsible for completing and retaining a Form I-9 for each individual they hire for employment in the United States, including both citizens and noncitizens. On the form, the employer must verify the employment eligibility and identity documents presented by the employee and record the document information on the Form I-9. Acceptable documents are listed on the back of the form and detailed under "Special Instructions." Most people give a copy of their driver's license and Social Security card, but a passport and other identification are also acceptable. No filing with the INS is required. The employer must keep the form either for three years after the date of hire or for one year after employment is terminated, whichever is later. The form must be available for inspection by the authorized U.S. government officials (i.e., INS, Department of Labor). If you are investigated and don't have proper I-9 forms on file, you may have to pay large fines.

Pay Rates

The pay rates for various jobs will vary depending on your location (urban or rural) and the job market. You may not believe that you can afford to pay someone $10 or $12 per hour to answer your phone so you can have a few hours off, but always remember that you may have more to offer an employee than just money.

You may start out using someone only part-time. Part-time work fits into many people's schedules easily. As stated earlier, if you are just starting out getting help, a wonderful pool of women exists who would love to earn a little extra money working part-time at your office or their home. If a woman can work for you with her baby in a carrier or on her hip, she may be happy to settle for minimum wage. You can discuss with any potential employees the nonmonetary benefits of the job, including the elimination of the need for day care.

How Do You Learn to Do Payroll?

An accountant or business counselor can help you get started with payroll management, and it is worth it to pay for this advice if it means that you get off on the right foot. Another good idea is to turn to another small business owner who has employees and ask to sit with the person who does payroll. Check out what you learn with your accountant for accuracy. I learned how to handle a payroll by paying my husband's employees at his veterinary practice. It is not as difficult as it may seem at first to write a paycheck and deduct Social Security, federal, and state taxes. Using the tax booklets is not difficult. Once you learn how, you may need an hour at the most to pay four or five people. If you have a computer program such as QuickBooks or Peachtree, you can pay 15 to 20 people in less than an hour. Then you must pay your withholding, Social Security, federal, and state taxes. Small businesses make these payments at least monthly, but sometimes the state withholding is due only quarterly. If you have already learned to pay sales taxes, then you have a taste of how to keep the necessary records.

Use some system to keep track of the employee's time or classes taught, consults done, miles driven, and so on. I use simple 3 × 5 inch file cards as time cards. Fancy time clocks are available in business supply catalogs and stores, and some computer business programs include time clocks. At my office each employee puts her name at the top of her 3×5 card and fills in the dates worked and time coming to and leaving work every day. If teaching a class, the instructor fills out a card with her name, date, and class taught. On payday I add up the person's time and pay each employee per hour, or for classes taught or consults done, and staple the time card with the stub or copy of the paycheck. I file these documents in my payroll file for the current year.

With business software, you will have payroll reports easily available for each employee. Many programs calculate your tax liabilities/withholding for you; you simply put in the employee's hours worked and rate of pay, and the program writes the check for you. If you cannot use a computer, get the tax withholding booklets from the IRS and your state government and buy some payroll forms from an office supply store or catalog. You will have to look up in your tax booklets the correct chart depending on how often you do your payroll (e.g., weekly, biweekly, monthly). Once you have figured the person's gross pay, consisting of the hours worked multiplied by the pay rate, you look at the chart for the amount of tax withheld given the number of deductions claimed (from the W-4 form). Next, you calculate the Social Security and Medicare deductions according to the instructions in the booklet. You will have a payroll form for each employee and record each paycheck you write to him or her with all the amounts: gross pay, Social Security, federal, state, and any other withholdings and the net pay (what the employee actually takes home). All should be in nice neat columns.

Taxes

Don't let payroll taxes scare you. If you get help the first couple of times you do payroll until you feel confident with the process, you will find it a regular chore, but not the impossible mystery that it may seem now. Paying an accountant to help you set up and get started on the right track is well worth the money. Once you learn how, the challenge involves remembering deadlines and paying the various taxes on time. You will receive a coupon booklet to complete and submit with your payments for federal and state taxes. If you are extremely busy or can afford it, businesses will do all of your payroll and your payroll taxes for you. You simply sign the checks once they are written.

U.S. taxes that you must pay if paying employees include the following:

- Social Security and Medicare—you deduct the tax from the employee's pay and you contribute an equal amount.
- Federal withholding—deducted from the employee's check.
- State withholding—deducted from the employee's check.
- Federal unemployment tax (FUTA—Federal Unemployment Tax Act)—paid by the employer, based on your total payroll, and often paid quarterly. FUTA provides for payments of unemployment compensation to workers who have lost their jobs.
- State unemployment tax—paid by the employer only.

You can electronically file your state and federal taxes by computer or telephone if you wish. This approach can make filing your withholding easy to do, and you may perform this task in the same session that you are writing the paychecks, or monthly, depending on what schedule is required for your business. To calculate the total federal tax deposit, multiply the Social Security tax withheld times 2 to include your contribution as the employer, add the federal tax you withheld for your entire payroll, and write a check for this amount to your bank. You include your tax ID number and fill out your ticket, in pencil, being careful to insert the number just as the instructions tell you within the little boxes. If your payroll exceeds $50,000 (at which point you ought to have a whole staff to handle your accounting), you may have to file every two weeks. Your state withholding may be due either monthly or quarterly, because your payroll will be small. You will be notified by the state and federal agencies of your filing deadlines.

Quarterly reports are due with summaries of all you owe and have paid. At that time you will pay any extra taxes due. Paying an accountant or business advisor to help you through this process the first few times will ease your apprehension.

To make life easier, you may choose to let an accountant figure your quarterly reports for your payroll taxes and your yearly income tax forms. In this case, you take responsibility for only the routine work of figuring and paying the withholding taxes, which becomes very easy after you have done it once or twice. Then all you do is supply your payroll records to the accountant.

Payroll Records

All employers are required by law to maintain complete payroll records of all employees. These records include:

- The employee's name and Social Security number
- The date hired, rehired, or returned to work
- The date and reason for leaving employment
- The state in which services were performed
- A schedule of work hours (your work schedule on a calendar, time cards, or computer records)
- Time lost when the worker was unable to perform his or her duties
- Wages paid, and dates covered for each pay period (time cards again)
- Tips
- The cash value of other forms of remuneration (e.g., gifts given as bonuses)
- Payments in advancement or reimbursement for business expenses

This recordkeeping is not as daunting as it may sound. If you keep a folder for each employee you can just jot down pertinent information. Keep her application and résumé, and add your notes about the date hired, pay rates, raises, evaluations, date leaving your employment, and reasons why.

What About Benefits?

Do you have to pay your employees benefits such as sick time, vacation time, health insurance, retirement, and 401(k) plans? That sounds like more than a beginning employer can handle. The truth is that these benefits are not required, especially if you are hiring part-time help and have fewer than 50 employees. Social Security is a benefit because you contribute an equal amount. You probably won't face the issue of paying these other benefits until your business has grown to the point that you have full-time employees. In that case, you and the employees should expect some reasonable benefits. As you gain experience being an employer, you will see that treating your employees well benefits both you and them.

It is a good idea to put in writing and point out the monetary and other nonmonetary benefits that you may provide to your employees. Possible monetary benefits include the following:

- Social Security
- Vacation and sick time (earned according to how many hours the employee works)
- Retirement accounts (Your business is unlikely to quickly reach the point at which you would offer this benefit, but you can check with your banker as *you* may want to save for your own retirement.)
- Health insurance (You can pay for a policy for your business including yourself and your employees, or give the employee a certain amount to be used toward paying her own health insurance policy.)
- Professional liability insurance
- Professional dues (ILCA, AWHONN, childbirth certification organizations, or other professional associations)
- Professional subscriptions (JHL, LLL, childbirth publications, AWHONN)
- Continuing education and certification expenses (conference registration, hotel, travel, recertification expenses)
- Uniforms (lab coat or scrubs)
- Name tags

Possible nonmonetary benefits include the following:

- Flexible scheduling
- Part-time employment that fits into a family's routine
- The possibility of working from home, even taking calls with a cell phone while away from home (Note: avoid cell phone use while driving)
- No day-care expense if you allow the employee to bring her child to work
- A pleasant, casual work environment
- Enjoyable work helping families and improving their health
- Buying things from you at a large employee discount (I offer my employees anything I sell for my cost including shipping, and they take advantage of this benefit frequently, buying for themselves and gifts for others.)
- Free consultations, if needed, for their own breastfeeding problems

INSURANCE

Worker's Compensation Insurance

If you hire employees, you need to obtain worker's compensation insurance. This insurance will pay if any employee becomes injured while working for you. One of my childbirth instructors, who was eight months pregnant, was preparing to teach a class at my office. She fell down a flight of stairs while carrying teaching supplies. Thankfully she was only bruised and spent one night in the hospital being monitored. The worker's compensation insurance paid her entire medical bill, which otherwise would have been a huge unexpected expense for my practice.

Most companies that provide business insurance can sell you a policy that suits your needs. Your premiums will be based on your yearly payroll and the type of work done by your employees. Most of the people you hire will be considered a low risk, doing office work, so your premiums should be minimal.

Professional Liability Insurance

Every professional, and especially one in a private practice, should maintain professional liability insurance. Ideally, you should already have insurance for yourself. If you pay another professional as an employee, you may need to carry additional coverage, even if she already has her own. You need to discuss this matter with your lawyer and insurance company. The amount of time that the employee works for you changes your risk of being sued for something she does under your employment. Any professional who works for you is at potential risk of making a mistake, and both you and she could be sued as a result.

If the professional works for you as an independent contractor, her own insurance may be adequate. Nevertheless, you should talk to a lawyer familiar with professional liability. If you decide to pay this and other professional fees, it represents another benefit to the employee and a business deduction for you.

Business Insurance

Business insurance protects you from fire, theft, other damage to and loss of your inventory, office equipment, and files at your office or in your car while being used for your work, and clients being hurt on your premises. A single incident could cost you huge amounts, so this coverage is essential once you enter into business. Shop around as you would for any insurance policy.

Evaluating someone is difficult for a first-time employer. It is especially challenging if you are unhappy with some aspects of the employee's work. This process will be easier if you have written policies and procedures, so you can compare her work to your already established standards of practice. Periodically, perhaps every six months or so, or more often when she is first hired, you can let the employee know, formally, how she is doing. Comparing her work to your written policies and procedures keeps you objective.

One of the worst habits to adopt is to be vague. You might know you are displeased with the employee but you must be specific to produce an improvement in her work. Saying "You need to be better with the clients" is so broad that it gives her no way to improve her behavior and no way to please you. Be more specific by saying, "Ellen, you've been working here three months. I've noticed that when a mother comes into the office and you are on the phone, you wait until the phone call ends to look at or greet her. I understand the situation, but as our policy and procedures manual states, I would like you to acknowledge her presence as soon as she comes in the door. You can look at her, smile, and whisper that you will be with her in just a few minutes. Motion to her where she can sit to wait or walk around to look at our merchandise, so that she feels welcomed and that you are not ignoring her. Do you think you can do that?" This approach opens the door to a discussion on how the employee can handle the situation better and gives you a place to start if the employee does not improve her performance.

Be sure to document each time you evaluate the employee in her file and note the agreed-on action to take in any situation. For example: "Discussed the math errors Betty has been making on the rental agreements, six errors this past month. Also, she has not made copies of the proper identification from the client on four rentals this past month. We agree that I will practice doing the math on sample rental agreements with her until she can do them without error, and she will work harder to remember to obtain the needed ID from every rental client. She says she is too shy and embarrassed to ask people for their ID. I stressed that this is our policy and she can tell the client it is required for our rentals. I also informed her of the purpose of obtaining this ID—we need to be able to locate clients who try to steal pumps or not pay. We practiced different ways she can ask the client for the ID. She agrees to get the ID from now on."

If Betty continues to fail to get the ID, you can revisit the issue: "Betty, we talked two months ago about your not getting the required ID from people who rent pumps. This issue appears to still be a problem because you have filled out five rental forms with no ID since then. How can we fix this problem? I need a receptionist who can get all the paperwork done correctly." This strategy gives Betty the ownership of the problem and the responsibility of deciding the solution. The needed behavior is clearly spelled out. If Betty cannot improve her performance, you are justified at ending her employment and have the documentation to show she did not comply with your company's policies and procedures.

Firing someone is probably the most difficult thing you will ever do, but it should be a rare occurrence if you take the time and effort to hire carefully, train well, and evaluate your employees on a regular basis. Everyone wants to know how he or she is doing in his or her work. Typically, your evaluations will include only praise of your employee's work. Don't think you shouldn't do an evaluation because you have nothing negative to say. That is the perfect opportunity to pat a good employee on the back and thank her for the many little things she does to promote your practice. Praise her, be specific about what you like that she does, and especially give her any compliments you have heard from your clients. Thank her for her accuracy, attention to detail, the way she keeps your office so neat, her updating of your client files and lists of interested people for classes, friendliness with clients, and anything else she does to promote your practice.

Raises can be given after a good evaluation or anytime. I typically give a small raise, $0.15 to $0.25 per hour, after the first three months and the employee is on her way to being fully trained. Six months and one year after hiring are also good times for raises. Don't discount the value of even a small raise to someone. Whenever you give a raise, write a small note recognizing the employee's good work and thanking her for her help and dedication. Everyone needs and wants encouragement. Frequently we get and give too little of this valuable emotional benefit.

Why would you want to allow an employee to bring her child to work?

- It sets a good example. If you have a wonderful mother who can breastfeed her child in a sling while waiting on your customers, it can say more to a new inexperienced mother than hours of classes and counseling on parenting.
- Many mothers are committed to what you do and are your best, most enthusiastic advocates and wonderful employees. They are or have been breastfeeding mothers and are willing and eager to assist you.
- You may pay less than if the mother came to work without her child and had to pay for child care. This policy is fair for both of you.
- You will find mothers with great education and skills whom you could not afford to hire other way. The mothers I have hired have included teachers, a medical technologist, nurses, a librarian with her master's degree, and one mother with a degree in finance. All were willing to work for minimum wage if they didn't have to leave their precious little ones.
- Mothers with children tend to be the most devoted and enthusiastic employees whom you can find. Usually it is more than a job for them, as lactation consulting is for most of us.

Disadvantages of such a policy include the following:

- The employee with a child in tow gets less done because she must stop and tend to the needs of the child.
- Children can and do get sick. You must have backup plans in case the mother must stay home with a sick child. Some days, you may not have a worker because of a sick child.
- Children have good and bad days. Babies can be teething or just grouchy. What will you do if your normally wonderful employee has been up all night with a teething baby? You must be patient and plan for substitutes or see if you can do without an employee on that day.
- It is difficult for the mother to work too many hours. Usually a four-hour shift is all a young child can take. If you need someone eight hours per day, you may need to hire another person to fill in or have a backup person or plan.
- Sometimes an employee works well until the baby begins walking, then the happy baby becomes an active toddler who destroys your office. If your child-proofing and redirecting efforts don't work, you may have to reconsider the work relationship and offer the employee the choice of not bringing the child to work anymore or finding other employment.

What Should You Do?

Although I am a strong supporter of mothers bringing their children with them to work, and I did it myself with my own babies, I have learned that this situation has to be managed well so that it benefits all parties. More than a dozen employees have brought their babies, from three months old to four years old, to work for me over the past six years, and I have learned a lot about this type of work relationship.

1. The workplace must be made child-proof. You will tear your hair out if an 18-month-old pulls your papers off the desk faster than you can pick them up, or dismantles your pump display and spreads pump parts all over your office. You need drawer and cabinet latches, gates, and barriers that are easily opened or removed so you and your clients can get through. Of course, the child needs to be able to see and have easy access to his mother or the situation won't work. You may rearrange your office so the desk, telephone, and paperwork are gated out, at the same time the child can be close to mother and easily supervised by her while she is working and he is playing.

2. The mother and child must fit your work situation. This does not work for everyone. It is not conducive to a professional atmosphere to have a miserable toddler who has been confined too long, screaming in the background when your receptionist answers the phone. A high-need child may not be able to adapt. The mother will either have to come to work without the child or find other employment that is more compatible with her child's current stage of development.

3. Hire people who share your philosophy of breastfeeding and parenting. Conflicts of philosophy will cause conflicts in the work relationship. Be sure to interview carefully and get to know the potential employee before committing to a long-term work relationship.

4. Teach your employees to give gentle, effective child care and discipline. A mother who slaps and shouts at her child, ignores his cries, doesn't anticipate his needs, does not know how to keep him occupied, or fails to provide acceptable activities will not work well for you. Remember—she represents you and your practice to your clients.

5. Begin every work arrangement by having a trial and probation period. Start with two or three days as a trial just to see whether everyone seems compatible. If things go well, hire the employee to begin a three- to four-month probation period. This span is a good amount of time to get to know someone and determine whether the arrangement is working for both of you; it also allows either party to terminate the relationship before she is an official employee. According to labor laws, she is *not* an official employee until the probation period ends. If you find a wonderful, smart woman who has a two-year-old who runs from one place to another creating disaster, screaming for attention every time the mother tries to talk to a client, you can honestly say that the situation is not working out. Write out policies and procedures that include guidelines for working with a child in tow. I talk with employees before hiring, telling them that I love babies and children and heartily believe that mothers should be able to work without being separated from their children, but that it has to work for both of us. The mother must be able to give appropriate care to her child *and* complete her work.

6. Give the mother consideration and time to take care of the child's needs, and encourage her to do so whenever things are quiet at your office. She shouldn't wait to change that diaper or breastfeed, especially if your office tends to become very busy, because as soon as the baby gets really hungry a customer will inevitably come through the door. Our office becomes very busy in the late afternoon, as people stop by to weigh their babies or pick up needed items.

7. Promote the use of slings or other baby carriers so that the mother can keep her little one content, interested, and supervised while she tends to the customer.

8. Provide space for the child to play and nap if needed. This portion of a room should be child-proof, have a VCR for entertaining tapes, and be easy to clean.

Over all, it has been a pleasure to have my employees bring their little ones with them to work. I hope that this option works for you.

SUMMARY

Getting the help you need can make a huge difference in how you feel about your practice, especially if you are close to burnout. Help and business advice are available in many forms. Hiring help can begin with volunteers, part-time help working from the employee's own home, part-time help in your office increasing as needed, instructors for classes, and others. Even the LC with the smallest practice can benefit from someone who knows how to keep the basic office running so she can have time off with her family. Don't be afraid to investigate and take advantage of the possibilities available to you. Keep your options open. Think positively. If you think you need help, start talking to people. Once others become aware of your needs, opportunities may present themselves to you. Keep an open mind and you will find just the help you need.

RESOURCES

Internal Revenue Service

- The Digital Daily: access to income tax forms, instructions, publications, regulations, including information on e-filing.
- By computer: www.irs.gov.
- By fax: (703) 368-9694.
- By phone: call for forms, publications, and automated information at (800) TAX-FORM. You should receive your order within 10 days.
- Walk in: some forms, instructions, and publications are at many post offices, libraries, and IRS offices.
- CD-ROM: Buy at www.irs.gov/cdorders for $21 or call (877) CDFORMS. Pub. 1796, Federal Tax Products on CD-ROM, gives current and prior years' forms, instructions, publications, and popular tax forms that may be filled electronically or printed out.

State department of taxation

State employment commission

Immigration and Naturalization Service

- By computer: http://www.ins.usdoj.gov/graphics/index.htm. You can download the I-9 forms from this site.
- Office of Business Liaison
  Fax: (202) 305-2523
  E-mail: office.business.liaison@usdoj.gov.
  Hotline: (800) 357-2099.
  Mail: INS Office of Business Liaison, Room 3034, 425 I Street, NW, Washington, DC 20536.

Other Good Sources of Help

- Small Business Association: http://www.sba.gov/. You can search for your local SBA.

- Check your phone book for your local business development center. It often has educational programs or courses, resources, and counseling to help new small businesses. It is usually well worth the investment of time and money.

- SCORE (Service Corps of Retired Executives): www.score.org provides business advice on-line and in person, counseling, e-mail counseling, workshops, how-to articles, business resources, and more. It has many excellent links for all your business questions and needs. SCORE Association, 409 3rd Street SW, 6th Floor, Washington, DC 20024, (800) 634-0245.

- Center for Women's Business Research: http://www.nfwbo.org/.

- American Small Business Association: http://www.asbaonline.org/.

- Business/office supply stores and catalogues where you can obtain employment applications, payroll forms, and computer business programs that include payroll capabilities. Computer programs such as QuickBooks or Peachtree cost about $200 to $300 and contain all the tables you need to do payroll. Updates can be obtained and included easily whenever the tax rates change.

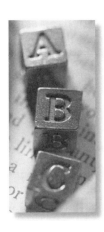

12 Information Resource Management, Computers, and the PPLC

Dennis L. Smith, MS

Managing the information in your private practice is ultimately your responsibility. It is complex and uncertain. While this chapter can't shoulder the responsibility, it is intended to help you deal with the risks and complexity. This chapter has two goals:

- To equip you with a practical philosophy about information management for the PPLC and the use of information technology, including computers, to meet your information management needs. The philosophy should help you make realistic choices in planning how you want to use computers.

- To get you started in selecting the information technology to economically implement your plans. The latter part of this chapter contains quick discussions of the many choices you will face if you decide to buy a business computer.

Whole careers, including mine, have been built on this process of implementing solutions to information management needs. A single chapter cannot possibly cover each step thoroughly. I'll simplify the task with these assumptions:

1. You are a friend of Linda.

2. You've talked to her about setting up a private practice, and she suggested that we have a chat about buying a computer.

3. You don't have time for the two-week lecture series I presented on a similar theme to management customers in Washington, D.C.

I'll cut many explanations, eliminate most of the reasoning for my recommendations, and just call it like I see it. With luck, in a single conversation I can prepare you to avoid the worst mistakes that first-time business customers make and equip you with some techniques and information to face new issues with good decisions. I offer a philosophy that will help focus your attention on the most critical needs in your practice and then in purchasing information technology.

Ted Nelson, the genius who conceived and named "hypertext," and who now operates HyperLab at Keio University outside Tokyo, Japan, inspired much of my philosophy. Ever since he wrote *Computer Lib* in the 1970s, Nelson has advocated updating the way people deal with information. He urges designing books so they can be explored as the reader's interest dictates rather than from front to back. Other than the section on information management immediately following and a section on Moore's law, this chapter is built in that fashion. If a section interests you, read it. If it doesn't seem to apply to you, skip it. That idea underlies Ted Nelson's radical concept of hypertext.

Nelson also saw the following obvious rule for applying computer power to real-world needs, which no one else seems to have noticed until he articulated it.

USING A COMPUTER SHOULD BE EASIER THAN NOT USING A COMPUTER

Let this statement guide you as you manage your private practice information and consider using computers. Savor the phrase: "Using a computer should be easier than not using a computer." It seems so obvious that it is easy to brush past, but we all have experienced situations in which it was not true. Don't let your private practice become another case of excessive technology slavishly applied. If information technology threatens to get in the way of your business by demanding time you should spend on clients, or if technology starts to consume resources you should use on professional education, challenge the technology. You don't need to be a computer engineer to expect that computers should meet your needs.

This reasoning explains why I use the term "information management" to cover the way you handle information in your practice, and I write about "information technology for your information tools" rather than discuss computers. You may not need the expense and learning curve of a computer and software for every aspect of your business.

Information technology represents technology that you apply to use, alter, store, and retrieve information. Computer hardware and software fit into that category. Information technology is not limited to computer equipment and software, however. A telephone is an example of information technology, as is a notepad on which you write down phone messages. The envelope back that Abraham Lincoln used to draft and edit the Gettysburg Address is a terrific example of information technology. He used it to store and manipulate information. This chapter introduces you to the process of selecting information technology, from cool laptops to Post-it notes, based on how the tools you choose can help you in your private practice lactation consultant role. Sometimes I'll seem almost anti-computer. That skepticism is meant to help you keep an open perspective, so you can critically evaluate the time and financial issues related to adding information technology to your practice.

As you consider information technology tools to assist in your information management tasks, keep in mind that part of information storage is information protection. Issues concerning information protection will be raised throughout this chapter in various contexts.

WHY WOULD *YOU* WANT A COMPUTER ANYWAY?

Another truth of applying information technology is that it is better to list information management needs and then shop for information technology to meet those needs than it is to buy a solution (e.g., a computer) and then begin looking for a problem. Before we go any further, jot down a list of how you do or might manage information in your practice. Create your list before you read the possibilities listed next. You need to list the information you need to manage (use, alter, communicate, store, and retrieve) and indicate how you need to manage it in your practice.

Here, in no particular order, is a list of items to compare with the list you just prepared:

- Manage (i.e., store, alter, retrieve, communicate, and use) names, addresses, and phone numbers for clients, their physicians, your associates, and your suppliers
- Manage sales and purchase records for tax calculation and to extract profit and loss information
- Draft and send consult letters to referring physicians
- Design and print brochures and business cards
- Keep track of phone calls and correspondence
- Address envelopes
- Track accounts receivable and payable
- Prepare and present new parent classes or in-service programs
- Present instructional video to clients and professionals, or even prepare and distribute your own original videos
- Make travel plans and reservations
- Keep track of business inventory
- Prepare client handouts
- Locate and buy reference books or other materials for your practice
- Gather and organize information on current issues related to breastfeeding, such as ways to help mothers or to help you advise physicians on what they can do to help mothers with breastfeeding problems that may involve more than physiology
- Exchange breastfeeding information with other LCs

The possibilities listed here are the result of a quick "brainstorming" session. They may exceed the needs of any particular private lactation consultant, but still may omit some information management need related to your unique practice.

Take a look at your list of private practicc lactation consultant information management needs. Have you written the words "computer" or "software" on it? Watch out! The assignment was to list what you need and want to do to use, alter, communicate, store, and retrieve information in your practice. If you've mentioned computers or software, you've moved on to selecting tools to meet your information needs. That step needs to be consciously done only after you have a solid understanding of your needs. Soon, we will discuss tools for information management, but you should continue to update your list of private practice information management needs regularly as you think through the issues raised in this chapter.

The value of implementing new information technology is only as good as the organization you apply to the information during the implementation process. On your list, mark the information and information management items that are the most important to your business. Identify the information management items that are the most frequent, easy, difficult, or unpleasant. The bad news at this stage is that chaotic information, such as random receipts and notes in a shoebox, will be just as random if copied into a computer without some planning; this concept is referred to simply as GIGO (Garbage In, Garbage Out). Now, with your new thorough perspective of the way you use, communicate, store, retrieve, and alter information in your practice, you can begin to consider what information technology might help you.

SOME USES FOR INFORMATION TECHNOLOGY IN LACTATION CONSULTANT PRIVATE PRACTICE

Computers can be great for drafting really pretty correspondence. Once you know how to use them, a computer, some word processing software, and a printer can make a prettier and better-spelled letter to a medical professional than most people could ever do with a pen and pad—at only 100 times the price of a good pen and a batch of quality printed stationery and business envelopes.

PCs are great for writing your next book, tracking your accounting, or expanding your knowledge and base of personal contacts through various Internet connections. With a good knowledge of database management, you can set up computers and software to manage your client files for 10 times the price of a four-drawer filing cabinet and paper supplies.

If you set up a pump depot, you may want to spend money on computer hardware and software, and spend time learning how to use your purchases, so that you can have fast, easy access to data about your pump business. Alternatively, you could buy a Trapper-Keeper student notebook and clipboard, saving a lot of up-front time and money, and keep your pump depot information at your fingertips. Add a flashlight and your Trapper-Keeper will be useful even when electric power, Internet, and phones are all unavailable!

Computer tools also can automate much of your telephone answering needs, saving your client from the sudden shock of your teenage son yelling, "Hey, Mom! Telephone!" They could give you six layers of touch-tone telephone that would provide your practice with the facade of a major corporation, rather than a home office. Impressive complexity is presented as a selling point with some computer accessories. As you are now focused on using information tools wisely, you may well consider an answering service or a $49.95 digital answering machine with clear voice recording to make a smaller friendlier impression.

Do you want to have information technology help you manage your business financial records? A number of software packages on the market can, once you understand how they work and take the time to load them with the ongoing details of your business, quickly accept sales and income tax data; they can keep you up-to-date on how rich or poor your business is making you. Some people prefer to solve their business financial recordkeeping problems by purchasing the part-time services of a Certified Public Accountant and likewise hiring a bookkeeper that the accountant suggests. The middle road is retaining an accountant and capturing your data with the accounting software recommended by your accountant.

You could also use another Trapper-Keeper, a filing cabinet with folders, or a properly equipped computer as information technology to maintain your client records.

MULTIMEDIA AND GAMES

You probably didn't put "play music, movies, and games" on your list. Even so, a family member, friend, or salesperson is bound to suggest PC entertainment products to you with considerable enthusiasm. You'd better think about that issue now. Ill-considered use of your PC for entertainment can be risky and expensive.

Music CD players and speaker systems come standard in all modern PC bundles, so, if you like music or environmental sound in your office, you're in luck. The speakers will give you some optional sound cues as you use your PCs and will be important if you play the instructional videos that are included on the CDs of some popular software tools.

Do you really need the free games and multimedia features that usually come bundled with computers? How important are they for your practice? Are they worth the headaches when they don't work or if you have to pry your 10-year-old or his father off the latest game running on your machine? (The last sentence deliberately used male nouns, because, until now, males have statistically been the dominant users of PCs for games, although we prefer to call them "simulations.") When you shop, be prepared with your prioritized list of business information management needs for which you are considering using a computer. Keep reminding the salesperson what you really want to do. Word processing, accounting, e-mail, and World Wide Web surfing can be done on low-cost, low-commission machines that a salesperson might not want to offer.

The biggest users of machine power and the most common sources of problems on shared computers are computer games. Game software demands extra power to maximize the thrills. To fully use computer power for game excitement, game programmers sometimes violate operating system safety rules; that technique can lead to later failure of your business software. Check with your tax advisor about the legality of deducting an entertainment PC (i.e., a game machine) as a business expense.

If you must share your computer with a gamer, expect problems and try to compromise. You reduce your risk by allowing only Microsoft® games on Windows® machines. If you allow other games, insist that they be certified on the packaging as Windows compatible. Games that require computer configuration adjustments will change the way your machine works for business, once the adjustments are made. Microsoft and PC Disk Operating Systems (DOS) are obsolete operating systems designed in the 1980s. If you allow DOS-based games on your computer, you run a substantial risk of future problems.

Finally, the casual sharing of computer games sometimes propagates computer viruses. More than one LC has found her business computer infected by a son's installation of a shared virus-infected game.

THE LIFE CYCLE OF ELECTRONIC EQUIPMENT

Before you purchase a PC, you should select those information management needs from your list that justify the cost of the tools you buy to meet those needs. What is a computer worth to you? No universal answers apply when calculating the value of a computer to your business. I use Moore's law to pare down a list of possible computer applications before shopping. Moore's law was originally stated in a concise but complex fashion by Gordon Moore (who co-founded Intel four years later). I rephrase Moore's law to say that the cost of the integrated circuits used in computers falls by 50 percent every 18 months. From this postulate, I conclude that *the dollar value of computer technology has a half-life of about 18 months.*

To at least break even on a computer hardware purchase, you need to get back half the purchase price in the first 18 months of use. If you don't expect to get that much value out of your system in the form of the money and time it saves you or the money it makes for you in performing the tasks for which you purchased it, then the investment won't be worth the money expended. When you think about this test for the value of automating a prospective information management task, don't forget to include in your cost the time required to set up the system and enter information to be managed with it, but realize that you can spread the cost of that time over the whole life of the machine. Also, you might want to assume that you will have a problem during implementation that will take you about eight hours of phone calls and research to fix. Ideally, Moore's law and conservative anticipation of the effort of setting up an application will help you avoid a low-payoff application. I once had an over-enthusiastic student who spent $2000 on a PC to manage his bachelor grocery list! He was very disappointed.

DO YOU NEED YOUR OWN PRIVATE "GEEK"?

I've chatted with many lactation consultants. An LC in Ohio said, "[Lactation consulting] is about empowerment. Women are reclaiming their knowledge of their bodies." While it's generally accepted that entrepreneurs should surround themselves with a "management team" including at least a banker, an attorney, and an accountant, some entrepreneurial and independent LCs may be reluctant to surrender the design of a system for handling their business information to advisors of either gender. Information management decisions are very personal, and letting someone else make them builds vulnerability into your business. On the other hand, time spent becoming a wise computer shopper is time lost to becoming a wise LC. If you are comfortable keeping salespeople focused on your needs or have a computer technology advisor who can act as your advocate, you probably can skip the following detailed discussion of computer specifications and computer shopping.

Some computer experts (self-designated "geeks") work as much for pride in their efforts as for money; therefore, finding a friend or family member volunteer from the computer world who is willing to share insight is one approach to building a safety net for your early information technology decisions. You are particularly fortunate if you can find a friend in a private practice similar to yours who has successfully implemented computer solutions to the information management tasks at the top of your prioritized list. Keep your information management priority list handy as you work with your geek. Experts may be proud of their successes and eager to share them even if they are not high on your needs list. Your information management list can help keep your guide's enthusiasm focused on your needs.

If you would like to control this aspect of your business without a geek, I suggest skimming these paragraphs, then visiting computer stores or store Web sites to get a feel for what sort of computer choices are possible and how they affect the prices of the available models. Then you can review these paragraphs as needed.

If you have special accessibility needs for your PC, you may wish to search for a geek with some experience in the many accessibility options available for PCs. It is possible that a computer users group in a city near you will have formed a special interest group (SIG) with the specific goal of assisting others with unique computer interface needs.

In some professions, such as lactation consulting, selecting a certified professional would be a wise move in choosing an advisor. The International Board Certificate represents an *unbiased* professional certification program. With the constant head-over-heels development in computer technology, the focus of certification has shifted from certifying expertise in the profession to certifying expertise in products. The prevalent certification program in the computer world today is run by Microsoft Corporation and certifies individuals in terms of their knowledge of specific Microsoft products. If you get advice from a certified Microsoft expert, realize that the advice will likely involve your purchase of Microsoft products. Caveat emptor.

To go shopping, you need three things:

- Your philosophy for approaching information management
- Your list of needs sorted into priority order
- A healthy dose of skepticism

Discuss your needs list with your geek, if you have one. You can consider selecting the computer hardware and software to help you with tasks that are difficult or time-consuming using simpler tools. This chapter will cover a lot of popular tools and concerns, but I will be terse with my rationale. Perhaps I won't anticipate your needs sufficiently. Use some common sense and test these thoughts as they apply to your unique situation when you are planning and purchasing information technology with your future business at stake.

Macintosh, Windows, or Linux: Choosing an Operating System

You must choose an operating system (OS). An OS ties together the hardware of a computer to make it work. Operating systems are essential, and each of the three major operating system families is incompatible with the other operating system families. The three OS families are Windows (which evolved from the now-obsolete DOS), Macintosh, and Linux. Proponents of these operating systems can be emotional in their beliefs and sensitive about challenges. Make sure your geek and you can agree on an operating system with which you feel comfortable.

Macintosh systems cost more money for the computing power delivered, but their followers insist that cost is paid back in saved time. Apple Macintosh computers have the hard-earned reputation of being the most user-friendly PCs. While true believers in the other operating systems will correctly point out that fewer products and programs are available in the Macintosh world, and that those available carry a premium cost, few have ever criticized the ease of setup and use of modern Apple Macintosh computers. Macintosh computers are generally acknowledged to have the most physically attractive designs. You may need less help setting up a Macintosh, but, if you do feel you need a Macintosh geek, such a person may be more difficult to find. Macintosh has a relatively small share of the PC market, so there are fewer Macintosh stores and experts.

At the opposite extreme from Macintosh in terms of user-friendliness is the Linux family of operating systems. No single company dominates Linux. Like the residents of a freewheeling nineteenth-century Wild West town, Linux users have the raw freedom to reprogram their operating system to perfectly match the application software they write. Some office software is available, but, so far, Linux has been employed more for Internet server centers than for general small business use. This is changing. If you are the pioneering type, you might be interested in this operating system with a promising future. Because much Linux software is nearly free, Linux is poised to offer its pioneer users breathtaking savings.

For the rest of us who want stability and the standardization of an operating system with about 80 percent market share, Microsoft Windows is the choice. Windows users must live with Microsoft, a corporation that more than once has been accused of abusing its monopolistic power to dominate its market.

Most PCs are built to run Windows. Most PC repair technicians know more about computers running Windows. Most stores sell PCs that come with Windows preinstalled. Niche market computer applications, such as a special-purpose pump depot application, are more likely to be built for Windows machines so they can reach the broadest customer base without having to support multiple OSs. When in doubt, choosing safety in the vast numbers of the Windows-based community seems a reasonable choice.

Palmtop, Laptop, or Desktop

Palmtop computers and pocket computers are cool status symbols equipping businesspeople with light and extremely portable information tools, but they are not designed to be primary business machines. They do much less and cost much more for what they do than your other alternatives. I'll say no more about them.

Laptops are also pricy portable tools for the businessperson of this millennium. A laptop may have a place in your business. As a general rule, expect to pay about twice as much for your laptop as you would for a similarly equipped desktop of comparable quality.

The laptop's advantage of portability around your home and during your travels can be impressive. A part-time LC and full-time parent could do LC "paperwork" at a swim meet; a business-traveling LC lecturer could make last-minute changes to a presentation while flying to a conference.

The cost of a laptop's advantages is its higher price and the greater risk of damage to hardware or loss or exposure of data. Some homeowner's policies cover the risks of theft or breakage of laptops, but others do not. Not much bigger than a purse, laptops are easy targets for thieves. In addition to the risk exposure that the value of the laptop creates, you must consider the effect of your loss of access to critical business information should your laptop be lost, stolen, or broken. Also, you must consider how the loss or theft of your laptop would affect your clients, if that laptop makes their credit card numbers or other personal information suddenly available to the thief.

Considering the higher risks and costs of laptops, this chapter assumes that the majority of PPLCs will start with desktop PCs. If your key information management tasks require mobility and can pay off despite the higher risks and costs of a laptop, you can still use the information given here. It is phrased for desktop buyers but is nearly always applicable to laptop buyers as well. Laptop buyers should pay particular attention to the discussion of extra-cost store warranties. A warranty that covers accidental breakage of a laptop's delicate and expensive screen could be really important, even as it could add as much as $500 to the price of the laptop.

W hen you buy a computer, compare the manufacturers' and stores' selling points with your information management needs list. Don't be surprised if the selling points don't seem to have anything to do with your list. These points tend to describe the tool and leave it to the buyer to fit the tool to a need. You must have brought your needs into tight focus, and then have the courage of your convictions when you meet the computer sellers.

In-store PC choices are overwhelming. If you've found a geek you trust, consider his or her favorite brands and suppliers. You could work out a budget first, and then let the geek take the lead in shopping while you come along to keep the focus on a PC for your needs (not games or cool technology).

When Linda and I shop, we use her needs list to keep perspective. We never buy computers on the same shopping trip in which they are first offered. That way we can have a calm discussion over a hot fudge sundae safely away from the salesman. You may honestly be told that the PC best for you is low in stock and may not be available if you wait. Remember Moore's law: That PC is probably being sold off to make room for an even better product.

Here is a review of some common types of computer stores.

WHERE TO BUY A COMPUTER

Custom-Assembled Computers

Small independent computer stores can, and even prefer to, assemble a computer specifically for you from the case up using highly standardized commodity parts. Assembly is straightforward. I personally select all the internal components for my computers from DALCO, a nationwide computer supplier and assembler, which happens to have its headquarters, its warehouse, and a small computer storefront near my home.

This approach of building custom machines is a common offering of local independent computer stores. If you don't want to specify what goes in, the salespeople, who may also be bench technicians, can offer a list of the most popular assemblies. They will be similar to the big brands down the street, but built from standard parts. Independent stores don't have the advertising budget of the big chains, so they must rely on their reputations to gain business.

Two main concerns arise in purchasing a custom-assembled PC. First, you need to trust whoever specifies what parts go into your computer. Second, you need to trust the seller/assembler to stand behind the work and parts.

If you have a smart advisor and a dependable store, you are indeed fortunate. Your machine built from "PC-compatible" (formerly referred to as "IBM-compatible") parts will be easy to maintain, because any reliable technician will recognize the parts and, for the foreseeable future, will be able to buy low-cost replacement and upgrade parts. If you or the store from which you purchased it moves, these advantages remain and become more important. Computer technicians nearly anywhere on Earth can service your machine, without needing to special-order parts from a brand-name corporation for a higher price and a longer wait.

"Big Box" Store Packaged Computer

Large electronics chain stores such as Best Buy, Circuit City, and CompUSA, to name just a few, offer another viable option. They will have ready-to-use computer bundles, often available immediately and "on sale!" You can select from consumer brands such as Macintosh or, for Windows shoppers, Sony, Compaq, and Hewlett-Packard, or numerous store and lesser-known brands. Some of the major manufacturers also offer more expensive business lines that differ more in terms of the higher-quality customer services department backing them than in performance. Most of these machines will have a mixture of standard and custom-engineered parts. They will probably be more attractive and have a few more cute buttons for extra features, but may be more costly to service.

A brand-name computer purchased from a reputable supplier such as CompUSA, or perhaps your favorite "big box" store, is likely to give you reliable performance. Unfortunately, when computer journalists test-shopped the local and national computer stores and their repair centers, they have found both good and disappointing stores varying from city to city. I can provide no general advice on this score.

Bargain machines purchased from high-volume outlets without repair centers probably will be just a little more likely to break down and, as you must then find a service center, may be a little more difficult to get repaired. If your advisor says you truly can save a lot of money buying that way, you may think of it as a bet you probably will win, assume that your advisor is correct, save the money, and spend your savings later if you happen to have a problem.

Some stores pay commissions to their salespeople or offer bonuses for pushing certain items. If your sales representative seems to be leading you toward a certain brand or bundle or offering superfluous items, be wary. There is an enormous diversity of salespersons in computer stores. I've met a few brilliant experts and a lot of naive youngsters. Unfortunately, unless you know how to filter farce from fact in technobabble, it may prove difficult to tell the former from the latter.

Computers from Mail, Phone, or Web Order Warehouses

Dell, Sony, Hewlett-Packard, CompUSA, and other computer sources have stores on the Internet. You could have your geek sit with you as you surf the Web and consider your choices or try to work out what you are buying in a toll-free phone call. If you have access to a PC for browsing the World Wide Web to a dealer's site, using the Internet to formulate your choices might be a good way to practice shopping before facing a live salesperson.

One of the biggest advantages of buying from a large, reputable Web sales operation is the relatively easy customization of individual orders. For example, Dell allows you to select a basic system model, then fine-tune it to your specifications by choosing particular memory, hard drive, operating system, bundled software, and accessories. If your hardware choices are overwhelming, just stay with one of the ready-made models and choose the software you want bundled with it. It is usually more economical to purchase an office suite such as Microsoft Office for small business preinstalled on your PC as an upgrade from Microsoft Works than it would be to buy the generally similar but somewhat more expensive Microsoft Office off-the-shelf product and install it yourself.

Keep in mind that if you order a PC from out of town, you may need to ship your PC out of town to deal with a problem. The seller will discourage you from returning a product, as it will prefer to protect the sale and send a technician to repair your machine, or have you deal with the problem on your own. You might find it reassuring to buy from a local store that you have confirmed has expertise available to get you through setup issues and new user difficulties locally. Do you know any satisfied customers of the out-of-town dealer you are considering?

If you have purchased an out-of-town dealer's machine with a local service warranty, note that the individual providing that service may not be a company representative. Use of third-party technical support services is not unusual. I once had a new employee of a third-party repair service show up at my home completely untrained. He had never seen my brand of computer before, despite the fact that it was a big seller that year!

I have learned the hard way to look at reference sources such as *Consumer Reports*, *PC World*, or *PC Magazine* and to buy only well-respected brands from reputable sellers; I also consider personal referrals from individuals I know and respect. That's how I found a lesser-known custom-assembly PC dealer that I now know from personal experience can be trusted.

WARRANTIES AND SERVICE CONTRACTS

Apart from the poorly trained technician concerns mentioned earlier, there are other reasons to avoid investing much in long-term warranties and service contracts. In particular, those items are high markup (profit) centers for the sellers.

Consumer-oriented sources consistently advise against extended warranties and service contracts for heavy appliances. PCs and laptops will become obsolete so quickly that soon you may wish you had the money spent on a service contract to instead purchase a brand-new machine.

Laptops are probably the best candidates for extra-cost warranties, because they are more vulnerable to physical damage in travel. Laptops are more difficult to upgrade and therefore tend to become obsolete more quickly; be careful not to pay a premium for a warranty that protects your machine well after your machine has become an antique. Consider Linda's 1998 laptop. When it was new, it sold for $2100. Four years later, laptops with at least twice the power sold for less than $1000. (That's Moore's law at work: In four years the laptop's price dropped by more than half and the new laptops available for that lower price were more than twice as powerful as the original expensive machine.) Three years after the computer's purchase, you may not care about a warranty on your old machine and may be more interested in a new laptop.

Wherever you shop, bring your geek and have the courage of your convictions in buying only features that you want and need or that come on all machines and are essentially "free." I've taken the main points from a random sales advertisement from my local newspaper and present its offering as starting point for discussion, translation, and explanation of the technobabble that you may encounter when shopping. If obvious guidelines exist for making a wise purchase, I'll offer them. Sometimes the choices you face don't have simple "bottom-line," one-rule-fits-all solutions. That's why you need to be equipped with a list of prioritized list of information management needs and a trusted advisor. Finally, every wave of new operating systems and software demands PCs with more resources. It generally doesn't cost a lot to go from smaller than average resources to the middle-sized average models, but buying machines with "bleeding edge" features can prove very expensive.

AN EXAMPLE COMPUTER "SALE" BUNDLE

Following is the text of a hypothetical computer advertisement. Moore's law keeps driving these numbers to change, but the rationale behind the discussions will persist.

- Intel Celeron processor 1.1 GHz computer
- Microsoft Windows XP Home Edition
- 256 MB Sync DRAM
- 20 GB Hard Drive
- 40X CD-ROM Drive
- Some software preloaded
- Free printer (after savings and rebates), $69: –$20 mfr. mail-in rebate, –$49 bundle mail-in rebate
- Free monitor (after savings and rebates), $159.99: –$20 instant savings, –$60 mfr. mail-in rebate, –$10 bundle mfr. mail-in rebate, –$70 store bundle mail-in rebate; 17" .27 monitor (16" viewable)
- Includes 3 months of on-line Internet service (3 mo. begin on date of purchase; to avoid being charged a monthly fee, simply cancel before promotional period ends.)

AMD or Intel Processor [N] GHz Computer

You'll see ads like this for Sony, Hewlett-Packard, and other Windows PCs. Macintosh's bundles are simpler because the brand of the hardware and the operating systems are the same and not a commodity. Macs have to compete only with Windows machines, not with essentially identical systems from other companies.

Intel makes most of the processor chips for Windows PCs. **AMD** also makes respectable and price-competitive processors for Windows machines. Both companies have excellent reputations. Use other criteria to select your PC.

[N] (where N is a number) **GHz** (gigahertz) refers to the clock rate, or how many billion clock pulses a processor ticks off in one second. It is useful in comparing processors within families, such as Intel Celerons with other Intel Celerons, Intel Pentium IVs with other Intel Pentium IVs, or AMD Athlons with other AMD Athlons. The clock rate is less helpful between families, because different families can do different amounts of calculating during a single clock pulse. For complex math or games and multimedia, Intel's Pentium line is faster for the same clock rate than Intel's Celeron line. AMD's Athlon chips are a little faster than Pentiums with the same clock rate, so AMD has begun to name its chips with model numbers that AMD (and independent testing agencies) believes are comparable to the clock rates of matching Pentiums. Apple Macintosh computers include different processor chips than the other devices mentioned here and cannot be compared with the other processors using simple clock rates.

Speed is not particularly important for routine-use business machines. PCs with higher clock rates may have other factors, such as hard drive speed limitations, that keep the higher processor speed from increasing performance as much as you would expect. As Moore's law hints, these clock rates differ from season to season. As the chips get faster, software builders inevitably find ways to use the power for cute features that force consumers to stay on this gigahertz treadmill. For business machines, buy as much speed as is economical, but below the very expensive speeds. The fastest machines cost disproportionately more for a few extra clock pulses. For example, a hypothetical PC with a 1.1 GHz processor might cost 5 percent more than a 1.0 GHz processor, while a 1.8 GHz machine might cost 10 percent more than a 1.7 GHz machine. If you decide to pay a little more for a little extra "nice-to-have" processor speed, watch out for the "price-to-performance ratio knee" where you begin paying a substantially higher price for a little more performance. On the other hand, if you plan on playing computer games, you will want as much extra speed as possible.

Microsoft Windows

Windows releases often ship with assorted problems, but most ready-made PCs probably have fewer problems than custom-assembled machines because the mass-production manufacturers theoretically can test their wares better. In any case, Microsoft usually follows each new release with an easy-to-install "service release" to fix many of the worst problems. A conservative shopper would either buy a PC with the previous operating system, or wait until the Service Release 1 free update was available before purchasing a Windows computer. Microsoft sometimes offers various versions of operating systems, such as "Home" and "Professional" editions. If you think the professional edition might be appropriate for you, get a comparison chart from the operating system aisle at your store or from a Microsoft Web page, and review how the extra-cost features will assist you with your information management needs. According to Microsoft, Windows XP Professional works more flexibly with other computers on home or business networks than does Windows XP Home.

[N] MB (Megabyte) Sync DRAM

For basic business PCs, I just pay attention to the "RAM" in "DRAM," which stands for "random access memory." In the computer world, "mega" can mean either 1 million or 2^{20} power, which actually calculates out to a little more than 1 million. A byte usually can hold no more than one alphabetic character or digit. Thus, if all you put in the memory were simple English characters, you could put in hundreds of millions of them. The memory in your machine is essential to hold and run the software and data you load and store on the hard drive. The operating system will want lots of memory, too. Memory chips are regularly redesigned to run faster; the current fastest memory "flavor of the month" matters more for games and multimedia.

Memory is cheap. A good "rule" is to equip your PC with *at least* double the memory the operating system manufacturer lists as a minimum requirement; quadruple the specified minimum would be even better. For example, a package for Microsoft Windows XP Professional instructs: "128 MB or higher recommended (64 MB minimum supported; may limit performance and some features)." Applying our rule, 256 MB would be a wise amount of memory, and 512 MB would be a very economical way to enhance the performance even more.

If your machine contains extra empty memory slots, you or your geek can easily add more of the same kind of memory later when Moore's law makes it even cheaper.

[N] GB (Gigabyte) Hard Drive

"Giga" represents either 1 billion, or a power of 2 that is approximately 1 billion. Hard drives for desktops usually come with more gigabytes of memory than laptops do. If you don't use multimedia, almost any popular size will suffice. If you plan to use your PC for video or sound, a hard drive with more capacity is better. PCs with middle-sized drives don't cost much more at initial purchase, and you will be amazed how much capacity the operating system and software use. With modern desktop PCs, you, the store, or your geek can easily add a second hard drive later. Thus if hard drive capacity is not important to you today, you can upgrade when it's cheaper next year. The same is not true with laptops, on which only the premium machines have much hard drive flexibility. An add-on internal drive would add weight to the laptop and would have to be compatible with the original manufacturer's designs. Also, note that external hard drives tend to be very expensive compared to the built-ins.

The more important issue with hard drives is speed. The bundled drive is probably a slower model, but speed is not listed in the advertisement and may be difficult to discover. You can ask your salesperson who may guess or make up a speed that pleases you. Sometimes manufacturer Web sites provide this information. In basic desktop hard drives, a motor spins a disk at 5400 revolutions per minute. For about $10 extra, the manufacturer or PC assembler could have built a PC with a hard drive spinning at 7200 rpm, capable of supplying data to the PC about 33 percent faster. If you have a choice, get a PC with a 7200 rpm hard drive with minimum 20 GB capacity and preferably at least 40 GB. Hard drive speeds improve only a little from year to year. Their capacities, however, race to get bigger.

40X CD-ROM (Compact Disk—Read Only Memory) Drive

As you purchase more software, you will need a way to put it into your computer. Today, software is generally distributed on CD-ROMs. You must, therefore, have a drive capable of reading CD-ROMs. Every PC sold for regular retail customer use will come with something that can read CD-ROMs. Virtually all PCs come with the capability and sound gear to play music CDs as well. (Watch out when you buy music—some music CD recordings on the market are specially designed to not play properly in PCs to discourage use of PCs to copy music CDs.)

The "40X" indicates how much faster the CD can spin when it is loading computer data than when it is playing music. You probably won't notice much difference between a 40X and a 12X drive in normal business use. I have an old PC with a 4X CD-ROM that does seem slow but still works adequately. If you load games, you will want the extra speed. The "read-only" feature, however, is a big drawback. In the past, people have stored their own files for backup or distribution to others on "floppy" disks, named for the flexible storage material inside the plastic case. To share and save the bigger files created by modern PCs, you should own a CD-R or CD-RW drive instead of a CD-ROM drive. You can use your CD-R or CD-RW drive to record your information on durable *recordable* CDs, which, unlike floppy disks, can't be erased. CD-R disks can hold a lot of data upon first writing or when you later add data on remaining blank space. Today, most CD recorders also have the ability to write on the less durable but also economical CD-RW *rewritable* disks.

The example machine does not come with a DVD-ROM drive, but you really should consider one or plan to add one to your desktop at a later date. While once commonly translated as "digital video disk," DVD is now referred to as "digital versatile disk." There is more value to a PC DVD player than just the ability to play videos and see those few extra features on the video DVDs that can be unlocked only on PCs. Some computer software is already distributed on DVD-ROMs, and you should expect more software and reference materials to be distributed on this medium in the future. DVD-ROM drives can also read CD-ROMs and can play CD recordings that are playable in CD-ROM drives.

Some DVD-ROM players in PCs can record on CD-R or CD-RW disks, so you may not need two drives. As a luxury, you can purchase a PC with a DVD record-capable drive, but such machines cost substantially more than the more practical choices listed here.

Some Software Preloaded

It probably won't be the software you want, but it's there. Also, if you are considering a PC bundle at a big-box store, the store has no choice about selling it to you. Think of it as free and worth about what you pay for it.

The preloaded software will probably be "teaser" items that are designed to raise your perception of the value of the PC package and to get you started on a basic software product that you will later want to upgrade for an additional charge. Common bundled items include multimedia demonstrations such as entertainment products, encyclopedias, and starter office suites such as Microsoft Works. Microsoft Money personal financial management software is also frequently included in bundles. Offers vary, so check before you buy. Note, however, that the presence of Microsoft Works on your machine may be important in qualifying you to purchase Microsoft Office as an economical upgrade rather than as a costly retail stand-alone license. Microsoft Office is discussed in more detail later in this chapter.

If you buy a PC from a custom assembler, you should not expect to get preloaded free software. You may get some software bundled with the devices, such as a CD-RW drive or a premium sound card, that you have the assembler provide and install. The big mail/phone/Web order PC sellers do give you more control over preloaded software. They are discussed more later.

Free Printer (After Savings and Rebates) $69: –$20 Mfr. Mail-in Rebate, –$49 Bundle Mail-in Rebate

Your free printer will be $69 plus tax and chosen by the store. You can then try to promptly and correctly file the very specific rebate form, which you may need to request and locate somewhere else in the store before a rather tight deadline expires. The stores can offer these kinds of rebates because they are sufficiently difficult to discourage the majority of customers from collecting. The $69 printer is probably a remarkably good deal if you don't print much, but you should keep some things in mind.

Inkjet printers are cheap to make, but the ink cartridges they use are often expensive. Low-priced inkjet printers can print attractive color work, but will be slow and costly to operate. Many ink formulas are susceptible to smearing if they are exposed to moisture. Some can fade upon exposure to light or some kinds of pollution. If you print a lot of black-and-white text, you may find that a laser printer saves you time and money in the long run.

Color printers designed specifically to print photographs use six color inks. A few printers need special, more costly paper to print good-looking color images. More expensive printers can often print good images on plain copy machine paper; they may have separate ink cartridges for each color so you won't have to replace a complex cartridge with four or six colors of ink when you have used up only one color.

Just because a color printer can print pretty pictures does not mean it can print an attractive business letter. Look at samples of the kind of information, text or image, that you intend to print. Printers today should be designed to connect to your new PC's USB (Universal Serial Bus) port. You eventually may be disappointed if your new printer needs to connect to the older but still available parallel port on your new PC. Note also that printer manufacturers tend to overstate the speed of their printers, especially the color image print speeds. Ask for a demonstration, or just brace for slower than quoted speeds when you print real documents.

Free Monitor (After Savings and Rebates) $159.99: –$20 Instant Savings, –$60 Mfr. Mail-in Rebate, –$10 Bundle Mfr. Mail-in Rebate, –$70 Store Bundle Mail-in Rebate

Your free monitor will cost $159.99 plus tax and be a brand and model chosen by the store. As above, collecting the rebate(s) will be a hassle.

17" .27 Monitor (16" Viewable)

The monitor in the bundle may be a deal breaker. If a bundled monitor seems like too good a deal to resist, ask yourself, "Would I be interested in free eyeglasses or dental work from a dealer who offers me no selection?" Protect your vision. Get the very best monitor that you can afford. Even if you decide to purchase your PC from an out-of-town dealer, you still might want to buy a monitor from an in-store display where you can actually view candidates and select the monitor best for your eyes. You are likely to spend much more time and visual effort looking at your PC monitor than you do examining the details of your TV's picture.

If possible, see how your choice of monitor looks when working with your choice of PC. If you are willing to spend $200–$300 on a visit to the optometrist and purchase of new glasses, seriously consider spending at least that much on a monitor that will be easier on your eyes. Don't pinch pennies when choosing a monitor. Make sure that you understand the terms of the store's return policy. Be prepared to return your monitor if it doesn't look as good hooked up to your PC in your office as it did in the display in the store.

The monitor mentioned in this advertisement is the absolute minimum that you should consider for business use. Like conventional TVs, the monitor is described in terms of its 17-inch diagonal screen. Don't expect conventional computer monitors to actually let you see all those inches mentioned in the ad. Some of the screen is covered by a plastic frame, leaving you able to view only some 16 inches of information.

The **17"** diagonal has evolved to become the minimum monitor size for reasonable business work. Microsoft Windows draws its name from the boxes of data and images that modern software splatters over your monitor. You are likely to be disappointed with the lack of space for windows on any monitor smaller than 17 inches. If you can afford a little extra cost, you will appreciate the extra windows space on a 19-inch monitor. Monitors larger than 19 inches tend to be considerably more expensive, however, so you might not want to go for a much larger screen.

The **.27** refers to the dot pitch. It provides a vague idea of how fuzzy the image, and especially the text, on your monitor will be. The .27 dot pitch is on the fuzzy side as monitors go; .25 would be better.

Flat-panel computer monitors remain expensive, but their prices are falling. They are pushing CRT monitors into obsolescence. Through the end of 2001, prices of the older CRT (picture tube)-based monitors managed to fall just as rapidly, keeping the CRTs as the best-buy choices. The display quality of modern flat panels is such that you often can pack the windows that would need a 17-inch CRT onto a 15-inch flat panel. (Likewise, you may be able to use a 17-inch flat-panel monitor instead of a 19-inch CRT monitor.) If, when you choose a monitor from the store selection display, you "fall in love" with a flat panel, you need to have a store technician show you how to connect it to your new PC, which may have an older connection for a CRT monitor. Be sure to get a "no questions asked" store return warranty that lasts long enough to allow you to confirm that you will be satisfied with your flat-panel display on your own PC. Laptop buyers may want to keep these flat-panel size recommendations in mind and be particularly cautious about laptop screens smaller than 14 inches. Watch out for a vocabulary slip: A "flat screen" monitor is a premium CRT, while a "flat panel" monitor is solid state and only a few inches thick.

All PCs come with some kind of **USB (Universal Serial Bus)** sockets. A few now have the newer USB 2, which is much faster than USB. When you have a choice of add-on accessories, including mice, printers, scanners, and monitor-top small video cameras, buy the USB models. You can increase the number of USB sockets by adding low-cost "multiplier" devices called hubs. If you need a hub, buy one with its own power supply.

While connecting **cameras** to your PC may be a topic of discussion, this sort of item does not need to be purchased at the same time as your PC. Today, USB is an easy and popular way to connect premium still cameras and basic video cameras to PCs. USB 2's transfer system is suitable for connecting USB 2 hard drives and USB 2 digital camcorders to your PC.

Today's digital **camcorders** use a connection called IEEE (Institute of Electrical and Electronic Engineers) 1394. Other names for this same standard are Firewire and Sony's i.LINK. IEEE 1394 was the dominant high-speed connection for computers in homes and home offices in 2001. As USB 2 is built into more PCs, future camcorders may begin to use it instead of IEEE 1394.

Other Accessories

Most packaged PCs come with a generic **keyboard** and **mouse**. If you have no special accessibility issues, just use the ones that come with the PC until you gain some experience. Large computer stores have displays with keyboards, mice, and mouse-substitute pointing devices such as trackballs or styluses that you can at least examine and perhaps test. For something as important to your long-term health as these interface devices, you should eventually upgrade to what best works with your body.

Some individuals have special needs for **accessibility**. Today's Microsoft Windows operating systems come with a generous supply of accessibility features built in. They can read text files aloud, although not as smoothly as Hal of Stanley Kubrick's *2001, A Space Odyssey* movie. Windows can be configured with type sizes, styles, and colors that assist individuals with limited visual acuity. Keyboard and mouse speed and behavior can likewise be tuned to the needs of users.

Speech input/output software and microphones are available and get better every year. Some versions of Microsoft Windows come equipped with text-to-speech "read aloud" software or even speech recognition features. Before you purchase add-on software, find out what is included in your operating system. Speech recognition software does not work as well as depicted in the movies; if you need to use it, stick with the best software available, not the introductory packages. For example, IBM offers Via Voice in a number of versions. As the price rises, IBM adds more versatility and increased compatibility with popular software. At the top of the line for a little more than $200, IBM's Via Voice Pro includes a well-designed microphone and dual-earpiece headset engineered to work well with the software. If you intend to use speech input, buy a more powerful computer. Speech recognition requires a lot of your PC's resources.

Scanners are cheap, so they represent a low-risk purchase. If you buy a scanner, select a USB-compatible model, not an older parallel port or SCSI model. The SCSI models may even be a little faster in scans, but USB is simpler to set up and you will find it easier to connect your USB-compatible scanner to other PCs in the future. The scanner will probably come with same photo retouching software, and you may find some image processing software in your office suite. You should probably see how you like included software before you purchase extra-cost photo-related software.

Modems and NICs (network interface cards) are used for connecting to the Internet and to other PCs. Several years ago, modems for connecting PCs to telephone circuits were standard with PCs. Now, even though phone modems work better than ever, more expensive Internet connection options are gradually pushing phone modems into the annals of history. More recent choices for connection to the Internet include ISDN, satellite, (A)DSL, and cable data services. Changing government rules, price regulations, and taxes, along with a dynamic technological and business environment, preclude a detailed discussion or recommendations on this front. Which service is appropriate depends on which options are available in your area, which have competitive prices, and which are supported by responsible providers; naturally, the service you select must match your needs well enough to be economically justified. Because the technology is ubiquitous, easy, and economical to add and later to remove, you might want to use phone service until you are ready to plunge into one of the more costly options.

You can buy a phone modem for about $50. It can be installed in your desktop or laptop, but a convenient desktop option is to add a USB modem. Most phone modems now offered are rated at 56 kilobits per second (Kbps). U.S. federal telephone restrictions, however, bring the practical capacity of the common modem down to 53 Kbps. Unfortunately the nature of telephone lines themselves often limit actual Internet connections to half of that limit—

say 26 Kbps. A convenient way to estimate what these numbers mean is to divide them by 10 and call the result "text characters per second." Thus, if you have a phone line with a typical level of background noise, you may be able to connect to the Internet and send or receive about 26,000 bits per second or 2600 text characters per second. That's not bad for e-mail with professional associates, but disappointing for multimedia or downloading software updates.

You will need an **Internet Service Provider** (ISP) to call when you want to connect your modem and PC to the Internet. Major Internet service providers such as AOL, Sprint, AT&T, MSN, Ameritech, and Prodigy really differ only slightly from one another. Among the major reputable national or regional providers, shop for a bargain. Another alternative for "homebodies" is a local ISP with a physical customer service office that you have the option of visiting when you need help.

Will you be traveling? Does the ISP you are considering provide easy-access phone numbers in the areas you may visit? Local ISPs probably won't, so wide-ranging frequent travelers should stick with a national supplier or they may face astronomical long-distance charges from motel rooms to their distant ISPs. Generous ISP service is available for $20 or less per month. You can save more if you have a realistic idea how often you might want to be connected each month. It is easy to underestimate your needs here, so, at least at the start, aim for more than you think you might need and avoid long-term contracts. If you don't mind dealing with e-mail and Web sites with extra advertisements, you may be able to get very-low-priced Internet services.

Watch out for purchase "discount" ISP packages from computer sellers, which include long-term ISP service commitments and often high monthly charges. These deals are not bargains—they are traps. Buy the computer you want from the computer store, and buy the Internet service you want from an ISP. Don't tangle the two up. Failure to heed this advice is nearly certain to cost you more in the long term.

Web site hosting now comes bundled with many ISP Internet access services. Before you publicize your e-mail or Web site address, you need to consider your long-term rights to use the address provided by your ISP. The e-mail address denny456@niftyisp.net and the Web site address www.niftyisp.net/denny456.htm remain good only as long as Denny stays with the hypothetical Nifty ISP company. If Nifty ISP goes out of business or Denny decides to change ISP providers, then Denny's e-mail and Web site address must change.

For about $40 per year to register and maintain registration of your own Web site name, and an additional monthly fee to your ISP for **alias domain hosting**, you can register a name of your own creation that can connect to your Web site and e-mail accounts and that you can take with you if you change ISPs. Your geek and the ISP representative can tell you more about this possibility. If you decide to create an alias domain name, make sure that it is registered with you, not the ISP, as the owner and administrative point of contact. Work with your ISP and advisor to select a responsible name registrar. There are some fly-by-night registrars that could cause problems.

LAN (local area network) connections also use NICs. You may be offered a variety of LAN gear. Modern Plug-'n-Play Ethernet cards are easy to install if you don't mind connecting your machines with wires. Avoid special-purpose home networks that use special nonstandard equipment.

Wireless LAN equipment is even easier to set up and connect. In fact, if you are kind enough to set up a wireless LAN, a computer enthusiast with a laptop driving by your office may be able to connect. Quality encryption is a new and important feature in wireless LAN products.

Do you really need a local area network at all? Check your information resources management list. Do you need to share Internet access or share printers or scanners across a LAN? Don't buy LAN equipment just because it is low-priced and easy to install. Don't set up a LAN unless you have a business reason, and be extremely cautious with the more expensive wireless gear, even if it is "way cool."

Protecting Your Computer

Did you know that while you are on the Internet, you are literally *on* the Internet! While you are visiting other computers, someone else "on the Internet" can also visit *your* computer. If you connect cable or DSL Internet service, you will be on the Internet whenever your computer has electric power and the Internet will maintain a permanent connection to your computer. Think how public you'll be! Imagine a hacker looking over your shoulder as you enter your business transactions. To protect your computer from the vulnerabilities, you need, at least, a **firewall** and **antivirus software**.

Firewalls are available as hardware for local area network Internet connections and as software for individual PCs. Consider Zone Alarm®, Symantec's Norton™ Firewall, or McAfee's Firewall. Zone Alarm is available on the Internet for free download for nonbusiness use, and for a modest charge for business use. Other options are available as well, but space precludes listing every available product.

UPS (uninterruptible power supply) devices and surge protectors are important accessories that protect your PC's delicate integrated circuits from occasional power utility problems. Surge protectors are economical. I don't pinch pennies on them, preferring to buy premium models in the $40–$100 range. Remember to protect all outside circuits that connect to your PC: power, phone, and LAN. My surge protectors have saved my PCs from destruction on at least two occasions.

UPS devices cost a little more and come with built-in surge protectors. Do not connect both the UPS and external surge protectors together. UPS devices include substantial rechargeable batteries and can keep your PC running for a short time even when power is off. They cushion failures long enough for you to save your work and shut your equipment off correctly. The better UPS boxes can also maintain the correct voltage levels for PCs even when a "brownout" affects incoming power. APS and TrippLite are two major manufacturers of power and surge protection products.

Backing up, or copying your important files to a storage medium such as CD-ROMs, is an important part of responsible information management. I've found that elegant backup hardware and software modeled after tools used by corporate Information Technology departments tend to confuse non-technically oriented users. You can simplify your backup tasks if you keep your data separate from your software and in easy-to-remember locations.

Some software saves setup information and data in the same location as itself. Usually you can choose this location. Store your data in one clear area on your hard drives; Microsoft Windows systems include a folder called "My

Documents" that is a good starting point for such an arrangement. Then make straightforward copies of your data on a regular basis, when their loss would be painful. This approach is easy with common CD-R or CD-RW drives.

I don't recommend purchase of special backup software or hardware. A potentially serious problem with these packages is that they "compress" the data to take up less space and place it in specially coded files, saving space and sometimes making the process faster; that approach requires special software to later remove the compression to restore and read the data. If, after an emergency, a problem arises with removing compression, your compressed backup data are useless.

It seems safer for a very small business to copy those important files that you always keep in your documents area to backup disks the same way you would copy any files in routine use. The cost of this practice is that your backups won't include data you forget to keep in your documents area or numerous user preference settings, which are scattered about your computer or stored in the operating system's "Registry." Those items cover a multitude of trivia, such as your choice of background color for your Windows desktop screen. To me, this cost seems small for a system that offers easy, regular backup of important business information. If you want to be more thorough, talk to your geek or computer dealer about backing up the Registry and using more comprehensive backup tools.

Any backup system is only as good as the use you make of it. Back up your data thoroughly and often. To protect your data from threats such as fire, flood, and burglary, you should consider off-site storage. Corporations set up off-site storage centers sufficiently far from their regular locations in order to keep their information safe from regional disasters.

Very economical Internet-based data storage centers seem to be growing in popularity. Keep in mind that a low-cost Internet backup service could raise its prices once you become dependent on it. I don't like to "protect" my personal information, or that of my customers, by giving a third-party access to it and placing it in an Internet-accessible location. A safe-deposit box for your backup CDs would be good (and simple) alternative.

Furniture

The position of your desktop's display and keyboard will tend to define how you sit when you use them. Staying in one position for extended periods can be hard on you. Consider your choices in computer desks and chairs so that you can have healthy postures and ease in changing positions from time to time.

The list of accessories could go on to include game and music devices that connect to the game/MIDI ports on standard PCs, but they seem beyond the scope of advice aimed at private practice PC buyers.

It's time to look at your information list again. What tasks did you mark as potential candidates for a PC? Perhaps word processing and accounting. Consider the candidates carefully. Unless you have chosen to be a Linux operating system pioneer, software will probably cost you more than hardware over the life of your computer.

If you are considering using your PC for accounting, discuss software choices with your CPA. Once you've selected the software, you may find

CHOOSING SOFTWARE

that it requires a specific operating system to run, simplifying your PC choice. Our accountant uses Intuit's QuickBooks. QuickBooks runs on Microsoft Windows machines, which is acceptable for us. Macintosh clients of that accountant would need to find a Macintosh application capable of sharing QuickBooks-compatible files. Mac users could use MYOB accounting software or find a way of running Windows on a Macintosh, which is possible. Of course, setting up a Mac to run Windows may be more costly than buying a Windows machine, and loses the benefits of Mac's premium features. Microsoft Money is a personal accounting program that frequently comes bundled with PCs. Linux users could use GNUmeric accounting software. Whatever accounting software you are thinking of using, make sure that your accountant can work with it and that it can work with your tax software.

Any PC you buy is likely to have some basic word processing software bundled with it. For example, the Windows operating system comes with Microsoft WordPad. If your information management list has only limited requirements for word processing, you may find that the word processor bundled with your machine is sufficient.

Prepackaged PC bundles may include a home software suite such as Microsoft Works. Some current versions of Microsoft Works now include Microsoft Word, a very powerful word processor. Microsoft Works also incorporates a good basic spreadsheet program, which is really handy for math and tabular analysis.

Microsoft Office XP is a family of suites ranging in retail price from less than $500 to nearly $1000. Even the lowest-level standard edition is a powerful package with more features than any sole proprietor business owner will likely use in their entirety. The components of the standard edition—Word for word processing, Excel for spreadsheets, Outlook for e-mail and contact management, and PowerPoint for electronic presentations—all dominate their fields in business use.

If you expect to communicate in the business world, you will probably need Microsoft Office. The market share held by these applications is so large in the business world that you may not be taken seriously without the ability to send and receive Microsoft Office files. This suite is available for both Windows and Macintosh operating systems. Although it is not currently available for Linux, the Star Office suite for Linux may offer sufficient compatibility.

Few people wind up paying the full retail price for Microsoft Office. Microsoft offers upgrade options that may apply if you already own an earlier version of Microsoft Office, Microsoft Works, or some competitive office suites. Microsoft sometimes offers its products to educators or students at substantial savings. If you are considering purchasing Microsoft Office or other expensive software products, be sure to investigate upgrades, competitive upgrades, educational offerings, and other sales discounts that may apply to you.

You're less likely to have odd technical problems in Windows if you work with brand-name software; Microsoft now so dominates the software world that it is possible to set up a simple business software system using only its products. Other reputable suppliers with market niches include Intuit for accounting needs, Adobe for art and publishing products, and Norton and McAfee for software security. Roxio/MGI offers an economical and powerful line of design and publishing software that has real value but lacks the name recognition of Adobe with commercial printing firms.

Even adding too much good-quality software may cause problems in your PC, just as running too many accessories on a car can cause problems with your automobile's power systems. Add what you need. A little general-purpose software, such as an office suite, can eliminate the need for many other special-purpose programs.

Special-purpose software for lactation consultants or pump depots is an option with advantages and risks, about which honest experts can disagree. Someone with some understanding of your business and its information management tasks usually builds special applications, so you may get a head start on organizing your information. On the other hand, that someone might be a part-time programmer who bases rather simple software on the needs of a very small field of LCs. In that case, you run a special risk that the programmer may lose interest in updating the software as operating systems evolve, leaving you locked into an old system.

If you've bought a good office suite and accounting/bookkeeping package, you may find that the tools you need for managing a client practice or depot are built into the customer section of the accounting software or the contact manager in your office suite. You probably will purchase and install accounting software and an office suite anyway, so you might as well make your investment work hard for you before you spend more time and money on supplementary products. For both the customer list in QuickBooks and the contact manager in Microsoft Outlook, you can add "custom fields" that might be sufficient for your needs. To see if your software supports custom fields or other customization, load the search window of your help function and search for the root word "custom."

A s noted earlier, you must protect the personal information you put on your computer, whether it is information about you or your clients. Purchase and keep your antivirus and firewall software (and sometimes hardware) up-to-date.

You can also reduce your exposure to hacker attacks and save valuable time by ignoring gag attachments to e-mails, even when they come from friends. I've had friends innocently forward virus-infected attachments such as cute screen savers, and I've received virus-infected attachments from associates whose e-mail contact lists were used by the viruses themselves to propagate farther. Because I routinely ignore such items, preferring to save time by simply reading mail from my associates and not looking at cute pictures and animations, my computer usually remains safe from basic attacks of this sort.

Some people protect the components in their PCs from the repeated stress of temperature change by always leaving their computers on. While this rationale has some merit, consider that the most delicate components of PCs often fail due to physical wear. Leaving a PC on can increase wear on hard drives and cooling fans, and significantly increases your exposure to hacker attacks. Even with power waste reduction features that "hibernate" the PC, leaving a PC on increases unnecessary use of electricity. I turn my PC off when I leave it for an hour or longer.

PRIVACY, CONFIDENTIALITY, AND SECURITY ISSUES

BACK TO REALITY: A BARE-BONES COMPUTERIZED PRACTICE

Some economists attribute the extended prosperity of the 1990s specifically to the growing productivity advantages gleaned from PCs. You probably have a personal computer and may decide to add another computer specifically for your business. Keep your priority list in your mind, and tackle one or two applications at a time. Installing an office suite would be a good start. A reasonable addition would be a good accounting package compatible with your CPA's software. Naturally, if you connect to the Internet or use e-mail, you need, at a minimum, the security software discussed earlier.

MAKING FRIENDS WITH YOUR COMPUTER

If you keep Ted Nelson's idea that "Using a computer should be easier than not using a computer" in mind, and progress slowly into new applications, you will find that each new one can build on your understanding of applications that you've previously mastered. In fact, the graphic user interfaces (GUI; pronounced "gooey") of both Microsoft and Apple Macintosh operating systems are designed to make learning of subsequent applications almost intuitive. Linux even offers you a choice of GUIs.

RESOURCES

Staying up-to-date on PC developments is challenging. If you choose to spend your time developing and using your skills as a lactation consultant, be prepared to always be "playing catchup" in the computer technology world. This lag is not as bad as it sounds. Just study your specific PC issue when you need to make a business decision that matters. The rest of the time, spend your energy on other more important areas.

To "get smart" on a new computer topic area quickly, I often start with the appropriate *For Dummies* book. These texts offer enough expertise to get going on a project. If you want to move beyond that level, major bookstores have contemporary selections of books that offer in-depth expertise. A number of fine publishers offer computer and information technology books, each with its own editorial style. Check the table of contents and the indices for the topics you want to study in depth. You will soon find that some publishers' text organization better fits your learning style. Comparing notes with your professional associates can be another good way to learn about new tricks or techniques for managing the information in your business.

FINALLY

Avoid geeks presenting information technology as an end in itself. Keep your business goals at the forefront. Drink lots of water.

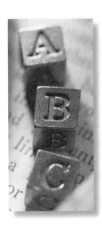

13 Promotion and Marketing

Debi Page Ferrarello, RN, BSN, MS, IBCLC

T he *most* important thing you can do to establish yourself in private practice is to practice with excellence. Be very good at what you do. Attend conferences, read journals, network with and learn from others. Treat each client with professionalism and utmost respect. Excellence is what you owe your profession, your clients, and yourself.

The *second* most important thing that you can do to establish yourself in private practice is to let the world know that you practice with excellence. Your marketing plan enables you to do just that. Your marketing plan provides for ongoing, dynamic communication with prospective clients and careful cultivation of your existing clients. You can use every bit of your creative energy in designing ways to get the word out that you have a lot to offer, because marketing never ends. Almost every contact you have with someone represents an opportunity to market your practice. So where do you begin? Let's start with your "corporate image."

YOUR CORPORATE IMAGE

Y our corporate image entails more than wearing wrinkle-free clothes and matching socks. It projects a sense of who you are, professionally speaking, through your dress and surroundings, your mannerisms, and even your stationery. When you walk into an office, pick up a brochure, and glance at a logo, you get a *feel* for the person providing the service.

Imagine a door with a name plate spelling out a practice name in rigid block letters. You recheck the address on the flimsy white business card you hold in your hand, confirm that you have the right place, and enter the room. The waiting room features a row of scuffed orange vinyl chairs, with bubblegum stuck under the arms. A few toys, all missing parts, lie strewn about the room. The cinderblock walls are dingy green and covered with outdated calendars, product ads, and a yellowing sign about not being responsible for valuables left behind. The staff is shielded behind sliding glass windows, which they open periodically to push sign-in clipboards and insurance forms onto the ledge. At regular intervals, someone in a white coat comes to a side door, calls out a name without looking up from a chart, and then disappears again with one of the people who have been waiting. What kind of *feel* do you have about this practice? I am guessing that your confidence in the quality of the service would be shaken, and that you would not feel welcome or nurtured.

Now suppose the business card was done in a soft hue with a well-designed logo. You recognize the practice door immediately because the same logo is posted on it. You enter the waiting area and are welcomed by the receptionist, who looks up with a smile, greets you by name, and asks you to have a seat in any of the available padded chairs. You notice the colorful play area for children, the current magazines on the coffee table, and the restful prints on the walls. The receptionist brings you some paperwork to complete, along with a pen, and asks if you would like some water. She also shows you where to hang your coat and points out the bathroom in case you need it. You are barely aware of the aroma in the air. Is it jasmine? Lavender? The faint scent, the fountain on the table next to you, the smile of the receptionist combine to make you feel cared for and relaxed. You feel much different about this practice, and you have yet to meet the practitioner!

As this example suggests, all of your senses are involved in forming your impressions. You can use all of them to your advantage as you develop your corporate image.

Think about the name of your practice. Some lactation consultants choose to use their own name for the name of their business. As long as you plan to remain a one-person practice, using your name works well. You will probably benefit from choosing a letter font to use each time you are printing something with the name of your practice. You may have heard about people with a "signature fragrance" or a "signature color." Your signature font will be similarly identified readily as yours whenever people see your stationery, business cards, or brochures.

Many other private practitioners choose to create a unique name for their business. Be sure that your business name incorporates not only what your practice is now, but also what you hope it will become. For example, I began with individual consultations, but planned to provide more comprehensive services in the future, such as lecturing, teaching health care providers, and contracting with hospitals to provide inpatient lactation services. I thought it likely that more people would work with me as my business expanded. For that reason, I initially chose a business name that would still be appropriate as I began realizing my long-term goals. Today, Breastfeeding Resources, Inc. is well known in our community and represents excellence in lactation consultation and education.

CREATING A LOGO

You are probably aware of the power of a logo. You already know that preschool children can easily identify fast-food chain logos long before they can read. Adopting a logo for your business can help the public distinguish you from your competitors as clients look for the familiar design on printed materials.

Many graphics are available in the public domain on Web sites and in clipart packages. Even so, I recommend using the services of a skilled graphic artist to create your professional logo. You want to be happy with your logo for many years to come. You want it to be unique, not one that will turn up on others' business cards or brochures. You want it to reflect who you are. Hiring an artist to work with you on this project can be one of your best investments as you launch your practice.

Years ago, my husband left his job to attend graduate school full-time. We had three small children and a mortgage at the time, and we needed income for little things like food and clothing. I needed to be serious about building my practice and wise about spending my limited funds. I chose to work with a graphic artist, and today, more than a decade later, I am still thrilled with the results.

How do you find an artist? Talk to people. Look at business cards all over town. When you see designs you like, ask who did the artwork. Talk to a local art school or university. Someone there might be able to recommend a student or to take on your work as a class project. Ask all your clients what they do for a living. The artist I chose was a client with whom I had developed a relationship.

When you do select a designer, make sure that the person understands what you do in practice. You will need to effectively communicate the image you are trying to create. It helps to collect business cards and brochures of other LCs. Share what it is that you like and don't like about each one. A good designer will give you several different prototypes and, with your input, modify one of them to give you just the right look. Remember that this image will appear on all of your printed materials, your Web site, and possibly signage outside your office, so you want to be very happy with it. It may never achieve the recognition of McDonald's golden arches, but referral sources in your area will come to associate your logo with you.

IDENTIFYING YOUR TARGET MARKET

As you develop your marketing plan, you will want to consider which efforts are likely to have the greatest impact. One thing to consider is *where* to direct most of your marketing efforts. For example, if you market directly to mothers, you need to reach many more people than if you market to potential sources of referrals. Direct marketing to mothers is unlikely to have the same effect as marketing to the pediatricians and nursing mother-support groups in your areas. Of course, new mothers usually keep in touch with other new mothers. Also, if you treat your clients with excellence, they are very likely to market your services to their friends and family. The marketing to prospective referral sources, however, you must undertake yourself.

Suppose that you've decided to make local pediatricians your target market. How do you begin? You will want to construct a list of all pediatricians practicing in your area. Be sure to obtain the correct spelling of their names and get current addresses. As you compile this information, enter it into a database on your computer so that you will have it in a usable format.

Next, you will want to learn to speak these providers' language. Many people compete for the attention of these busy health care workers, so you will need to package your message in such a way that it catches their attention and meets their needs. I observed sales representatives from pharmaceutical and formula companies, and then used them as models to fashion myself as the "breast rep." I would go into an office with food and make a quick introduction. If I had recently worked with one of the physician's patients, I would use the name as an "in" to tell the office personnel that I came to introduce myself. I would leave information about my services and ways that I could help them meet the needs of their patients while saving staff time. My goals were to let them know that I could help them by freeing up time spent working with breastfeeding mothers and babies, while simultaneously enhancing the practice's image in the community. Mothers appreciate a physician who understands their needs and refers them to an expert to help meet those needs. Right away, you want to let potential referral services know what they have to gain by recommending your services.

Other potential referral sources include hospitals, obstetricians, midwives, companies that employ large numbers of women, maternity shops, and mothers' support groups. Take the time to identify your target market, then use creative ways to reach them with your message.

Some of the most effective means of spreading the word about your practice are also the least expensive. Large ads in the Yellow Pages and glossy four-color brochures take a sizable bite out of your budget and may prove less effective than word of mouth or a Rolodex card with your name and number. You can cultivate clients in innumerable ways. Hold a brainstorming session and have fun dreaming up ways to let people know you are available. Here is a list to help you get started.

IDEAS TO MARKET YOUR PRACTICE

To Physician Practices

- Offer to do an in-service program for the staff on a breastfeeding topic of their choosing. This offer demonstrates that you want to help them meet their own perceived needs, and your excellent presentation will increase your credibility. Be sure to bring referral information with you.

- Develop prescription pad–sized referral slips. Visit the office frequently to restock them.

- Always send a consultation report after you have worked with one of the physician's patients. This report represents a wonderful way to market your services while meeting your own standards of practice.

- Periodically send pizza to staff, from the mothers and babies you have worked with. Include a note that says, "We hope you enjoy your lunch as much as we are enjoying ours. Thanks for referring our moms to (*your practice name*.)"

- Bring a decorative jar with your business card attached with a tag or tape. Stock it with candies or chocolates, and return often to restock it.

- Refer others to your referral sources. If a breastfeeding-friendly practice sends clients to you, be sure to let expectant parents know.

- Buy or create handouts for breastfeeding mothers to eliminate the temptation to give out formula company "educational material." Make sure that your contact information appears on the handout.

- Remember the practice staff at holiday time with a card and small gift. In fact, celebrate everything! Send in treats for Mother's Day, Halloween, Valentine's Day, and, of course, World Breastfeeding Week.

- Send in Roladex cards with your name, logo, and contact information.

- Create magnetized business cards, which are easy to stick on file cabinets for ready reference.

- Reward breastfeeding-friendly practices. Create an award that you give quarterly or annually in recognition for outstanding care to breastfeeding families. Everyone wants to be recognized for doing something good, and by presenting this reward, you are helping these practices with their own marketing.

- Shower them with gifts! You don't need to spend a lot. A copy of *Medications and Mother's Milk* or other inexpensive breastfeeding text helps staff members in their practice and makes them appreciate yours.
- When patients are very pleased with your services—and of course they will be—ask them to share their good feelings with their physicians.
- Offer to serve as a resource for triage nurses. Be someone they can call when they have specific breastfeeding questions. Establish yourself as their expert.
- Send a newsletter with "the latest" news and reports about lactation. Make it eye-catching and easy to read at a glance.
- Keep your name in sight by giving away pens, coffee mugs, and notepads with your name and number.
- Thank practices for sending you referrals.
- Teach classes for their patients. Some topics might include "Off to a Great Start," "Back to Work for Breastfeeding Mothers," and "Vacationing with Your Breastfed Baby."

To Nursing Mother-Support Groups

- Offer to speak at a meeting.
- Buy advertising space in a group's newsletter.
- Write articles for its newsletter.
- Ask groups to send you referrals.
- Thank groups for sending you referrals.
- Sponsor one of their fundraising activities.
- Make a donation.
- Donate a book to a group's lending library, and put your logo on the book-plate.
- Be a resource person for counselors to call with challenging questions.
- Refer your clients to the group for ongoing support after your consultation.
- Develop or buy handouts groups can give their mothers. Make sure that your logo and contact information appears on each one.
- Host a tea for counselors. Affirm them for what they do to support breast-feeding. Let them know how you can complement one another as you work to promote, protect, and support breastfeeding.

To Other Potential Referral Sources

- Do cooperative advertising with practitioners in other fields, such as massage therapists, chiropractors, and doulas.
- Develop a rapport with childbirth educators. Can you teach the breast-feeding class? Give out your brochures? Come up with an inexpensive gift for expectant parents with your name on it?
- Let the local hospital know how you can be of service. It can free up nurses who field phone calls from postpartum patients by referring them to you. You can give those nurses accurate, noncommercial breastfeeding information to pass on to their patients.

Directly to Mothers

- Advertise in targeted publications, such as parents' newspapers or nursing mothers' newsletters.

- Place a classified ad.

- Be a guest speaker at a nursing mothers' support group meeting.

- Teach breastfeeding classes, either in your own home or office, through a community adult education program, through physician practices, or at your local hospital.

- Produce coupons or gift certificates.

- Do cooperative advertising with baby shops and maternity clothing retailers.

- Make up gift packs to be given to expectant or new mothers through childbirth classes, hospitals, physician practices, or support groups.

- Place an ad in the Yellow Pages.

- Have a booth at a baby fair or expo.

To the Public—Be Your Own PR Department

- Write a press release. In fact, do so every time you do anything impressive, such as speak at a local meeting, attend a conference, or complete a course. Try to submit some information to your local paper every month. Enclosing a photo increases the likelihood that your press release will be published.

- Create a press kit with your professionally taken photograph, description of what you do in the exciting world of lactation consultation, a list of your credentials, qualifications, and accomplishments, and your contact information.

- Get known as "The Expert." When something related to breastfeeding hits the news, call the news editors of the local newspapers and television stations.

- Sponsor a community girls' softball or soccer team.

- Join the Chamber of Commerce. This will help you to hone your business skills, network with other small businesspeople, and provide opportunities to promote your business in ways that are completely new to you.

- Participate in a health fair.

- Write letters to the editor about anything remotely related to breastfeeding.

- Get yourself invited to be a guest on a talk show. Some radio talk shows look for new topics and interesting personalities. A "health talk" program would be ideal.

- Celebrate World Breastfeeding Week in a big way. Fly balloons outside your office, give away promotional materials, and serve food.

- Ask to address a Kiwanis, Rotary, D.A.R., or other similar group. Never underestimate the influence of grandparents!

- Use a metallic sign or customized licensed plate to promote your business every time you drive your car.

- Use your business address stamp and stationery for routine correspondence.

- Always keep business cards on hand.

- Write articles for newspapers, newsletters, magazines, and other publications.

- Prepare a catchy, one-line description of what you do. Share it at every possible opportunity.

- Donate items to charity auctions and raffles.

- Wear a polo shirt or baseball cap with your logo.

- Use personalized note paper for all of your informal correspondence.

- Leave your pens at the bank, supermarket, and everywhere else people write checks.

- Open your doors! Throw an "open house" party with lots of food, promotional material, and prizes. Of course, send out press releases and a picture after the event.

- Get interviewed. Call your local newspaper and tell the staff there that you are opening a practice and would love to tell a reporter all about it.

The more you market yourself, the better your results; marketing has a cumulative effect. If people hear your name all over town, they are likely to feel that you are The One with whom they want to work, and are often willing to pay a little more to consult with The Expert. Also, not everyone responds to the same type of promotion. Many women would never think to check the Yellow Pages for something so intimate and important as their breastfeeding needs, while others turn there first. Be creative.

We often think of marketing as our efforts to attract new clients. Taking good care of the clients that you already have, however, can be even more valuable. Cultivate relationships with your referral sources, thank clients who refer their friends and neighbors, and remember clients at holiday or birthday time. You want to demonstrate that you value your relationship with them and want to build on it. Remember—referral sources deserve care and feeding!

You may find it difficult to find time for marketing activities. In fact, if you decide that you will work on marketing when you have some free time, you will never do it! Some of the most successful private practitioners set specific working hours, right from day 1. Any time that they do not have a consultation during those "working hours" is time spent building the business. They use that time to visit practices, drop off brochures, write "thank you" notes, and submit articles. You will find that this is not time spent; it is time invested!

USE AVAILABLE RESOURCES

Look to your professional association for help. ILCA and IBLCE recently engaged the services of a marketing consultant firm to assist IBCLCs in marketing the profession and themselves. Check the ILCA Web site (www.ILCA.org) and the IBLCE site (www.IBLCE.org) for the *Self-Promotion Workbook* and updates on marketing ideas. The workbook, aptly subtitled, "Mastering the Art of Unabashed Yet Tactful Self-promotion," is a primer in promotion and marketing specifically designed for IBCLCs.

SUMMARY

Practice with excellence, and let the world know that you practice with excellence. Establish a corporate identity, and weave your identity throughout all business papers, cards, stationery, office, and other visible aspects of your business. Identify your target market, and develop specific strategies to reach each segment of that market. Use available resources for marketing strategies, including those developed specifically for lactation consultants by IBLCE and ILCA. Your successful marketing efforts will be creative, focused, and ongoing. Watch your practice grow!

RESOURCES

Books

Beckwith, Harry. *Selling the Invisible: A Field Guide to Modern Marketing*. New York, NY: Warner Books, 1997.

Blanchard, Ken, and Bowles, Sheldon. *Raving Fans*. New York, NY: William Morrow, 1993.

Edwards, S., and Douglas, L. C. *Getting Business to Come to You*. New York, NY: Putnam Publishing Group, 1991.

Holtz, H. *How to Succeed as an Independent Consultant*. New York, NY: John Wiley & Sons, 1988.

Korn, I., and Zanker, W. *Starting a Home-Based Business (Full or Part Time)*. New York, NY: Citadel Press, 1993.

Pollan, S. M., and Levine, M. *The Field Guide to Starting a Business*. New York, NY: Simon & Schuster, 1990.

Sohnen-Moe, C. M. *Business Mastery*, 3rd ed. Tucson, AZ: Sohnen Moe Associates, 1997.

Williams, B. *In Business for Yourself*. Chelsea, MI: Scarborough House Publishers, 1991.

Web Sites

www.breastfeeding.com lists private practice lactation consultants online.

Other Resources

Medela, Inc. manufactures electric breast pumps for lease and purchase. If you rent or sell Medela equipment as part of your private practice, the company can help you with advertising in print media and through direct mail to health care providers. Its toll-free number and Web site can also refer potential clients to you for lactation consultation.

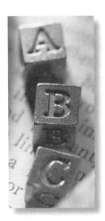

14 Pitfalls Related to Business

Linda J. Smith, BSE, FACCE, IBCLC

This chapter looks at the dark side of lactation-related businesses. We all begin this noble work with the best of intentions. However, as the poet Robert Burns wrote, "The best laid schemes o' mice and men, Gang aft a-gley." In other words, your careful plans can go astray, so that you suddenly face legal, financial, and/or other messy disasters. Serious attention to planning and an ongoing commitment to seeking and heeding sound legal and accounting advice can avoid some or all of these problems.

WHEN GOOD FRIENDSHIPS/ RELATIONSHIPS GO BAD

Many people from around the country have offered feedback about problems they have experienced in business partnerships or small corporations. Barbara Wilson-Clay writes:

> These problems are not necessarily unique to LC partnerships, but are, perhaps, intrinsic risks of linking one's fortunes to another's no matter what the circumstances. Because our choice of a partner (in business as well as in marriage) may be influenced by patterns of behavior, ideas, insecurities, and beliefs about ourselves that may not always be emotionally healthy, these partnerships themselves may not always be healthy. Just as some churches now require marriage counseling prior to the wedding, maybe individuals entering into business partnerships would profit from some joint counseling prior to entering into financial contracts. Because (just as in marriage) it is the differences in communication style, issues of dominance, and inequities in power sharing and work, rather than the business issues themselves, that sabotage partnerships.

Poor communication and interpersonal relationships can cause business problems, and vice versa. Poor business practices can also jeopardize friendships. If you're tempted to go into business with your best friend, be sure to "take care of business" by doing thorough legal and financial planning up front, before the first customer or client enters the picture. Business disasters have struck even such mother-friendly businesses as lactation consultant practices. Take a look at the checklist on the following page. How would you resolve each of the situations on the list?

It is crucial to realize at the start of your business venture that business relationships may affect your social relationships. Do not assume anything about your business partner—spell out everything in written documents. I strongly recommend engaging the services of an experienced, unbiased corporate attorney from the outset. Even though the nature of the business—professional lactation support—may be unique in your community, starting a business is not new, and a good business advisor will be familiar with the myriad ways in which new businesses can fail.

- What if you and your business partner disagree over practice philosophy? One of you is committed to alternative therapies; the other feels strongly that alternative therapies are not sufficiently researched and therefore outside the scope of practice for IBCLCs.
- What if a partner consistently kept inadequate or incomplete charts?
- What if a partner did not make a written or verbal report to a referring health care provider?
- What if you are one of the owners of a corporation, and another owner takes most of the company's client files, documents, and other proprietary information and sets up a competing business? What if the other person drastically undercuts your prices?
- What if one of your company's partners diverts most of the work to others, effectively shutting you out of the business?
- Are you prepared for unethical or even illegal actions on the part of your partners?
- What if a company officer disagrees with the decisions of the board of directors, and uses the company's money to establish a competing business?
- How would you handle a partner who did not provide a fair share of effort to the administration and management of the practice?
- How would you handle a situation in which other partners refused to hold a board meeting and began making independent decisions, effectively cutting you out of the business management of your practice?
- What if your business partner has an extramarital affair with your husband?

Consider hiring a business consultant, too. As Karen Evon says,

Business consultants help organize the business to increase profitability. Some offer complete package deals or simply target specific areas of concern. Others specialize in opening a new business starting with site selection and lease negotiations, through buildout, merchandizing, and grand opening. The money spent on the consultant's start-up and monthly consulting fees is well worth it when you considering how much money could potentially be saved by avoiding simple mistakes. Contact more than one consultant, conduct interviews, and choose one who shares your business vision and understands your mission.

COMPETITION: FROM WHOM? IS IT REALLY COMPETITION?

Competition is not necessarily a dirty word. Rather, it is usually healthy and appropriate, because the world is always eager for a better mousetrap. The LC profession arose out of the need for a new concept in health care: a professional who thoroughly understands and specializes in breastfeeding care and services. The existing health professions had ignored breastfeeding (or even discouraged it), and skilled volunteer mother-support group leaders were just that—volunteers. For a profession to grow from zero to 10,000 certified members worldwide in just 15 years is astounding, and speaks to the obvious need for IBCLCs.

Some LCs strive to become "the only game in town," viewing volunteer mother-support groups, pediatric clinics, hospital-based services, and other PPLCs as competition. Often, this attitude is unproductive at best. So many different contexts, situations, and mothers exist that there is certainly no *one right way* to help all mothers and babies. In one sense, then, there's really no such thing as competition until every mother everywhere has full access to breastfeeding care and services. Even in some areas with "a private practice on every block," some mothers still fail to get needed and timely help. Having a competitor in the area can give you someone to whom to refer occasionally and keeps you on your toes. But be careful of how you compete. You do not need to put someone out of business!

A colleague writes:

> There is an LC I know and to whom I referred clients if they lived closer to her. I started hearing from my clients that if they crossed paths with her and she found out they were renting a breast pump from me, that she would suggest that they return my pump to me and that she would rent to them for a cheaper rate, sometimes almost as low as her own cost! This kind of situation has long-reaching ramifications. Of course, I did not feel like I could trust her, and so I stopped referring people to her practice. What surprised me was the response from my clients! They were outraged! Not only did they not return my pumps, but they were bad-mouthing my competitor to their friends, their doctors, their nursing mothers groups. She has lost a lot of respect in the area for her short-sighted, mean-spirited practices.

In another sense, however, competition is real and the playing field is not level. Hospitals can hide the costs of professional breastfeeding care and advertise their services as "free." As hospital-based lactation services become more prevalent, private practice LCs may be forced to abandon their existing model of business. LCs with deep financial resources can undercut others whose practices need to be self-supporting. Storefront operations may draw more clients than home-based practices.

Part of your business plan should include a thorough analysis of the existing services available in your community. Find out what others are not doing, and build your practice to fill that gap in services. Be prepared to expand, shift your focus, and add or delete services as the market shifts in your community. Maintain a list of all sources of breastfeeding care or equipment in your community, and a list of providers of similar or related services. Update both lists yearly. This type of collaboration is appropriate and will help avoid conflicts of interest and business crises.

HOLDOVERS FROM VOLUNTEER WORK, OR HOW TO AVOID GIVING AWAY THE FARM

Whether you have been volunteering as a mother-support group counselor or working on salary for a health care institution, going into private practice means that you must think about money—early and often, and in virtually everything you do. Charging too little (or giving away too much) means that the economic burden of providing breastfeeding care falls onto your paying customers (or your family). We know that sufficient time is needed to uncover all factors contributing to a breastfeeding problem, yet a day contains only so many hours. Determining the amount of your time needed for an initial consult is a business decision as well as a clinical decision.

You can still donate some of your time, of course. You just need to be aware of the cost of doing so in the overall context of your business.

Today I spent about two hours on the phone and e-mail helping colleagues and mothers without receiving any payment. I don't mind sharing a copy of a good letter I've written or a link to a new research article, and I'm generous with my consulting services. However, I draw the line at doing someone else's research. It's a constant fight to keep "free work" to a minimum. I consider some of this donated time to be a contribution to my community or my professional responsibility to colleagues.

For clients, my stated limit is to provide no more than two free phone calls of 10 minutes or less, or two free short e-mails. If the problem isn't solved by then, I charge a fee or refer the mother to someone else who can help her within her financial constraints. I never give away equipment unless I'm field-testing a new product; even then, the client must agree to provide me with feedback on the product. In actuality, the mothers and colleagues who pay me for my services are subsidizing the "free" consults. Remember—the "free" services to individual clients require the same documentation as those for which you're paid.

Secrets and Intellectual Property

Diane DiSandro writes:

> Sometimes I think there are unrealistic expectations in our field regarding how a business is developed and run. Like most lactation consultants I know, I am committed to building our profession, and I donate many hours in person, on the phone, and via e-mail to helping others set up their practices. However, new people in the field sometimes expect more established colleagues to help to the detriment of their own businesses. I have worked very hard over the past 20 years to build my business to what it is today. While I am glad to share what I have learned, and glad to help others get started, I am *not* glad to give my own business away!
>
> I am always willing to steer others to where they can find the information they need. Giving a second opinion on a tricky clinical situation or even helping guide another lactation consultant who is setting up her computer is one thing. But I have actually had people ask me how to set up parts of their business, openly admitting that they hope to bid against me and turn some of my business their way! Then they nervously laugh and say that after all, I have a thriving business and why should I "hog" it all? I frequently hear how "lucky" I was/am, to be "in the right place at the right time," with total disregard for the long hours of work I have put, and continue to put, into building my business and my reputation.
>
> If a person has a unique idea to build into a niche in the community, that is the individual's intellectual property and no one has a right to expect the person to give it away! In the corporate world, this information is called "business confidential." And yet I have felt first-hand the scorn of colleagues who felt I was "holding back" information. Mind you, I am happy to encourage and point people to the things that have helped me get where I am. I am just not willing to actually develop a business plan for another LC, put in the time involved in setting up that person's practice, and give away every detail of what makes my practice unique.
>
> I have had several people over the years offer to become my partner. A full partner in my business. For free. Not an offer to buy into the business, just an offer to "help me out" by taking off some of the load. These people do not understand. They are insulted if I offer to hire them. They want a partnership. In my hard-earned business. For free. And again here I have experienced the backlash of negative feelings directed toward me for denying others a way into the business! They forget the offer to hire, and remember that I didn't want to give away a partnership.
>
> Once a person establishes a good reputation in her community, her practice has a value of its own that needs to be respected and protected. Protecting my own business is not stinginess! It is business. Discussing and guiding others is a nice thing for a successful LC to do—it is not her duty. And it is frustrating to be willing to be that guide, willing to help, and getting nasty comments for not giving away the farm!

Formula, bottles, teats (nipples), feeding devices, and breast pumps are, by definition, used only when the baby is not directly breastfeeding. Thus these products compete with direct breastfeeding. The ethical approach is to view these items as tools, with each having a limited and temporary therapeutic purpose, and to use the least amount of intervention for the shortest time to establish or restore direct breastfeeding.

A vigorous debate continues among LCs about using equipment to "assist" breastfeeding. Some advocate avoiding equipment at all costs; others are very quick to bring out the latest in technological solutions. Putting this idea in another context: Swimmers must compete without equipment, but they often use a variety of tools—fins, hand paddles, and pull buoys—to improve their technique during training. This use is good coaching—to pick the specific training aid to accomplish improved performance. To do so, the coach must thoroughly analyze the deficit in performance, select a device that will correct the error, and know exactly how long to use it and when to stop. Use of the wrong item or technique will not improve performance, and can even magnify the error. Good results begin with thorough knowledge of the optimal performance and a critical thinking process on the part of the coach.

Breastfeeding assistance equipment and products—yes, even bottles, teats, and formula—are all tools. They are designed for a specific purpose and work best when (1) they are safe and effective, and (2) their use remains limited to specific situations in which other approaches have been ineffective. There is no substitute for clinical judgment regarding when to use a gadget. Equipment can interfere with the mother–baby relationship, the baby's ability to obtain milk at breast, or the mother's supply if used incorrectly. Before you employ any gadget, obtain informed consent from the mother. Because the end goal is direct breastfeeding, gadgets should be used as a last resort and for the shortest possible duration to reach or return to that goal.

That principle doesn't mean that one should always "go without." Devices are not inherently evil. The problem lies in how they are used—too soon, too often, without a thorough analysis of the problem, without thinking of the consequences. Using the right device at the right time constitutes appropriate use of technology. Conversely, throwing a gadget at a problem because someone doesn't want to think through the issues or thinks that always using a gadget is fine is inappropriate. Always keep your eyes on the end goal—direct breastfeeding. Exclusive breastfeeding, like competitive swimming, by definition is "without equipment."

This point brings up the issue of profit. It takes time and money to purchase, lease, store, track, and handle equipment, so it is reasonable for an outlet to recover costs and make a profit. The manufacturers' recommended retail prices on most breastfeeding equipment include a decent profit margin. It is unethical to over-recommend such equipment, especially when you make money on its sale: This situation is a type of conflict of interest. One way to avoid this dilemma is to provide your clinical clients with a printed list of other rental or retail outlets in your community. My Statement of Professional Ethics appears on my price lists:

> I pledge my support of the World Health Organization's International Code of Marketing of Breastmilk Substitutes. I accept no money or gifts from sources whose goals are in conflict with direct breastfeeding. I have a financial interest in the products I carry and will be happy to supply a list of other sources for products. I rec-

GADGETS, VENDOR RELATIONSHIPS, AND THE INTERNATIONAL (WHO) CODE

ommend the use of breastfeeding equipment to solve problems only as a last resort and for the shortest time possible. My intent is always to protect and nurture the breastfeeding relationship, restore and enhance direct breastfeeding, and assist the mother in fulfilling her breastfeeding goals. I work as a member of the health care team.

THIRD-PARTY REIMBURSEMENT

At best, third-party reimbursement is a confusing mess. Some PPLCs hire a staff person to bill insurance companies; others insist on payment directly from the client and let the client fight it out with her insurance company. Reimbursement for breastfeeding care and services is often inconsistent even within a given company or for a given diagnosis. Some clients pursue the fight with their carrier (Diane Wiessinger observes that some companies reject the first three claim submissions, so be sure to try at least four times) and eventually get paid; others give up and resign themselves to paying out of pocket, as they would pay for baby furniture or children's shoes. Medela, Inc. has developed a helpful packet of information on reimbursement tailored to its products (see www.medela.com/NewFiles/reburstmt_pro.html).

In the United States, reimbursement for breastfeeding care and services ranks high on the list of priorities for national committees and organizations. (See the Foreword to this book.) When and how that recommendation will translate into individual PPLCs actually getting paid appropriately and consistently from third-party payers is anyone's guess. Insurance companies *should* pay for our services, of course—health costs for artificially fed babies and women who don't breastfeed are far higher, with precise data just starting to emerge. I truly believe that when insurance companies understand the real picture of infant feeding outcomes, they will quickly cover lactation care and services. Until then, keep trying to get reimbursed for your services, track what works for you and your clients, and encourage ILCA and IBLCE to pursue this issue at policy levels.

OTHER BUSINESS-KILLERS

- *Failure to establish "business hours" and dressing too casually.* It's tempting to wear old, comfortable jeans and sneakers when you're just doing paperwork in your home office, saving your "nice" outfits for when you expect clients or plan to leave the building. Don't! Establish some regular work hours, even if you don't pick a typical "9 to 5" schedule or your hours are very limited, and dress for work every time. If nothing else, dressing for work helps keep you focused on your practice. List your hours on your advertising materials, client handouts, and business cards. If a client returns a pump or stops by unannounced during nonwork hours, it's acceptable to be seen wearing old jeans and a sweatshirt if you really are cleaning the garage that day.

- *Letting your children, pets, family, or friends intrude on your business time or space, except in emergencies.* We're not talking about meeting the needs of little nursing babies here—that's a given. Don't let your children answer your business phone, take in pumps, or play with your clients' children. Clean your office and all business products thoroughly before work hours every day, especially if your dog sleeps under your feet while you're working at the computer in the evening, or if your cat thinks your display of slings is her private nest. Pet dander is a common allergen, which may present a serious problem for some clients. (*Note:* If you are allergic to animal dander or cigarette smoke, home visits may pose a health risk to *you.*) Even if your home office takes up a small corner of your living room, enforce the concept that when you're at work, you're at work—just as if you traveled elsewhere to work for someone else. That being said, however, it is completely appropriate to plan your work schedules around your family commitments, especially while your children are young.

- *Ignoring your marketing strategies and not tracking results.* Find out what brings you business, and do more of it. One company spent $6000 on a professionally designed, elegant brochure for a mailing, only to get a handful of responses. Word of mouth actually brought in more responses for the same event as the expensive mailing. Another company spent $4000 just for the *design* of a company brochure that was never even printed. Overspending on ineffective marketing strategies eventually forced this company out of business. A related issue is establishing reasonable pay rates, so that payroll does not consume all your income, leaving no cushion for administrative functions.

- *Failing to track equipment and/or failing to report accurately and promptly to vendors and taxing authorities.* You don't want a huge bill from a vendor for a leased pump that was lost 18 months ago, or a nasty letter from a government agency assessing back tax, penalties, and interest on income that you did not report appropriately.

- *Being unavailable, even for a short period of time.* This issue is a particularly difficult one for a solo practice. Diane DiSandro says

  There are times that we really need or want to pull back on our businesses and devote more time to our personal issues. At times like these, if I were someone's employee, I could cut my hours, take vacation time, or take a leave of absence, knowing that my job would be there when I returned to it. There would also be others who would keep the company running while I focused my attention elsewhere temporarily. In private practice, we must always keep aware of growing our business. To start turning away business means that the particular source of referrals may turn elsewhere. That's especially true in our work, where we do not get a lot of repeat business: A mother comes in, we help her, she moves on. We need sources of continuous referrals. Our referral sources do not keep track of the comings and goings of our lives. If it registers to them that we are not accepting new business, it can take a gargantuan effort to persuade them to reverse that thinking.

- *Thinking you can succeed in private practice on the basis of your clinical skills alone.* One more time: If you don't want to deal with the business aspects of a private practice, you should either volunteer your time as a mother-support group leader or peer counselor, or pursue employment at a hospital, clinic, or medical office. Successful PPLCs are entrepreneurs. That's why Part B on business skills precedes Part C on clinical aspects in this book.

- *Making jokes about what you do for a living.* We are *professional* lactation consultants, experts in helping breastfeeding mothers and babies. We work with mothers and babies in some of the most vulnerable moments of their lives. Uphold the dignity and grace of our profession in all you do and say!

CAN YOU REALLY MAKE A LIVING BY PROVIDING CLINICAL SERVICES ONLY?

The answer is a resounding *yes*! Many PPLCs make a decent living by providing clinical breastfeeding care. Some of their stories appear in this book. Many others happily thrive in their communities. An attitude of commitment, strong business skills, and superb clinical skills make the difference between operating a hobby practice or "lemonade stand" and running a financially viable, thriving, successful business providing lactation care and services. You can do it!

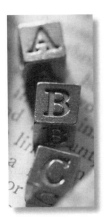

15 Realities of Private Practice

Roberta Graham de Escobedo, BA, IBCLC
Eve Moeran, RN, IBCLC

I practice in Merida, Yucatan, Mexico, a city of almost 1 million people. I am currently the only IBCLC within a 600-mile radius. Approximately 85 percent of my consults are house calls or hospital visits, although the corporate lactation segment of my practice is expanding rapidly.

ROBERTA GRAHAM DE ESCOBEDO, BA, IBCLC

If our goal as lactation consultants is to do everything in our power to assist mothers during breastfeeding, then surely you have felt some degree of frustration when you see mothers cutting short their breastfeeding experience to return to the workplace. When asked for reasons why they have chosen to formula-feed their children during the work day, most mothers will respond that the situation in the workplace is not conducive to either bringing her child in for breastfeeding breaks or for pumping and storing her milk. Forced between choosing to breastfeed at home or returning to work, many women sadly feel compelled to choose money over milk due to their economic reality. Should mothers be forced to make this heartrending choice? Of course not.

Recommendations encouraging exclusive breastfeeding for the first six months of life have been issued by the World Health Organization (WHO), the American Academy of Pediatrics (AAP), and other institutions around the world. Unfortunately, our shared reality of short or nonexistent maternity leave, paid or otherwise, does not contribute to attaining the goal of six months exclusive breastfeeding, not to mention the ideal of 12 to 24 months of sustained breastfeeding once complementary foods are added to the infant's diet.

As lactation consultants, we need to sit down and do an inventory of the resources available to us as we encourage working mothers to successfully combine breastfeeding with a work schedule. Your country, community, and practice setting surely presents unique challenges with which only you are familiar. By sharing what each of us has found useful in assisting our mothers to enjoy the breastfeeding experience, we all benefit. In this spirit, I offer a few concrete examples of how a lactation consultant might better help her working mothers.

WORKSITE LACTATION PROGRAMS: SUPPORTING BREASTFEEDING IN THE WORKPLACE

In Mexico, we are fortunate to have a national labor law that provides for three months of paid maternity leave—six weeks prenatal and six weeks postpartum. This law is patterned after the International Labor Organization's (ILO) Conventions for maternity protection in the workplace.

LABOR LAW AND LIFE'S REALITY

Mexico's national labor law states: "During breastfeeding you have the right to two half-hour breaks to breastfeed your child in an adequate and hygienic place designated by the company." On the upside, these two 30-minute periods are paid breaks, and the law does not specify for how many months these breaks may be taken, implying that an employee can take them for as long as necessary. On the downside, the majority of working women remain unaware that they have a right to breastfeeding time, as provided by law, and most employers do not fulfill their part of the bargain. Therefore, my first task has been to inform working women of their legal rights and prerogatives as breastfeeding mothers. The local press has proven exceedingly cooperative in this regard, publishing many articles on the topic of women, work, and breastfeeding over the past three years. In addition, several local radio stations have given airtime to promoting the concept of corporate lactation. Step by step, the public is becoming aware of the importance of supporting women in their dual role as mothers and as members of the work force.

As a private practice lactation consultant, over the past 15 years I have observed a steady increase in the number of mothers participating in the work force. According to national statistics, more than 50 percent of Mexican women are employed. I asked myself, Where should I begin? How can I best invest my time and energy to have the greatest effects? If what I hope to promote in the area of work-site breastfeeding support is to have a snowball or domino effect, which work setting will make the greatest impression on my community? As you analyze your community and explore the possibilities around you, you will discover which door is best to knock on first. In my case, the factory setting served as my starting point.

BREASTFEEDING SUPPORT AND SUPPORT BRAS

Don't you find it fitting that the first company to initiate a formal corporate lactation program in my area was an assembly plant that manufactures bras? I did. The firm began its lactation program in February 1999. In the first two years, more than 100 women participated. The program includes a prenatal group consult, in which employees are informed of the benefits of breastfeeding for both mother and baby, shown how to prepare for a return to work, and provided additional information about the breast pump they will use. The employees are given, free of charge, a double-pumping kit, and two electric breast pumps are available in the lactation room in the factory. Currently, approximately 18 women pump twice daily in this factory, which employs approximately 1000 employees, 70 percent of whom are young women of childbearing age. According to the factory nurse, who helps to coordinate the lactation program, so many mothers have participated at this point that the peer pressure has had a positive effect on returning mothers. All mothers automatically enter the program upon return from maternity leave, because their colleagues encourage them to participate.

To date, seven factories have added lactation programs to their employee benefits. As this number increases, so does the pressure on other companies to do the same. Thus knocking on the door of the factory segment of the labor market produced a noticeable effect in my area of practice. The best is yet to come.

I am always on the lookout for that door begging to be opened, and soon the next key opportunity presented itself. What better target than the newspaper with the largest circulation in southeast Mexico? When the director of human resources at this prestigious newspaper returned to work after having her first baby, I knew my next goal had been chosen for me. Working closely together, this young mother and I created a program tailored to the specific needs of the company. An electric pump, a double-pumping kit, and a prenatal orientation meeting with employees who were due to go on maternity leave constituted the key elements, complemented by a lovely lactation room for the use of the participants. The addition of this newspaper to the list of "mother-friendly businesses" was a key element in my next step toward making positive inroads in the community for working mothers.

PRINT AND PUMPS

O pportunities to promote breastfeeding lurk at every turn. We must simply remain alert and move quickly to seize the moment. When my city held elections for mayor last summer, I knew another door had been flung open. Upon returning from the annual conference of the International Lactation Consultant Association (ILCA), I was able to make a formal 45-minute presentation on corporate lactation to our new mayor, key officials in charge of women's affairs, and several city council members. Upon learning that not only seven factories but also the local newspaper had implemented similar programs, the mayor indicated that the government would seriously study the proposal and that approval was highly likely. She was good on her word; breastfeeding support for women working for the city government has become a reality, with lactation rooms being established in multiple locations because the government's offices are scattered across the city.

GOVERNMENTAL AND EDUCATIONAL INSTITUTIONS

Finally, consider one last example of how a community becomes mother-friendly on yet another level. In my practice, I frequently counsel mothers who find that a return to the university setting poses challenges slightly different than those faced by the working mother. Class schedules are not as flexible as work hours, and a paid maternity leave does not exist when you are in the middle of a semester or, worse, near a crucial exam period. The need for a quiet place for staff and students to pump and store milk became more than evident to me, so the next door presented itself. Was there a name on that door? Most definitely.

The administrative director of a private university was renting an electric breast pump from me. The pump enabled her to manage her duties at the university without having to abandon breastfeeding. This woman was instrumental in setting up a formal meeting with the university's dean, to whom I made proposal for a two-pronged program: pumping equipment and prenatal consults offered to the administrative and teaching staff, paid for by the university, and access to a lactation room offered to the students, who would be responsible for purchasing their own equipment.

The dean responded in an unexpected way that demonstrated a most enlightened and humane perspective. He said that the university existed solely because of and for the students; because the university considered the family to be of enormous importance, according to the dean, it did not seem logical or fair to pay for pump equipment *only* for the staff. The university would offer this support for both staff and students alike! This amazing response left me thrilled and speechless. Two other large universities are now on my list of prospective institutions where lactation programs would benefit more babies of staff or student mothers. Once more, the domino effect will come into play, as one university sets up a program, the others will certainly have to follow suit.

WORKSITE BREASTFEEDING SUPPORT ALSO SUPPORTS YOUR PRACTICE

As you explore opportunities in your community where your expertise can most definitely improve conditions for working mothers, keep in mind that LCs are above all promoting breastfeeding, not pumping equipment. When making a formal presentation to the director or general manager of a company, I offer several options from which he or she may choose, stating clearly that, as a lactation consultant, my goal is to assure exclusive breastfeeding for as long as possible:

- Option 1 is to simply create an adequate place for the mother to pump and store her milk, and to allow for the two 30-minute breaks as the labor law requires.
- Option 2 includes a manual pump for each employee.
- Option 3 includes a double-pumping kit with an electric pump.

All of these options include prenatal counseling for the employees prior to their maternity leave. In Mexico, because not all people may have telephones (especially women working in the factory setting, who often come from outlying small towns), follow-up phone consults may not always be possible. As mentioned earlier, you need to tailor your program to your own setting and the needs of your community.

When approaching businesses and other institutions, remember to be direct, concise, and clear when making a proposal. Time is at a premium when you have been given 30 minutes with a company executive. Learn to present the benefits of a breastfeeding program with clarity and in terms that are understood in the business world: reduced employee absenteeism, lower employee turnover, increased loyalty toward the company, and positive corporate image. Increased productivity and return on investment are key concepts to stress. Save the warm and fuzzy qualities for your mothers when helping with that first latch.

As more breastfeeding programs are established, I remain constantly amazed at how worksite breastfeeding support programs adapt themselves to the setting they are designed to serve. Thus far the factory, newspaper, city government, and university settings are all doing well.

I wonder which doors will open next?

EVE MOERAN, RN, IBCLC

I am in my sixties, and lactation consultation is my second business in this lifetime. The first was a large service company, which enjoyed great success. That business gave me the experience and background in generating mistakes needed to run a small company. My first business was a carpet cleaning business, which also dealt with flooded carpets, provided carpet repairs, sold new carpeting, and did fire damage restoration. At night, I taught childbirth classes because one of my basic trades was as a midwife. After 18 years, I returned to the health care field as an LC.

K now what you intend to do with the business before jumping in. Will you sell your business or let it run down? Exactly what do you propose to do?

I reached my initial goal within three months. I intended to pay the commercial rent, health insurance, mortgage, and all other sundry bills while keeping the place stocked.

You'll need to lay out these costs and determine what needs to be done to get you there.

- Rent so many pumps.
- See so many mothers for a consult.
- Teach so many classes.

I always reached my goals, but not always from the source I expected. My current goal is to continue to build my business and then to sell it.

Hint: Answer the telephone. Keep thanking the client for her business.

GOALS

I was a registered nurse from New Zealand who became a head nurse in orthopedics. I then went to Australia, where I trained as a midwife at the Royal Women's Hospital in Melbourne. My closest friend and I then went into what was termed the Australian Outback, working in a tiny local hospital doing our own deliveries. If we needed a surgeon for a cesarean, a doctor was flown in for the operation. This experience occurred so long ago that the instruments came wrapped in cloth and I would not have suprised if Florence Nightingale was watching from around a corner.

My major background toward becoming an LC involved 30 years of teaching childbirth classes at a major hospital in the United States. During the last 10 years of my career at the hospital, I established a breast pump rental program and worked on the floor as a lactation consultant.

I enjoyed working with mothers and their babies so much that I decided to specialize in lactation. I found a great introduction to the subject with Chele Marmet in Los Angeles at The Lactation Institute. At that point, I decided to spread my wings and took an IBCLC preparation class with Linda Smith. I was the only person who did not take the board examination after that class. I followed this course with the Lactation Consultant Program at the University of California at San Diego. The 160 clinical hours were very helpful as I observed great lactation consultants sharing their expertise on a daily basis.

After I passed the IBCLC exam, my certification gave me the confidence to strike out on my own. However, it was Linda Smith who said, "With all those years and experience working with new mothers and babies, you could go out on your own." I was grateful for the confidence she showed in my skills. Needless to say, I was very proud for her to see my store a year or so later, especially given that it stocked many of her educational tools for teaching new mothers.

Hint: Answer the telephone. Keep thanking the client for her business.

EXPERIENCE COUNTS

I started my business with a loan of $25,000. Doing this again, I would recommend starting off with greater funding, $50,000, to provide more flexibility. I calculated how much product I would need initially and what I

FINANCES

wanted to keep as my base amount in my loan account. I continued to order more product as necessary, which allowed me to maintain my loan account at a decent level.

PRODUCT

I am a Medela rental and retail outlet. I find the company's pumps and products to be the best and easiest to replace if a problem arises, which is very rare. Most products in my store come from Medela, but not all. I carry a local brand of baby slings, Mother Love products out of Colorado, and "My Brest Friend" breastfeeding cushions.

I started with three rental breast pumps, and increased that number to 50 in 24 months. I also teach childbirth classes and do some doula work. I have created a small, very specialized business without a broad base of products and clothing, which has worked out very well for me.

PRICE

Every product I sell carries a price label. The label shows the price, tax, and total charge. This method has allowed me to complete each sale quickly and efficiently, as all the work has been done previously. It also enables the client to be on her way quickly, instead of waiting for me to determine the total.

The price on lactation consulting must match what the market will bear. I can discuss many aspects of this issue until the cows come home, but if the client will not pay the price, all discussion is wasted. The client must experience value, perceive value, and be given value for services rendered. I settled on a price for 1 1/2 hours of service that might be considered low, but I make up the difference on product and repeat business. Another aspect of providing a lower price is that it enables me to answer the phone or treat another client at the same time. When I take two clients at the same time, it is obvious that my hourly rate increases, even as I provide excellent service to the clients.

LOCATION

Fortunately for me, "location, location, location" won in the decision of choosing a commercial space. I was able to find an office next to three obstetricians. Originally I was tempted to rent a small commercial space in a tiny shopping mall. Had I done so, I likely would not have prospered. My success has come from being next to these doctors. Approximately 10 obstetricians and 10 pediatricians practice within a one-mile radius from my store. The location is further enhanced by being within 5 miles of three major hospitals and within 15 miles of two others. The referrals are made by hospitals that strain to offload work for their lactation staff and by doctors who are grateful for the safe expertise in the neighborhood. When the doctors remember, they will refer their clients to me. You cannot always bank on such referrals, however, as they are often busy weighing subjects other than your business and its success. Having your door open into an attractive business setting helps draw the mothers in.

QUALITY

Set a high standard for the appearance of you and your business. Keep everything beautifully arranged, very clean, and brightly polished. Would this setting draw you in? Your personal appearance is also very important, white coat or not. Choose the appearance that you want to give to the world.

Hint: Keep answering the telephone. Keep thanking the client for her business.

I use a purchased report generation software program that standardizes the end results and looks very official when completed. Because of the medical codes and the documentation that I give to mothers, it helps them prove to their insurance companies that breastfeeding reduces the cost of health care. Most of my mothers are reimbursed by their insurers.

Answer the phone! Answer every call. I built my business on a cellphone and did not put in a land line for more than 12 months. I have never turned off my cellphone unless I was required to.

Cards

I print my own business cards. My card shows a photograph of a baby on the scale, which was scanned in for use.

Fliers

I have found photographs available to use for my fliers, which I also print myself.

Three-Folds

I have yet to design a three-fold brochure.

I send out 10 marketing pieces with every lactation report, including my business cards, a list of services rendered with prices listed, and some laminated marketing materials that can be posted in a doctor's office. I also deliver marketing pieces every month to hospitals that do not have breast pump rental programs.

When do mothers buy a breast pump? Many people would say after delivery, but I have wondered about the validity of that assumption. I decided to conduct my own survey as the months went on by asking every mother with whom I came in contact when and where she bought her pump. Of 100 mothers, 30 percent bought pumps prior to their delivery.

Many mothers buy pumps from major department stores, often because friends and family members purchased gift certificates from these businesses. Several mothers bought pumps on eBay, which do not include a warranty.

You need to know the sources of your business. Most of my sales come from the following:

- Prior relationships from my childbirth preparation classes
- Referrals from clients and doctors
- Returns of rentals
- Medela's toll-free phone program

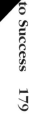

- Baby magazines
- Yellow Pages ads
- My Web page, www.breastpumpsandiego.com

Why does a client purchase from you? This question seems odd until you give it some thought. Many clients tell me that the answer is because I am so friendly. It is actually important to ask, "Why are you doing business in this store? What brought you here?"

UNIQUE SELLING PROPOSITION

I also believe in the concept of the unique selling proposition (USP). I learned about it from Jay Abraham's book, *Getting Everything You Can Out of All You've Got* (St. Martin's Press, 2000).

A USP states what you do and what is unique about your business:

- "Breast pump rentals 7 days a week."
- "One-year warranty on every pump sold, and a free rental if it breaks down, while it is being replaced."
- "Return your pump if you are unhappy. I will refund your money cheerfully within the first year."

I can hear your breath drawn in while you read the last statement. In two years, however, no one has asked for her money back. The question is, Can you afford a dissatisfied client? Medela does not want an unhappy client so it pays the airfreight for replacement pumps.

You need to explore and attractively format the reasons why you are the superior choice. What makes your service and your company better than the competition? Why did the client come to you? After all, a client can purchase a breast pump at numerous other places.

My USP follows a suggestion from Jay Abraham, "Take away the risk clients face by doing business with you. Make it easier to say yes than it is to say no." If you remove the emotional, psychological, or financial risk factors that are attached to the breast pump purchase, you make it easy for a client to stay with you.

YOU CAN NEVER THANK THE CLIENT ENOUGH

I send a "thank you" card to each client with the paid invoice, which I personally sign and write "thank you" on. The card reminds the client of the year's warranty and the free rental if the pump breaks while Medela ships a new pump.

Additionally, I send a birthday card one year later to each client, congratulating the baby by name for organizing his or her parents for one year. These cards are printed and filed at the time of the original transaction. I do receive calls thanking me for the birthday card, and it generates more business.

I call and follow up on all breast pump rentals and sales to confirm that the client is satisfied and happy. This follow-up gives me the opportunity to verbally thank the customer once more.

You need happy, excited clients who enjoy doing business with you, clients who will tell their friends. Thank them for coming to your business, considering the distance they had to drive and the time it took. Remember—they can go shopping in many other places, and you want them to remember your store as the best experience they ever had.

Of course, by now you will have guessed that I always thank the client for her call and her business. Customers are your business, and without them you won't be in business long.

I also thank Medela for being there and turning out a high-quality product. If the company did not, I would not have my successful business today.

Hint: Keep answering the telephone. Keep thanking the client for her business.

BOOKKEEPING

If you choose to use a computer bookkeeping system, I would recommend taking a course to fully understand such a program. You will want to meet with your accountant to set up the program correctly so that the end-of-year tasks become easier. Of course, you can hire experts to assist you if your budget goes that far. Once the system is set up, your life will be uncomplicated as you generate purchase orders, receive supplies, do your state board of equalization (sales) taxes, and generate all kinds of reports. Of course, it will take a long time and patience to enter all the activities that go along with running your business.

A credit card machine is essential—two-thirds of my payments are processed that way. We certainly did not anticipate how important this factor really was to our overall success.

COMMENTS

Eve Moeran's case study provides a small commentary on one woman's perception of her own company. The ability to have a stream of customers and to keep a stream continuing is certainly a talent. The author would be delighted to consult with you and can be reached at (619) 325-1630 or e-mailed at milkmade@home.com.

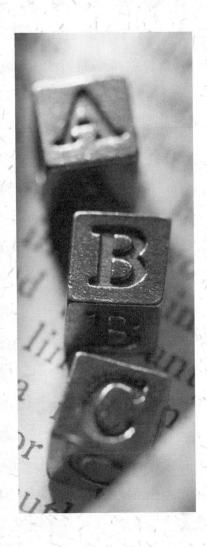

PART C

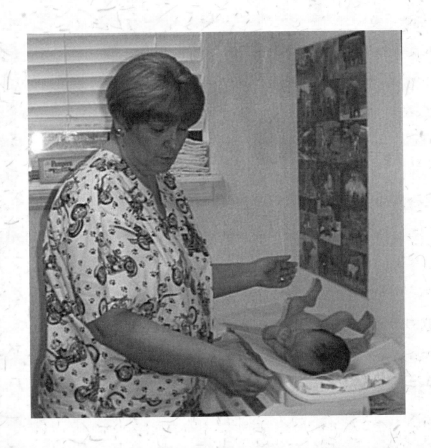

Managing the Clinical Aspects of Private Practice

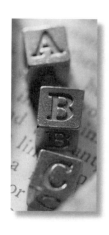

16 Overview of Clinical Practice

Linda J. Smith, BSE, FACCE, IBCLC

D o you have what it takes to be a successful private practice lactation consultant (PPLC)? In Part C, covering clinical practice, we explore how to actually do the work of the PPLC—the clinical care we provide.

Success in clinical practice means that you and your clients are confident in your clinical skills, you find solutions to the majority of the breastfeeding problems encountered, you incorporate evidence-based practices in your work, you enjoy providing breastfeeding care to a wide variety of clients, and both clients and health care professionals are satisfied with the results of interacting with you and refer others to your practice.

Part C addresses management of the clinical aspects of a private lactation practice. First, the ABC Protocol in Chapter 17 provides a sequential philosophical and practical framework for quickly getting to the root cause of a breastfeeding problem. Chapter 18 walks you through a typical interaction with a mother, from first contact to closure. Chapter 19 provides suggestions for setting up and running breastfeeding classes. Chapter 20, on pitfalls related to clinical practice, reminds you of our limits and some behaviors to avoid. Chapters 21 and 22, on professional responsibilities and other aspects of PPLC work, explore your practice in the broader context. Finally, Chapter 23 provides two more examples of successful practices.

A caveat needs to be added here. This book will not tell you how to handle specific clinical situations. Here are some reasons why:

1. Each mother and baby is a unique dyad. Therefore . . .

2. Each clinical problem might call for a slightly different approach.

3. We are consultants, remember? The mother ultimately decides what she is willing to do for a particular problem. (Rules 2, 3, 4, and 5)

4. One-size-fits-all, "cookbook" approaches to solving breastfeeding problems are rarely appropriate. This principle is especially true for the complicated situations that often end up in our private practices.

5. New research emerges constantly, steadily adding to our base of knowledge. Sometimes new research confirms our common understandings. Sometimes it may completely change our approach to a clinical situation.

6. Many excellent sources of clinical management exist that you should already own and have digested before you reach this point. Many of the best reference books are listed in the appendices to this text.

7. Even highly skilled and knowledgeable people disagree on some management strategies. I'm not about to add fuel to that fire!

✔ I have the skills, knowledge, and abilities to help mothers and babies with a wide variety of breastfeeding questions and problems.

✔ I always keep Rule 1, "Feed the Baby," as a guiding principle and highest priority.

✔ I practice in full accordance with ILCA's *Standards of Practice* and IBLCE's *Code of Ethics*. I have a system in place for obtaining and acting on feedback about my practice from clients, colleagues, and other professionals in my community.

✔ I use evidence-based practices where they exist, and theory-driven strategies where research is lacking.

✔ I obtain informed consent from the mother before I begin working with her, and I clearly identify closure when the client interaction is finished. I carefully, thoroughly, and accurately document all interactions with clients and retain clinical records for the legally required length of time.

✔ I maintain a clean, inviting area where I interact with clients, and I send reports to my clients' physicians promptly after the consult.

✔ I use the least amount of intervention for the shortest time to establish or restore direct breastfeeding. All equipment and products that I sell or rent are safe, effective, and reliable, and are covered by product liability insurance.

✔ I purchase sufficient books, periodicals, and literature to meet the needs of my clients and to remain up-to-date on clinical and business issues.

✔ I keep my knowledge and clinical skills updated by maintaining membership in ILCA, regularly attending conferences, seminars, and courses, and participating in other relevant educational programs.

8. Solving difficult breastfeeding problems is part science and part art. You're not going to learn the art from a book—that's why you need many hours of experience and preferably supervised clinical instruction from a skilled mentor or preceptor.

9. Many—perhaps most—clinical situations call for collaboration and cooperation with other care providers, especially the mother's primary care provider. I do not want to convey the idea that only the LC has all the answers. That's Rule 4 again.

Your desire to provide direct one-to-one clinical support of individual mothers is probably the reason you wanted to go into private practice in the first place. Part C provides a structure, an overview, and specific suggestions to launch your practice.

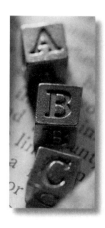

17

A Clinical Framework: The ABC Protocol[1]

Linda J. Smith, BSE, FACCE, IBCLC

As a PPLC, how do you know where to start? How do you know which mothers or babies are in immediate danger and must be referred to their doctors or an emergency room? What problems can be handled adequately over the phone? How do you get to the bottom of a breastfeeding problem quickly, using the least of your resources, while placing the least stress on the mother and baby? I've thought long and hard about these questions and developed the following schema, the ABC Protocol, which is modeled on American Heart Association's *Basic Life Support* (Cardiopulmonary Resuscitation) protocol. The steps are sequential and increase in complexity. This protocol works both as a prevention model and as a plan or template to use for solving problems by increasingly skilled providers.

In private practice, we often see the "train wrecks"—mothers and babies who have fallen through the cracks of other support systems. Often several other people have tried unsuccessfully to get breastfeeding working smoothly. Mothers come to us (enter our "system") at the last step, already in crisis mode. Our immediate concern is to keep the baby fed while we identify the underlying causes of the problem and help the mother implement strategies that will get the baby to (or back to) the breast.

Although this schema does not address every breastfeeding problem, it is a starting point for the vast majority of problems I've seen in 30-plus years of LC work.

INTRODUCTION

Most early breastfeeding problems occur because of poor milk transfer from the mother to the baby. They present as breast and nipple problems (damaged nipples, engorgement, mastitis) and/or infant hunger issues (jaundice, poor weight gain, crying, lack of stooling).

The cause of inadequate milk intake is almost always either (1) a behavior issue—the baby is not at breast ("the baby isn't in the restaurant"), or (2) a mechanical issue—the baby is at breast but not feeding ("the baby is in the restaurant but not eating"). It is tempting to think all breastfeeding problems have a behavioral origin, because much has been written on cultural and psychological aspects of breastfeeding.[2] Nevertheless, physical and mechanical problems also occur even when psychosocial factors are optimal. This problem-solving strategy addresses quantity (behavioral) issues first, and then carefully investigates quality (mechanical) issues.

Nearly all breastfeeding problems are best solved face-to-face. Early feeding problems carry significant risks: The baby is at risk of dehydration and caloric deprivation, the mother is at risk of engorgement and mastitis, and the dyad is at risk of early cessation of breastfeeding.

Any and all rules for infant feeding that restrict the baby's access to the breast interfere with adequate caloric intake. These include, but are not limited to, scheduled feedings, pacifier use (zero calories!), use of artificial nipples and manufactured milks, and social issues. These issues relate to *quantity* of time at breast. Behavior issues can be discussed via the telephone.

Of course, you cannot see a sick baby over the phone! If the problem is not completely resolved in one to three days, a health care provider competent in breastfeeding management should see the baby in person. One sensible approach is to limit telephone help to one or two 10-minute phone calls. If more help is needed or the problem does not resolve completely, a home or office visit should be scheduled.

Early nipple pain and breast refusal are mechanical issues that *must* be visually assessed. A common myth states, "If the baby is at breast, she must be eating." This is not true! A baby can be happily at breast, but not actually taking milk. This issue relates to *quality* of time at breast. Mechanical issues mandate a direct observation of feeding with careful evaluation of the milk transfer process.

Rule 1 is always "*feed the baby*." Next, try the easy solutions that do not involve equipment. If they don't work, then use your best critical thinking to determine which equipment or technique is best suited to resolve the problem at hand. Stop when the mother and baby decide that successful breastfeeding has been achieved. The goal is staying at or returning to Step 1, effective feeding directly at breast.

STEP 1. FEED THE BABY AT THE BREAST
Time frame: 1–3 days

The goal here is to rule out behavioral issues and minor mechanical issues. The first step is working with the mother and baby together.

First, assure enough time at breast. If the baby isn't near the food, she can't eat! To obtain enough calories, the baby should be at breast at least 140 minutes per 24 hours, or an average of about 11 minutes per hour.[3] Most babies cluster feedings into 20- to 30-minute sessions, using one or both breasts, at least every 1½ to 3 hours. After six weeks, babies may have one 4- to 6-hour sleep stretch per 24-hour day. Other acceptable patterns may also develop.

Signs of Trouble
Red flags[4] include the following:

- Consistently fewer than 8 feedings per 24 hours
- Feedings are consistently less than 5–10 minutes per breast
- Mother removes baby from breast at a predetermined time
- *Any* pacifier use[5]
- Mother worries that baby "isn't getting enough"

What to Do
Get the baby to the breast!

FIGURE 17.1 ABC Protocol ▶

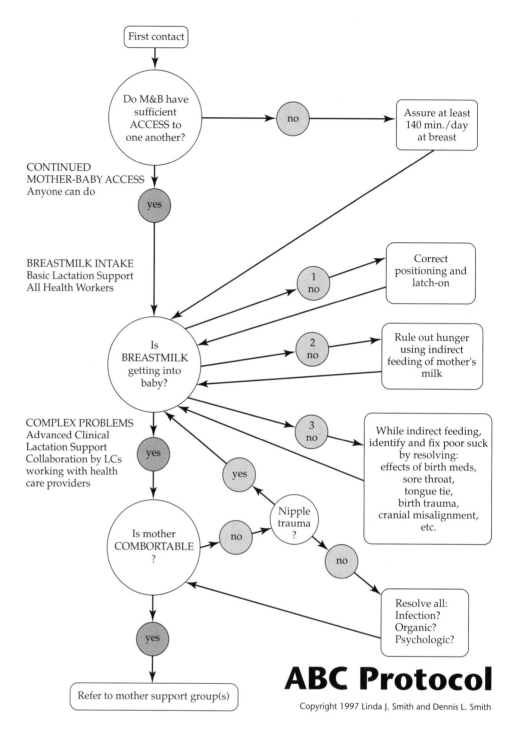

ABC Protocol

Copyright 1997 Linda J. Smith and Dennis L. Smith

- Keep the mother and baby in constant skin-to-skin contact for 24–48 hours.
- Maximize the amount of time during which the baby is at breast, keeping it as continuous as possible.
- Stop *all* pacifier and bottle (artificial nipple) use.[6]

Warning! If the mother refuses to bring the baby to breast frequently *for any reason*, the baby is at immediate risk of inadequate caloric intake. Follow Rule 1, *feed the baby*, with any reasonable source of nutrition—by any method—while addressing this issue! Breastfeeding is impossible without frequent breast contact. That's why it's called *breast*feeding. Stop here and explore why the mother is unwilling or unable to bring the baby to breast frequently. If this issue cannot be resolved and the mother continues to limit the baby's access to her breast, a reevaluation of her expectations and the therapeutic goals is necessary.

Second, assure good milk transfer: The baby can be near food, but not actually eating. Audible swallowing should be heard for most of the feed (10-plus minutes per breast) at a rate of about one swallow per second, with pauses between bursts of swallows. *Look* at the temporal-mandibular joint (in front of the ear) for movement, *listen* for gulping, and *feel* for movements of the lower jaw and swallowing.

Signs of Trouble

Red flags include the following:

- Consistently fewer than 8 or more than 16 feedings per 24 hours
- Feedings that are consistently shorter than 5 minutes or longer than 30 minutes
- Rapid sucking with little or no swallowing that occurs most of the time
- Baby sucks three to four times, falls asleep, *stays there*, and repeats this pattern
- Mother's nipple is creased, cracked, flattened, or painful after feeding
- Breast fullness that does not change as a result of feeding

What to Do

Make sure milk is getting from the mother to the baby!

- Assure deep attachment (grasp) at the breast/nipple
- Assure good alignment of the baby's body
- Assure that baby is properly sucking and swallowing

When to Go to Step 2

- Corrected positioning *does not* result in gulping or swallowing
- Corrected positioning *does not* eliminate nipple compression or pain
- The baby pulls away from the breast, screams, or cannot stay at breast
- The baby does not come off the breast spontaneously in less than 20–30 minutes with obvious satiety

The goal in this step is to continue to feed the baby while correcting suck problems, nipple preference or confusion, or oral motor disorganization, often manifesting in reverse or uncoordinated tongue peristalsis. Since feeding at breast is not effective, working with the mother and baby separately is necessary. Poor sucking results in inadequate milk intake for the baby, and in milk retention, engorgement, and subsequently lowered milk supply in the mother. Hunger may cause a poor or disorganized sucking response, resulting in a self-fulfilling vicious circle. Step 2 breaks this cycle by assuring adequate calories for the baby while maintaining or increasing the mother's milk

STEP 2. FEED THE BABY, BUT NOT NECESSARILY AT THE BREAST

Time frame: 1–3 days

supply. The feeding method used in Step 2 should correct early interferences and/or avoid compromising future direct breastfeeding. A disorganized suck caused by hunger may resolve in two to five days if artificial nipples are completely avoided and the baby receives sufficient nourishment; feeding at the breast can then begin again.

First, *get milk.* To increase milk supply, *remove milk from the breast more frequently and thoroughly*. Use a hospital-grade electric breast pump,[7] preferably with a double collection kit. Hand-expression is an excellent method if the total collection time remains the same. Collect milk at least 140 minutes per 24 hours, just as the baby would have nursed: A typical pattern is about every two hours during waking hours and once or twice at night. Do not let milk stay in the breast more than four to five hours at any time. At each session, collect until the milk flow changes from spraying to dripping, or about 10–15 minutes per breast, then for 2 more minutes. Longer sessions do *not* result in more milk collected; more frequent removal sessions signal the body to maximize production. If milk begins dripping or leaking at any time, *collect immediately*.

Signs of Trouble

Red flags include the following:

- Supply does not increase after two to five days of determined pumping/expressing
- Nipple or breast pain occurs or continues
- The mother is taking hormonal contraceptives
- The mother has *ever* had surgery on her breasts

What Does Not Matter to Milk Supply

- Mother's fluid intake, food quality, or food quantity
- Telling the mother to "rest" and "relax"

Second, feed the baby with anything *other than* an artificial teat (nipple). The goal is to provide calories while permitting or encouraging anterior-to-posterior tongue peristalsis and discouraging tongue thrusting. Feed the baby with a small cup, dropper, spoon, or medicine spoon. "Fingerfeeding" with specialized feeding tubes taped to a finger may help a baby organize her suck. Use of a feeding tube device *at breast* is not included in Step 2 of the protocol.[8]

To calculate the baby's needs: Multiply the baby's weight in pounds by $2\frac{1}{2}$ to 3. An 8-pound baby needs about 20–24 ounces of milk per 24 hours, an average of about one ounce per hour. A week-old baby's stomach holds about two ounces—the size of a golf ball. If the amount collected is less than the baby needs, consult with the baby's care provider regarding obtaining pasteurized donor human milk from a milk bank or an artificial feeding product.

To cup feed, sit the baby upright. Touch the lower lip with the edge of the cup until the baby opens her mouth or licks the edge. The baby will begin to sip or lap the milk. Continue giving a little at a time until the baby is obviously satisfied and sufficient total calories are obtained.

Third, keep attempting to breastfeed baby for comfort. After giving one to two ounces by an alternate method, try breastfeeding. You could experiment with a thin silicone nipple shield. Assure meticulous latch-on and positioning. Breastfeeding should be comforting and is desirable even if few calories are obtained. *Also, keep track of intake by monitoring baby's stools and urine!*

When to Go to Step 3

- Breastfeeding causes nipple pain, compression, soreness, or damage
- The baby continues to be unable to latch on and feed from the breast
- The baby's suck does not improve after two to five days of increased calories
- The baby has a difficult time feeding from a cup, dropper, or tube/finger

---

STEP 3. FIND OUT WHY THE BABY CAN'T GET MILK AT THE BREAST

The goal is to identify and fix the *cause* of the underlying suck problem. *Continue to feed the baby* with mother's milk, using any feeding device that accomplishes effective, nonstressful feeding. Follow Rule 1, *feed the baby*. Consider the sufficient *volume* of milk first, then the *type* of milk, then the feeding *method*.[9] Help the mother maintain her milk supply in the most efficient manner. At this point, the baby's feeding problem has persisted despite previous strategies, therefore further investigation is needed to identify whether this baby has a disorganized or dysfunctional suck. Disorganized and dysfunctional suck problems are not corrected by using artificial nipples. An artificial nipple (teat) should be used only as a last resort for feeding. Many parents are at the "last resort" stage if Step 3 becomes necessary.

Step 3 includes a complete and careful medical evaluation. Breastfeeding does not cause sucking problems. However, sucking problems may jeopardize the baby's nutritional status. Inadequate nutrition exacerbates virtually all infant problems, including poor oral-motor response. Ineffective or inappropriate feeding practices may further compromise undernourished babies with feeding problems. In nearly all situations, human milk is best even if direct feeding at the breast is impossible or must be modified. Maintaining the mother's milk supply is usually the easiest part of managing Step 3 problems. The lactation consultant can continue to help the mother maintain a good milk supply and preserve and enhance whatever at-breast feeding is possible.

POSSIBLE CAUSES AND CONSEQUENCES OF POOR SUCKING PATTERNS

The reasons and remedies for suboptimal sucking responses in otherwise healthy babies[10] have not yet been thoroughly studied. The underlying causes of poor sucking patterns may have long-term consequences to the baby that are unrelated to feeding. The lactation consultant is expected to work closely with the primary care provider and other members of the health care team as appropriate. The following possibilities are areas to be explored *in cooperation and collaboration with the entire health care team*.

1. Effects of birth medication. Administration of narcotic analgesia, epidural anesthesia, and general anesthesia can affect the baby's sucking and alertness for several hours to several weeks after birth.

   To identify: History of birth medication.

   Remedy: Time. If the baby cannot suck well, use a good pump or hand-express milk to maintain the mother's supply. Feed that milk to the baby by an alternate, nonteat method until the effects of the medication wear off.

Noticeable improvement should occur within one week, even if total reso-lution takes longer. If no improvement appears in a few days, seek further evaluation. In my experience, these babies are very susceptible to nipple mispatterning or preference several weeks or longer.

Cost: Pump rental and patience.

2. Sore throat from suctioning or intubation. Vigorous suctioning or intuba-tion may cause swelling or result in soreness in the mouth and/or throat. Some babies will react by biting, clenching their gums, or tongue-thrusting to protect their airway.

   To identify: History of suctioning or intubation.

   Remedy: Time and gentle, respectful oral experiences. A suctioned baby may not want anything in his mouth for a while, not even a breast. Cup feeding seems to work well for many of my clients. The baby's strong urge to suck may overcome this aversion if nothing firmer or more threatening than a breast is offered. Do *not* use pacifiers, artificial nipples, or finger-feeding in this situation.

   Cost: Pump rental and patience.

3. Head insult or injury during birth. The use of forceps or vacuum extraction, prolonged pushing, excessive or persistent molding, or cephalohematoma may cause head pain and motor inhibition.

   To identify: History of events during delivery and immediate postpartum.

   Remedy: Time, gentle patience, and posture changes. Treat the baby as if he has a severe headache. Reduce sensory input by reducing noise and music, light, touch, and excessive motion. Try keeping the baby upright against a parent's bare chest, kangaroo-style, in a quiet, darkened place. These babies seem to feel and feed better when the "sore side" of the head is higher than the unaffected side. If the baby can nurse effectively in one position, use it frequently without trying for variety. Cool cloths on the baby's head may help. Cup feeding of pumped milk may be more comfortable for the baby than feeding directly at the breast.

   Cost: Pump rental and patience.

4. Oral structural problems, especially tongue-tie (ankyloglossia). A short or tight lingual or labial frenulum can inhibit or completely prevent anterior-to-posterior tongue peristalsis and proper lip position.

   To identify: Visual clues: heart-shaped or square-tipped tongue, tongue cannot extend past lower lip, lingual frenulum attaches less than one-half inch from tip of tongue. Functional clues: tongue peristalsis absent or re-verse, tip cannot rise at least to mid-mouth, mother's nipples are creased and cracked across tip or have unhealed wounds on tip, tight labial frenu-lum prevents upper lip from rolling upward, the baby cannot latch deeply and obtain milk at breast.[11]

   Remedy: Evaluation and possible treatment by qualified provider such as a dentist or physician. The dentist/physician will clip the frenulum (freno-tomy) with sterile scissors and immediately have the baby put to breast. Anesthesia and suturing are usually not required unless the frenulum is very tight; bleeding is very rare. A simple frenotomy procedure can be done hours after the baby's birth. The mother often notices immediate and com-plete pain relief and effective sucking.

Cost: Medical/dental outpatient surgical treatment, may be covered by insurance.[12]

5. Misalignment of cranial bones related to birth (including persistent molding) that has not spontaneously resolved. This may put pressure on sensory and motor nerves as they pass through the foramina in the infant's skull, which in turn can affect sucking, swallowing, and digestion. The vagus nerve can also be affected.

To identify: Gagging, persistent poor tongue peristalsis with posterior humping or bunching, weak suck, and/or tongue thrusting after nipple confusion is corrected; facial asymmetry; postural asymmetry; head molding persisting past one week; arching; plugged tear ducts; asymmetric head mobility; palpable ridges along cranial sutures.

Remedy: Evaluation and possible treatment by a doctor of osteopathy or other qualified provider trained in manipulative therapy on infants.[13] This therapeutic modality is subtle and gentle, and has produced remarkable results.

Cost: Osteopathic or other structural evaluation and treatment;[14] may be covered by insurance.

6. Other medical or health problems in the baby. These include cardiac abnormalities, neurological problems, severe allergies, fungal or other mouth infections, metabolic abnormalities, and so on. Some providers suggest that "feeding behavior is the first thing to go wrong" when a severe problem is developing in a baby. *Collaborate with the baby's primary care provider whenever Step 3 becomes necessary.*

These steps are sequential. The goal is to remain at or return to Step 1. Any policy and procedural barriers must also be addressed if they interfere with any of these steps.

SUMMARY: A QUICK CHECKLIST FOR SOLVING BREASTFEEDING PROBLEMS

Step 1. Feed the baby at the breast. Keep the mother and baby together.

   a. Assure sufficient time at breast (quantity issue).

   b. Assure effective feeding at breast (quality issue).

Step 2. Feed the baby with mother's milk indirectly. Keep the mother and baby together even if direct breastfeeding is not possible.

   a. Maintain or increase the mother's milk supply.

   b. Feed the baby in a way that safely encourages proper tongue movement.

   c. Continue attempts to breastfeed directly.

Step 3. Find out why the baby cannot obtain milk from the breast. Keep the mother and baby together even if direct breastfeeding is not established yet.

   a. Continue feeding the baby with mother's milk while causes and remedies are investigated.

   b. Support the mother's milk supply, her efforts, and her motivation.

   c. Collaborate with other providers!

NOTES

1. © Copyright Linda J. Smith, BSE, FACCE, IBCLC. Used with permission.

2. These quantity/quality problems seem to occur at a ratio of about 80:20, with 80 percent of them related to "not at breast" issues. If the baby is at breast enough, the rest of the problems are mostly mechanical issues, yet often prove more difficult to resolve. Research is especially lacking in this area.

3. Feeding sessions should be at least 134-138 minutes per 24 hours. The volume of milk obtained and the frequency of sessions vary inversely; more milk is obtained with more frequent sessions than with less frequent sessions. DeCarvalho, M., et al. Effect of frequent breastfeeding on early milk production and infant weight gain. *Pediatrics* 1983; 72(3).

4. Not all "red flags" indicate a problem. However, most problems have at least one "red flag." Investigate all "red flag" situations very carefully before deciding that no problem is present.

5. Pacifiers may be part of Step 3 of the protocol for specific therapeutic purposes as recommended by a qualified oral motor therapist. Pacifiers are by definition excluded from Step 1, direct breastfeeding. Sucking is designed to bring calories to the baby. During sucking, digestive enzymes and hormones are released in preparation for food intake. The consequence of gastrointestinal responses in the absence of expected calories is unknown but may be of concern. Providing any other sucking object moves the dyad to Step 2 of the protocol.

6. Bottles and artificial nipples/teats may be part of Step 3 of the protocol, feeding of human milk by any successful method. They are by definition excluded from Step 1, direct breastfeeding. By definition, breastfeeding happens when baby is *at the breast*. Providing milk to the baby in any way other than directly from the breast moves the dyad to Step 2 of the protocol.

7. Weak and/or inexpensive pumps may not remove sufficient milk to increase milk supply.

8. Feeding tube devices at breast may be part of Step 3 of the protocol, depending on the cause of the sucking problem and the therapist's recommendations. During Step 2, the goal is to remove milk from the breast and get it into the baby indirectly. Feeding tube devices do not remove milk from the breast. If a baby can't get milk out of a breast filled with milk, it is unlikely he can get it out of a tube placed at breast either. Other feeding devices may have lower risks than tubes. Research is lacking in this area, however.

9. Muscles, including those used in sucking and swallowing, need nutrients to contract sequentially and properly. Denying a baby food to "improve the suck" is unjustified. Babies must receive adequate and appropriate caloric support while oral motor problems are solved.

10. These principles were developed for otherwise normal, full-term babies. Different protocols may be developed for premature babies or babies with significant diseases and handicapping conditions.

11. Messner, A. H., Lalakea, L., Aby, J., et al. Anklyoglossia: Incidence and associated feeding difficulties. *Arch Otolaryngol Head Neck Surg* 2000;126:36-39; also, Mukai, S., Mukai, C., Asaoka, K., Anklyoglossia with deviation of the epiglottis and larynx. *Annals Oto Laryngol* 1991;100 (suppl 153):1-20.

12. Both medical and dental procedure codes may apply. Insurance reimbursement varies.

13. Dr. Judith O'Connell, DO, and others used this treatment effectively on more than 100 babies in Dayton, Ohio in the past decade. Most babies' problems resolved with two to four treatments over a four- to six-week period. Further research is planned.

14. Fravel, M. M. P. R. A pilot study: Osteopathic treatment of infants with a sucking dysfunction. *AAO Journal* 1998:25-33.

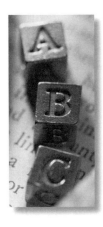

18 The Lactation Consult

Linda J. Smith, BSE, FACCE, IBCLC

Legal issues intertwine with clinical decisions and actions in nearly every interaction with clients. Before you read any further, stop and read (or reread) Chapter 31, "A Legal Primer for Lactation Consultants," in *Core Curriculum for Lactation Consultant Practice* and follow the author's recommendations in every aspect of clinical work.

This chapter covers some general concepts. First and foremost is *know what is normal*, and clearly point it out to the mother. An excellent and useful framework for identifying and describing the normal can be found in *Maternal and Infant Assessment for Breastfeeding and Human Lactation*.[1]

Other core concepts are as follows:

- Find the cause(s) of the problem(s) before suggesting any remedies.
- Behavioral problems need behavioral solutions.
- Mechanical problems need mechanical solutions.
- Infections need medical diagnosis and treatment.
- If it ain't broke, don't fix it.
- If something is working, do more of it or keep doing it.
- If something hurts or isn't working, stop doing it.
- Be as committed to breastfeeding as the mother is, and slightly more.

I'm serious about these principles! Too many novice lactation consultants jump right in trying to fix a problem when they haven't taken the time to thoroughly investigate the root cause(s), or they don't recognize normal. A primary feature of PPLC work is sufficient time to thoroughly analyze a breastfeeding dyad's situation.

Mothers usually come to us already in crisis with a specific complaint. Often the LC is not the first person who has attempted to help her, which may have made the situation worse. Once we start working with her, we frequently find more than one problem, or a cascading series of issues that will need to be addressed to help her achieve her goal.

Help the mother pick which problem is the highest priority for her, making sure the baby is fed and her milk supply is supported. Fix what you can at the time of the visit. Send her home with a few (2–3) things to work on over the next several days. Schedule a follow-up visit or phone call for about three days later. At the follow-up contact, figure out and reinforce what's working, stop whatever isn't working, and adjust the plan accordingly. Identify and set some long-term solutions into motion. Ideally, actions and conversations that take place during the first visit will resolve much of the presenting problem.

INTAKE AND RECORDKEEPING

The first contact with the mother starts the LC–client relationship.[2] This initial contact often occurs by phone.[3] In those few minutes, you must decide whether to work with the mother by phone, refer her immediately to a physician or emergency room, or see her in person. The minimum documentation includes the date of the call, the mother's name, the baby's name(s), her phone number, who referred her, her statement of the problem, what you told her, and any referral made.

A word about charting: *How* you document is important; *that* you document every clinical contact is absolutely mandatory. You can use the forms in this book or in *Breastfeeding and Human Lactation*; purchase forms from the Lactation Institute, Childbirth Graphics, or other sources; or design your own.

If you work with the mother by telephone, document your conversations. The longer I practice, the less I like telephone work because I can't see the mother or the baby. If I can't get to the bottom of a problem in one to two conversations of less than 10 minutes each, I stress the need for an in-person visit. If the mother won't come in for an office visit or schedule a home visit, I refer her back to her doctor or to another source of help and document the interaction.

THE INITIAL VISIT

This description covers a typical LC office visit. If you have office staff or are doing a home visit, there will be minor differences before you begin work with the client.

First, welcome the mother (and anyone else with her, including the baby) and thank her for coming to seek help. Discuss what the visit will be like:

> I'm going to ask you many questions. You may wonder why some of them are asked, but please humor me by answering all of them. I'd be glad to explain why I ask these. When your baby shows signs of needing to nurse, we'll stop whatever we're doing and feed the baby right then. Before I touch you or your baby, I'll wash my hands and put on gloves. If you think of something relevant, add it at any time. We'll weigh your baby too. Before we get started, I need to get your permission to work with you and your baby.

Subjective: What the Mother Tells You

After the mother signs the consent and release form, begin filling out the intake and history questionnaire. The lactation history should include, but not be limited to, the following items:

1. Name, address, number of children, previous breastfeeding experience, general health

   a. This pregnancy—facts, her feelings, events

   b. This baby's birth—facts, feelings, events

   c. Early (first 1–3 days) breastfeeding history with this baby

   d. What's going on now—facts, feelings, events

   e. The chief complaint—what she wants fixed

   f. Her goals for this interaction, this baby, and this breastfeeding experience ("If you could write the perfect script for your breastfeeding story, what would it look like?")

2. Risk factor screening

   a. Breast surgery, infections, trauma to the breasts or chest wall

   b. History of any abuse (physical, sexual, emotional), abortions, eating disorders, addictions, depression

   c. Chronic illnesses, accidents, hospitalizations

   d. Her entire birth story (This interview may be the first time she's been able to tell her birth story to anyone who will really listen and validate her. Physical and emotional events during labor and birth can have profound effects on both mother and baby.)

As you go through the history, try to maintain frequent eye contact with her while you write. If her emotions are strong, stop and validate her feelings immediately, and continue offering specific support until she's ready to move on. I use a lot of counseling skills while taking the birth and lactation history. Talk to the baby, too—she's a partner in this equation. Take your time. Taking a thorough history is 80 percent of the job. Keep going until the mother has told you everything. Taking a detailed history is one reason why an effective consult takes 90 minutes or so.

Objective: What You Discover with Your Examination/Observation

I always put on a clean "clinical" jacket before I touch the mother and baby. If you haven't already washed your hands and put on clean exam gloves,[4] do so now. Use safety precautions and document what you observe. Your physical examination should include the following:

1. The mother's breasts:

   a. Visual assessment: symmetry, color, shape, unusual features

   b. Physical assessment: weight (full breasts feel heavy); nipple/areola texture and elasticity; feel for lumps; express some milk

2. The baby:

   a. General behavior and demeanor, mood

   b. Weight (naked) on an accurate scale; sometimes pre-feed and post-feed (see Appendix C for sources of clinical scales)

   c. Oral exam (suck exam)

3. A complete feed. Watch at least one entire feeding episode, as long as it takes. Pay close attention. You're looking for the following:

   a. Baby's cues, especially rooting and a wide gap; mother's responses

   b. Positioning—how the mother holds the baby

   c. Depth and effectiveness of the baby's latch and seal; mother's sensation during latch

   d. Signs of milk transfer: suck rhythm, rate, swallows, duration, bursts and pauses

   e. How and when the feed ends; baby's state and mother's comfort level

   f. Nipple shape and condition immediately post-feed

4. Documentation of all of these issues, plus whatever else you observe or discover.

Analysis—Assessment: Baby, Mother, and Their Relationship

Clearly state all the problems and contributing factors, including the mother's chief complaint. Include what is going well: "Cracked nipple skin, probably due to baby's disorganized tongue motion with thrusting." "Suppressed milk supply because of unrelieved, prolonged milk stasis when baby sleeps through the night." "Severe edema of the breast, nipple, and areola with milk stasis."

Immediate Intervention: On-site Care

As you go along through the visit, be sure to reinforce what the mother or baby is doing well. Modify, fine-tune, or correct positioning and latch. If the baby can't or won't latch, make sure he is fed with expressed milk or the mother's preference for artificial baby milk during the course of the visit. Discuss options for indirect feeding with the mother. Don't just pick a device arbitrarily. Care for her breasts, including pumping her breasts with a sterile pump kit. Begin treating any breast edema with cold cloths or other evidence-based strategies. Begin any nipple wound healing with evidence-based strategies that are within your scope of practice.

Plan: What You Will Do About the Problems

List solutions for the chief complaint first, then all the actions needed to resolve the entire situation. With the mother's feedback, rank them in order of priority, with only about three high-priority changes. (Listing more than three "top" priorities may be overwhelming.) Include the following factors, at a minimum:

1. How to feed the baby, how often, and with what (be specific)
2. Breast care and supporting/increasing milk supply (be specific)
3. Mother–baby relationship: massage, kangaroo care, talking to the baby

Make sure that nothing you've suggested or recommended has any potential to make the problems worse. We need to be constantly on guard to prevent future short- and long-term breastfeeding problems!

Evaluation: When and How You Will Know the Problem Is Fixed

Schedule a specific day and time for the first follow-up, usually in two to three days. The more complicated the problem, the more in-person follow-up visits likely will be needed. Simple problems may need only a phone call for follow-up and closure. In any case, you need to follow the client until some kind of closure exists. You cannot ethically abandon a client.

THERAPEUTIC OPTIONS

Your guiding principles include "First, do no harm" and "Use the least amount of intervention for the shortest time to establish or restore direct breastfeeding." Within that framework, you will need to become intimately familiar with the operation and features of breast pumps, feeding devices, and other equipment. There is rarely *one* perfect device or technique for all mothers or babies—remember Rule 5. Finding the best solution for a particular mother–baby pair is the art of PPLC practice.

It's sometimes tricky to use a device for a specific therapeutic purpose, without having it spill over into social or casual use. Bottles and teats/nipples are the best example of this risk, but even pump use can become a barrier to direct breastfeeding. Choose your solutions carefully.

Counseling Skills

Throughout the consult, listen and respond to the mother *so that she feels heard and understood.* This point is vitally important! Listening to the mother, establishing rapport, helping her express her feelings, and giving emotional support explains why initial consults take at least an hour. Breastfeeding is incredibly, terribly, agonizingly, wonderfully important to women. When it works, breastfeeding is one of a woman's most joyous, profoundly satisfying, empowering experiences. Strong emotions are also associated with the dark side of breastfeeding, however. "Our culture does not recognize the profound loss women feel when they can't make breastfeeding work. It hits you in the gut," observes Valerie McClain, IBCLC. Anguish, fear, guilt, bitterness, disappointment, anger, despair, frustration, betrayal—all are powerful emotions that can easily surface when a mother experiences breastfeeding problems.

How we deal with these strong emotions may mean more to the mother in the long run than any technique we might suggest. Again, I strongly urge you to take La Leche League's Human Relations Enrichment course, read the chapter on counseling in the *Breastfeeding Answer Book* and/or *Counseling the Nursing Mother*, or take a similar counseling skills training program. Use these skills throughout every interaction with your clients. Appropriate breastfeeding care isn't about gadgets, tools or techniques. It's about whether and how the mother is supported and validated. This distinction marks one of the huge differences between supportive and nonsupportive breastfeeding care.

Equipment to Assist Breastfeeding

Equipment (devices) and techniques fall into four general categories: to collect milk, to feed the baby, to "fix" the breast or nipple, or to "fix" the baby. Often these tools are used in pairs: one strategy to collect milk, and a companion strategy to feed the baby. Carefully analyze the problems first, based on the baby's problem. Consider the mother's preferences, and discuss the pros and cons of each device or technique with her. Reevaluate the situation within about 48 hours and every few days until the baby is at breast or back to breast (or the mother has opted to pump over the long term).

Equipment to obtain milk includes the baby (always the first choice, and not really a piece of equipment!), hand-expression, and breast pumps. Pumps should be comfortable and effective. Know what equipment is available, and know exactly how each device works, and pros and cons of each.[5]

Needing equipment to feed the baby is by definition a problem, because the baby isn't at breast!

- Outside-the-mouth devices (cups, spoons, bowls) have a long history of use, are easy to clean, may be less threatening to aversive babies, are recommended worldwide, and may encourage front-to-back tongue peristalsis. On the other hand, there may be more spillage, more risk of aspiration or too-fast feeds, no sensory input to the infant's palate, a suck response may not be triggered, and they are not fully researched for safety and effectiveness.

- Inside-the-mouth devices (teats/nipples, nipple shields, tubes, syringes, finger feeding) also have a long history of use, may help organize the baby's CNS, provide sensory input to the palate and the inside of the mouth, and have less spillage. On the down side, they are more difficult to clean, more expensive, may have a higher risk of too-fast or too-slow feeds, may risk oral motor "confusion" or mispatterning, may threaten orally aversive babies, and are not fully researched for safety and effectiveness.

Devices to "fix" lactating breasts are also poorly researched. They include absorbent pads for leaking milk, thermal treatments, nipple shields and breast shells that allegedly prevent injury or alter the nipple shape to facilitate latching, and products that are supposed to prevent or treat injuries, wounds, or various types of pain. Keep up-to-date on research in this area, don't rely on anecdotal remedies, and adjust your practice as new research is published. For example, no clinical research supports the use of heat for "engorged" breasts, even though that suggestion has been made for many years.

Devices and techniques to "fix" a baby's ineffective suck are poorly researched in the lactation literature, yet many of your clients will experience such a problem. Remedies for suck problems can be complex and very sophisticated, requiring far more knowledge and clinical skill than basic positioning and latch techniques. Don't be tempted to try the "fix of the week" presented at a workshop! The goal of any intervention is to help organize the baby's suck-swallow-breathe responses and feed the baby while you investigate the causes and therapeutic options. Meeting this need may mean taking additional training and becoming certified in another field (in addition to your current credentials), and/or collaborating with and referring to others in your community. These "others" could include osteopathic physicians, chiropractors, massage therapists, speech therapists, oralmotor therapists, neurologists, psychologists, and more.

Document which interventions were suggested, and why, and thoroughly explain the rationale for techniques that are not considered "standard." Reread *A Legal Primer for Lactation Consultants*.

REPORTING TO THE PRIMARY CARE PROVIDER

"The job's not finished until the paperwork is done," says the cliché, and PPLC work is no exception. Writing up the consult and sending a report to the mother's primary care provider is almost the last step of the consult. As with the principle of documentation, *how* to report has options; *whether* to send a report does not. The appendices of this book provide some examples of physician reports.

Finally, you deposit the client's payment in your business account, making sure the bookkeeping is done, too. I never deposit the client's payment until the doctor letter has been sent. (Florence Rotundo suggested this practice at a workshop many years ago, and it's served me well ever since.)

The interaction with the client eventually ends, and you need to get closure. Reread *A Legal Primer for Lactation Consultants* on what constitutes closure. You can't abandon a client. This doesn't mean if she calls again, you can't work with her! Open a new file, and start back at the beginning, almost as if she were an entirely new client.

CLOSURE

Equipment

- Digital scale with carrying case, calibration weights, scale pads (see Appendix C for vendors)
- Footstools, pillows (shaped and standard, various sizes and firmness)
- Padded table or other safe surface for examining the baby

CONSULT SUPPLIES AND EQUIPMENT

Supplies (Purchased in Sterile Packaging)

- Breast pumps: manual, electric, sterile single and double kits; parts for kits; extension cords and adapters.
- Feeding devices: small feeding cups (rigid and flexible, SoftCup feeder), spoons, #5 French tubes with 50 cc syringes, Hazelbaker™ FingerFeeders, SNS and Starter SNS, plain syringes, orthodontic syringes, Haberman™ feeders (regular and mini), Volu-feeds and 4–5 oz. bottles. Optional: teats (nipples)—several designs and shapes.
- Nipple shields: silicone, several sizes and designs.
- Gloves, both latex and nonlatex (vinyl, nitrile), preferably nonpowdered.
- Lab coat, scrub jacket, or other clean cover-up, preferably with pockets.
- Tackle box or other container(s) for various parts and small items.

Optional Items

- Bra pads
- Plastic ruler to measure wounds, scars, and other features
- Slings and/or other soft tie-on baby carriers for sale or to loan
- Books and handouts for loaning/giving to clients

The lactation consult proceeds in an orderly manner from the mother's first contact with the PPLC to closure of the mother and baby's "case." Each consult includes a thorough lactation history, information that the mother tells you, your observations and discoveries during your examination of the mother and baby, an analysis of what's going on, some immediate steps to make things better for the mother and baby, a plan to determine whether the initial steps are helping, follow-up, documentation, and reporting. Use the least amount of equipment for the shortest time possible with the goal of establishing or restoring direct breastfeeding. The mother is in charge—she guides and determines what options she will try. Document all aspects of your encounter with the mother and baby, and stay in communication with the physician or primary care provider.

SUMMARY

NOTES

1 Cadwell, K., Turner-Maffei, C., O'Connor, B., and Blair, A. *Maternal and Infant Assessment for Breastfeeding and Human Lactation*. Sudbury, MA: Jones and Bartlett, 2002.

2 Bornmann, Priscilla G. A legal primer for lactation consultants. In *Core Curriculum for Lactation Consultant Practice*, edited by Marsha Walker, 2002.

3 Wheeler, Sheila. *Telephone Triage*. Albany, NY: Delmar, 1993.

4 Regarding wearing gloves: ILCA's *Standards of Practice* 1.3.2 states, "Exercise principles of safety and universal precautions." However, "contact with breast milk does not constitute occupational exposure as defined by OSHA standards" (AAP, 1995). Furthermore, "gloves are not recommended for the routine handling of expressed human milk; but should be worn by health care workers in situations where exposure to breast milk might be frequent or prolonged, for example, in milk banking" (WHO, CDC).

AAP. Human milk, breastfeeding, and transmission of human immunodeficiency virus in the United States (RE9542). *Pediatrics* 1995;96(5):977-979.

Centers for Disease Control and Prevention. Recommendations for assisting in the prevention of perinatal transmission of human T-lymphotropic virus type III/lymphadenopathy-associated virus and acquired immunodeficiency syndrome. *MMWR* 1985;34:721-732.

Lawrence, R. *A Review of the Medical Benefits and Contraindications to Breastfeeding in the United States* (Maternal and Child Health Technical Information Bulletin). Arlington, VA: National Center for Education in Maternal and Child Health, October 1997.

World Health Organization, UNICEF, and UNAIDS. *HIV and Infant Feeding: Infant Feeding Options*. Geneva: World Health Organization, 1998.

World Health Organization, UNICEF, and UNAIDS. *HIV and Infant Feeding: Guidelines for Decision-Makers*. Geneva: World Health Organization, 1998.

5 ILCA's *Evidence Based Guidelines for Breastfeeding Management During the First Fourteen Days* is an excellent source of information. Other resources appear in the appendices of this book.

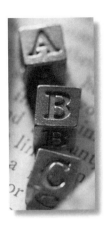

19 Breastfeeding Classes and Educational Services

Linda J. Smith, BSE, FACCE, IBCLC

As part of your practice, you may want to offer breastfeeding classes to parents or continuing education to professionals. Of the two types of education, parent education is usually quicker and easier to implement, provides a steadier stream of income, and exposes more potential clients to your practice.

LOGISTICS AND ADMINISTRATION

You'll need a room large enough to hold at least 10 people comfortably, allowing a minimum of 35 square feet of space per student. Have enough chairs and a few tables, and room for car seats and diaper bags. Set up the room to convey a warm (literally and figuratively), friendly atmosphere. Have some nutritious snacks and beverages, including water, available. Advertise a "babies welcome" message at every opportunity, because part of what you're doing is modeling a new paradigm. Don't just "allow" babies to come—make sure clients know that you specifically *want* them to bring their nursing babies.[1]

Combine teaching methods so that you use visual, auditory, and kinesthetic methods, active and passive strategies, and a variety of approaches. No one approach will work well for all audiences. Look for more teaching tips and specific activities in *Coach's Notebook: Games and Strategies for Lactation Education*. Keep each session short—no longer than two hours, and preferably a bit shorter. Start on time, and end a little early.

CONTENT OF BREASTFEEDING CLASSES/MEETINGS

There are three primary, "survival" messages for all basic breastfeeding classes for parents and professionals:

1. *Making enough great milk is easy.* Devote at least one-third to one-half of the class time to how milk is made, using new research and avoiding or explaining old myths. The most important process in ongoing milk synthesis is frequent and thorough milk removal. The mother's diet, her fluid intake, and her stress level play only negligible roles in determining milk quantity and quality.

2. *Breastfeeding should be comfortable for both mother and baby.* Teach this concept prenatally (or to professionals) with dolls, because positioning and latch are kinesthetic skills. Spend at least one-third of the class time on ways to hold the baby. The baby's mouth should be wide open and deeply

"latched" onto the breast, with the nipple tip well back near the hard-soft palate juncture; the baby's body is aligned with its head to preserve and protect the baby's airway. If breastfeeding is painful, something is wrong and needs careful evaluation.

3. *Help is available for questions and problems.* If you teach points 1 and 2 thoroughly, this message can be short and sweet, reinforced with a handout.

Once you've covered the basics thoroughly, continue to reinforce these primary messages in other and subsequent sessions. Include plenty of "why" messages to reinforce the decision to breastfeed and continue breastfeeding.

The five central messages of "why breastfeed" are as follows:

1. Human milk is species-specific nourishment for the baby.
2. Human milk produces optimal growth and development.
3. Human milk provides substantial protection from illness.
4. Lactation is beneficial to the mother's health.
5. Breastfeeding biologically supports a special mother–baby relationship.

The five central concepts of "how to breastfeed" are as follows:

1. Nurse early and often, within the first hour after birth.
2. All sucking should be at the breast; the length and frequency of feedings are determined by the baby.
3. Position the baby so nursing is comfortable and milk transfer is maximized.
4. Watch the baby's urine and stool output for assurance of supply.
5. Problems have solutions. Help is available.

Understanding the primary causes of lactation failure helps prioritize the information presented to mothers. In order of frequency, the causes of breastfeeding failure are as follows:

1. Perceived or actual milk insufficiency, caused by inappropriate feeding practices, rooted in lack of understanding of the process of lactation and lack of knowledge of infant behavior
2. Pain during breastfeeding, caused by nipple trauma from inappropriate technique or practices; breast pain from inappropriate technique; and/or nipple or breast pain from pathological organisms
3. Lack of support or undermining the decision from family and friends, health professionals, and/or employers and school administrators

The five central causes of breastfeeding problems in the first six weeks are as follows:

1. *Too few nursing sessions per day.* A normal pattern is 8–12 sessions per day; more are fine. Watch the baby for hunger cues.
2. *Nursings too short, ended by mother.* The nursing session length should be unrestricted. Let the baby end the session.
3. *Overuse of pacifiers and bottles.* Nipple confusion or preference can lead to breast refusal. Use of supplements decreases milk supply.

4. *Poor attachment, causing nipple pain and low milk transfer.* Breastfeeding should never hurt the mother. Investigate any pain associated with breastfeeding.

5. *Blaming breastfeeding for normal newborns' need for closeness, cuddling, holding, and so on. All* babies need frequent feeding, carrying, and comforting.

Use this information to guide the content of your classes. Weave in plenty of information on how to prevent the most common causes or problems in creative ways. Please don't just lecture—it's the least effective way of teaching.

SPECIAL TOPICS

Developing special classes on less frequently encountered issues will depend on your clientele. Ask for suggestions, study the problems that bring mothers to your practice, and plan accordingly. A support-group format often works better for single-topic sessions than does a formal class or lecture. Some common special-topic sessions focus on twins or triplets (be sure to have mothers of multiples available to facilitate these discussions), premature babies, or toddlers. A back-to-work class may also prove popular.

Conducting or hosting mother-support groups is a very important service, even though it's not always a huge moneymaker. Mothers learn from their peers in ways different from, and sometimes better than, learning from a professional. If you are a La Leche League Leader, you already know how to manage such groups. If you're not, the best reference for establishing and conducting mother-support groups is La Leche League's *Leaders Handbook.*[2]

COMMUNITY RESOURCES

If you don't want to, can't, or aren't in a position to set up classes or run a mother-support group, then find out where they are available in your community. Take the time to attend one session to see how the group is run and to make personal contact with the teacher or leader. Follow up with a one-on-one meeting with the instructor or group leader to discuss mutual referrals and communication pathways/strategies. Ideally, you will find one another mutually supportive.

PROFESSIONAL EDUCATION

Teaching health professionals about breastfeeding is often more of a remedial exercise than primary education in a new subject. Unlike parents, who are usually eager participants, health care professionals may be a "captive audience" and prove resistant, defensive, or even hostile to your message. A detailed discussion of "how to teach health care professionals about breastfeeding" is beyond the scope of this book. I've found that professionals are less resistant to "how to" messages than "why" messages in the early stages of their conversion to being breastfeeding-friendly.

If you have an opportunity to present in-service education to local professionals, start with the same core concepts listed earlier: (1) how to make plenty of milk, (2) positioning for comfort, and (3) resources available for help. Alternatively, use UNICEF's Baby-Friendly Hospital Initiative resources for ideas. (See Appendix B.)

SUMMARY

Offering breastfeeding classes for parents and/or presenting continuing education for professionals may be a productive aspect of your practice. Parent education classes are usually quicker and easier to implement, provide a steadier stream of income, and expose more potential clients to your practice.

NOTES

1. This concept is part of the *Innocenti Declaration* and models attitudes that support breastfeeding.

2. *New Leaders Handbook*. Schaumburg, IL: La Leche League International, 1998.

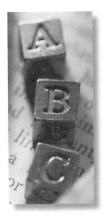

20 Pitfalls Related to Clinical Issues

Linda J. Smith, BSE, FACCE, IBCLC

Before you read this chapter, read *A Legal Primer for Lactation Consultants*. Again. Also read ILCA's *Standards of Practice for Lactation Consultants* and IBLCE's *Code of Ethics*. Again. And ILCA's *Scope of Practice and Education Guidelines*. Again. Remember—first, do no harm. Make sure everything you do or suggest is safe, even if you're not positive it will be effective.

"DIAGNOSING" WITHOUT DIAGNOSING

Problem identification is probably the trickiest and most frustrating part of private practice. The difficulty often arises when the mother or baby has a medical problem that surfaces as a breastfeeding problem or affects breastfeeding, but the problem has been overlooked, ignored, dismissed, disbelieved, or mismanaged by a licensed health care professional. You've done your homework on the condition and have read the medical literature thoroughly. You're fairly sure what the problem is, yet you're not supposed to label what it probably is (that's diagnosing) or suggest remedies (that's prescribing). In particular, you're not supposed to give the mother something to help fix the situation (that's dispensing). You've just spent 90 minutes with the mother and baby, accurately and thoroughly documented your observations, figured out what's wrong, and developed a plan for how to start resolving the problem. However, the mother is still hurting, and she came to you for help with this problem after other resources failed her, including her doctor. Now what?

Ideally, you would do as much as you can legally do on site, then send the mother and baby and your careful documentation of the symptoms back to her primary care provider for diagnosis and treatment, whereupon the doctor would quickly and cheerfully admit the oversight or mistake, accurately diagnose the problem or concur with your assessment, and treat the condition with evidence-based strategies that preserve and support breastfeeding.

Right. Don't laugh. This really happens in some places.

In the rest of the world, we must follow standards of practice and laws that *exclude* diagnosing and prescribing. That is, the standards assume that you possess no other credentials that allow you to make a medical diagnosis and prescribe treatment for a medical condition. If you have such credentials, you *know* what you're allowed to do and you probably don't need to read this chapter.

Take the high road here, because LCs are part of the health care team. Do not—I repeat, do *not*—disparage, ridicule, badmouth, or otherwise criticize other health professionals, no matter what you hear or how inappropriate the alleged action or inaction. Practice finding ways of validating the mother's feelings and giving her accurate, evidence-based information without attacking the giver of erroneous information. I know exercising restraint can be very difficult. Do it anyway.

Midwives may not be lactation consultants, but PPLCs are most definitely midwives in the linguistic sense—"with the woman." We walk *with* the mother through the process of figuring out what's wrong and deciding what to do about it. We act as a sounding board and source of information at each stage. While it isn't legal for us to diagnose, it's perfectly legal for the mother to self-diagnose. The decisions are hers, the power is hers, and the responsibility is ultimately hers.

You can give the mother published information on the problem from reputable sources, such as *Breastfeeding, a Guide for the Medical Profession* or articles published in the *Journal of Human Lactation* or other peer-reviewed journals. You can share possibilities with her and discuss how well she thinks her situation fits each of them in turn. You can share your own uncertainties about what may be going on, discuss treatment options, and outline "if, then" plans.

Once you and the mother are fairly certain of an appropriate starting point on addressing her situation, you can suggest ways for her to approach her primary care provider. Your own documentation and report letter can be very thorough, including references to medical texts and even research articles on the subject, and can even be very pointed—"Please evaluate XXX and confirm or rule out any infectious or other pathological condition that may be causing these symptoms." You can contact the primary care provider yourself and discuss your observations, as you've already obtained the client's permission to do so during the intake part of the consult. Perhaps LCs should consider ourselves "midpractitioners" as well as "midwives"—we walk with the physician, the occupational or physical therapist, or the obstetrician, sharing our expertise rather than forcing our point.

At this point, education and networking enter the picture. You need to start (or continue) addressing the larger issues of establishing and fostering competent breastfeeding care across all health care providers and systems. You can write two-page "teaching" reports to the primary care providers with footnotes and attached research articles, as I've done for many years. You could provide some brown-bag teaching lunches for local medical offices. I keep extra loaner copies of *Medications and Mothers Milk* by Thomas Hale, *Breastfeeding, a Guide for the Medical Profession* by Lawrence and Lawrence, and other references on my office bookshelf so that mothers can take this information directly to their doctors. You could copy or download articles from the medical literature and send them to the providers in your community or to the mothers in your practice. (Obey international copyright laws if you use this strategy.) You could keep business cards of supportive ancillary providers in your community, and send them to the primary care providers and/or your clients. These providers might include, but not be limited to, osteopathic physicians, chiropractors, dermatologists, cranial-sacral therapists, massage therapists, oral-motor therapists, mental health providers, dietitians, social workers, gastroenterologists, pharmacists, allergists, dentists, and ENT specialists.

Of course, even this strategy has its pitfalls. Some primary care providers become outraged when a lactation consultant "takes matters into her own hands" and refers a mother directly to, say, a licensed pediatric dentist who will assess her baby's lingual frenulum and treat it if necessary. One pediatrician told me, "If you ever refer one of my patients directly to a dentist again, you can forget about getting any more referrals from this practice." (*Note:* This physician does not believe that a baby's short, tight frenulum has any effect on breastfeeding, and would rather a mother stop breastfeeding than even discuss the effect of tongue-tie on an infant's ability to feed and speak normally, despite being provided with much professional literature on the subject.)

The mother has a right to know that evidence-based options exist. She has a right to a second medical opinion. The lactation consultant does *not* have the right to deliberately withhold information on a condition or evidence-based strategy for resolving a breastfeeding problem to "protect" the mother or her primary care provider. Read the *Code of Ethics for International Board Certified Lactation Consultants* in the *Core Curriculum*. Again.

Whatever you do, remember that you are a lactation *consultant*. Leave all decisions and treatment options squarely and firmly in the hands of the mother. Explain what you think is the root of the problem, and describe several options for resolving the situation. The mother picks the one she's willing to try, even if that means total, permanent weaning. Remember Rules 2, 3, 4, and 5!

"TREATING" WITHOUT TREATING

As of this writing, many interventions (fixes, solutions, remedies) for breastfeeding problems fall into the "common practice" area in the conceptual diagram as shown in Figure 20.1. As more research is done, some strategies will move into the core of evidence-based practices (for example, applying cabbage leaves to engorged breasts). Other strategies will be tossed out of the middle ring if research establishes that they are neither safe nor effective (for example, applying hot compresses to engorged breasts in the early postpartum period). The safest pathway is to use core strategies. Many of them are summarized in ILCA's *Evidence Based Strategies for the First Fourteen Days*. Do your homework early and often for all common problems, and stay alert for new research on these issues.

If no good research applies to a given clinical situation, then the next best strategy is to use critical thinking and pick a solution with a sound theoretical and physiological basis. Document it thoroughly, follow the mother closely, and stay in communication and collaboration with her primary care provider.

Some PPLCs might ask the mother if she uses "alternative" therapies for various problems, supporting those if they seem to be helping, while documenting her decision to try a nontraditional approach. *Warning:* Be aware that you are going out on a legal limb when *you* suggest or support nontraditional or "alternate" remedies.

The incredible ease with which herbal supplements can be purchased might lead some LCs to believe that it is safe to suggest that their clients use them, particularly because no prescription is necessary. Unless there is evidence to support the use of a particular supplement, however, making such a recommendation has the potential to subject an LC to liability for professional negligence.

Currently, the peer-reviewed research basis for recommending herbal remedies appears to be virtually non-existent. In addition, many (if not most) herbal supplements

FIGURE 20.1 Core practice diagram ▶

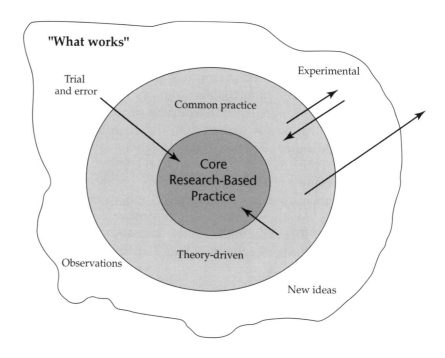

continue to be inadequately tested, inadequately labeled, and poorly made, causing dosages to vary greatly. For example, in the United Sates, the Dietary Supplements Health and Education Act of 1994 (DSHEA) has left the Food and Drug Administration (FDA) impotent to regulate these processes, so the suppliers of these substances are free to make health claims about them for which there is little or no scientific proof indicating their effectiveness (or the absence of side effects).[1]

Experimental ideas are just that—experimental. I don't have any easy answers to whether or not, or how much, you should explore innovative, alternative, experimental, nontraditional therapies for various situations. Sometimes the most critical observations and best thinking occur in community-based private practice, and I certainly don't want to squelch or discourage innovative thinking.

However, PPLCs work with vulnerable mothers and babies, and we have a sobering legal and ethical responsibility to provide *safe*, effective care. *How* you discuss innovative strategies with a mother, colleague, or primary care provider is critical. Be careful, do your homework, document what you do and why you do it, and remember Rules 2 and 3.

INADEQUATE CHARTING/ DOCUMENTATION

Nikki Lee, RN, MSN, IBCLC, CIMI, CCE, reminds us:

When you get a deposition or a subpoena to testify about a mother or baby, how will you find the specific chart you need? Is it filed chronologically? Alphabetically? By whose name—the mother's, or the baby's? What if the mother changes her name or moves?

When you read your notes (maybe several years later), can you remember this mother and baby? Can you hear her voice, see her face, and/or remember some specific detail of her home or living situation?

Are all your entries signed and dated? Are all the notes and records for that client in one place? Are any referrals and recommendations clearly described? Is your charting style consistent, and any acronyms or abbreviations defined? Are you prepared to have your documentation scrutinized in a court of law by the parents, prosecutor and defense attorney, expert witnesses, and a judge?

You should be able to answer yes to all of the above.

Working without feedback from clients and colleagues is a bad idea. Your training and education should have included working in a group setting with other lactation consultants well before you launch out on your own as a PPLC. If you are not part of a group practice, establish a peer support and review system with colleagues as a fundamental feature of your practice. Arrange to be observed periodically, and arrange to observe someone else periodically. Form a formal or informal "professional review board" for discussing clinical aspects of your practice. Attend conferences and coalitions, especially those that draw other private practice lactation consultants. Send "client satisfaction" surveys to your clients and referring colleagues, and act on the feedback you receive.

LACK OF PEER REVIEW AND CLIENT FEEDBACK/EVALUATION

Don't do it. Don't try to be the lactation consultant for your sister, cousin, daughter, or other relative or close friend. If a relative or close friend asks a pertinent question, of course you will answer her questions just as you would answer any mother (or anybody) who asks you a question. The sticky issue arises when you spot problems that the mother has not noticed or observe behaviors that are less than ideal for long-term breastfeeding. In those situations, do everything you can to get the mother into someone else's care while you continue to be her friend, sister, or other relative. It's almost impossible to wear "two hats" for very long, and your therapeutic relationship will quickly color (or discolor) your social relationship.

WORKING WITH FAMILY MEMBERS

At the very least, no mother or baby should ever risk being harmed or getting sick because they contacted you. If you are sick, don't see mothers and babies until you are completely well. Period. This mandate applies to you, your staff, and your immediate family (especially your children, who likely bring home infectious diseases all the time), and includes emotional and mental illnesses. If you are allergic to pets or cigarette smoke, doing home visits may pose a problem for you. Part of your responsibility as an IBCLC is to arrange coverage for your clients if you are unable to practice, for any reason.

EVEN LCS GET SICK

Occasionally you'll be the first to notice or pay attention to a serious condition in the mother or baby. Even if you're not sure what the problem is, you may notice that something "isn't right" or is very wrong. This reason explains why you get permission from the mother before working with her—so you can discuss this issue with her and her doctor immediately. Trust your instincts when something isn't quite right, and bring it to the mother's attention first. Depending on her response, bring her partner and/or physician into the discussion. You may even need to call an ambulance (paramedics, rescue squad) or help get the mother and baby to the nearest hospital emergency room.

For example, during one office consult, an eight-day-old baby turned blue (cyanotic) during nursing. The LC called the baby's doctor immediately and accompanied the mother and baby to the hospital, where a serious heart condition was diagnosed. In this case, not a single health professional had ever observed the baby *during* a feed.

THE SCARY MOTHER OR BABY

Have the courage and integrity to point out ominous findings to the mother. Don't hide your concerns out of fear that you will frighten her. Be honest, tell the truth, and help her find appropriate care for conditions that are unrelated to breastfeeding and/or exceed the scope of practice of IBCLCs. Stay in close contact with the mother's primary care provider(s). Comply with local laws regarding reporting dangerous situations to the proper agencies.

SUPPORTING THE MOTHER WHO STOPS BREASTFEEDING

The LC should not be the first person to suggest abandoning breastfeeding to a mother. However, the LC's job sometimes includes helping mothers stop breastfeeding comfortably. Perhaps the baby's suck problem cannot be remedied, or the mother's breast pain is just too severe, or her social/cultural situation is too overwhelming. Helping her wean gracefully may make or break her next breastfeeding experience, her feelings about this baby, and her advice to friends and relatives. Mothers and babies deserve our best information and support for gentle weaning. At the same time, as Diane Wiessinger noted in an earlier section of this book, we "take our clients to bed" with us. It's sometimes difficult to manage our *own* grieving when our daily fare consists of trying to rescue a steady stream of breastfeeding disasters. Finding a way to process our own feelings is part of taking care of ourselves so we can continue helping mothers.

Clinical options for an overwhelming breastfeeding problem might include long-term expressing or pumping milk and using alternate feeding devices, realistic and evidence-based information on human milk substitutes and/or family foods, and care of the breasts during weaning. Emotional support and counseling are vitally important. Remember, breastfeeding was important to the mother, or she wouldn't have started and you probably wouldn't have been working with her in the first place. Help her work through the painful feelings of her loss. If she changes her mind or the baby does not tolerate other feeding products, helping her build up her supply again is reasonably easy for several weeks after stopping, regardless of when she stops. Congratulate her for *any* breastfeeding, even just one feeding! Help her to grieve over giving up something that was important to her, but didn't work out the way she planned. It's normal to be sad or regret having to stop breastfeeding. If the mother is very sad for many days, help her find professional counseling. Remind her to keep giving her baby plenty of *time and touching*. In the long run, those elements are the most important things!

I like the way Pat Gima, IBCLC, sums up the PPLC role:

Show up.

Pay attention.

Tell the truth.

And let go of the outcome.

SUMMARY

You can avoid most clinical pitfalls by working conservatively and abiding by the *Standards of Practice, Code of Ethics*, and other professional guidelines. Achieving this goal means functioning as a consultant to the mother, her doctor, and other professionals, not as the primary caregiver. Cooperation, collaboration, and teamwork are the guiding principles of LCs' work. And finally, remember the legal principle of "first, do no harm"—practice safely at all times.

NOTES

1. See Appendix 31-C from *Core Curriculum for Lactation Consultant Practice*, by Priscilla Bornmann.

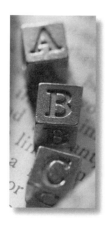

21 Professional Responsibilities Revisited

Diane Wiessinger, MS, IBCLC

As an IBCLC in private practice, there are certain things that you *must* do, and certain things that you *may* do if you choose. It's not an idle distinction. As allied health professionals with a responsibility to the public, we owe it to everyone, the profession included, to maintain a certain standard. Anyone performing those basic duties is doing enough, although many of us may want to do more. It's not possible to substitute those optional responsibilities for the mandatory ones; the optional ones, however, must always be "in addition to." For this reason, it's worth taking a look first—as we will in this chapter—at what an IBCLC *must* do. Chapter 22 describes some of the activities that go beyond the basics.

Is it *enough* to do no more than the basics? Certainly! Skip Chapter 22 if you like. Never feel that, in caring for mothers one at a time in a responsible way, you are not doing enough. You are the backbone of the profession, and you are changing the world.

MAINTAIN YOUR IBLCE CERTIFICATION

When I picked up my college diploma, I thought to myself, "Here is something that no one can take away from me. No matter what happens, what I do, or where I go, I will always have this degree." That's not true for your IBLCE certification, which is as it should be. A health care professional who falls behind the times presents a hazard to others. We have the great honor of belonging to a health care field that keeps its participants on their toes. You attained a certain level of competency to take the exam in the first place, and you must maintain at least that level to keep the initials you have earned. Some LCs may take the exam because their workplace wanted them to, because they wanted the initials for their records, or because they were required to. Those LCs will probably leave the field in five years' time, because they won't bother to collect additional education credits. But at least they're not *more* than five years behind the times before they lose their credentials. These LCs also don't represent the typical IBCLC in private practice.

Expect a certain proportion of your income to be used for the conferences you must attend, or continuing education independent study modules you must purchase to maintain certification. While you could potentially acquire enough continuing education credits through study modules alone, attending conferences at least occasionally brings the entire profession to life for us, in all its varied forms.

In the early years, you'll learn new things at every conference, meet people whose names you've read, take copious notes. You'll come away feeling ever so much smarter. As the years roll along, you'll sometimes sit through entire sessions without putting pen to paper, sometimes hear speakers with whom you disagree, and sometimes choose your conferences according to whether you want to hear those topics "again." A few more years will pass, and you'll realize you're hearing very little that's brand new to you. Are the conferences still as important to you as they were in the early years when you soaked up new information like a sponge? Absolutely! It's vital that you hear the same old information; it's the only way that you can know for sure whether anything has changed. No one will ever write to you, saying, "The following changes need to be made in your information base." No, the only way to find out what has changed is to listen to a session and hear nothing new. The experience may not be as exciting as hearing the information the first time, but you'll come to realize that having information confirmed is every bit as valuable as having information instilled. And now, in ways that were not true at the beginning, those conferences offer a place to meet "old friends." It's amazing how much camaraderie can exist among people who have actually met only once every year or two for only a handful of years. Conferences are an essential part of our work. And they're also food for our souls.

At about the eight-year mark, you'll begin to obsess about having to take The Exam again. Just before the 10-year mark, you'll buckle down and try to study. Some LCs will find the time to do so in earnest. Some LCs will do no more than flip through a few favorite books, dust off a few books that they have ignored in recent years, or never get further than simply intending to study. Most likely, LCs who have been active in the profession will pass without a problem. I found taking the exam for the second time to be a totally different experience from the first time: My eyes were dimmer and my bladder smaller. More importantly, I understood the larger rationale behind specific questions. I filled my scrap paper with "yes, but" responses, where initially I had felt a need to respond in writing to only one or two points. The exam itself felt like a hotel room chat with conference friends—a comparing of cases, a pondering of problems. I felt competent. That is what 10 years of conferences and clients and honestly trying, one mother at a time, will do for you.

Other health care professionals don't have to take a recertifying exam every 10 years; why should *we*? (I hear you whining.) Ah, but think what the quality of our MDs would be if their degree and license to practice evaporated without regular testing! Today, nearly every new allied health profession and medical specialty includes mandatory periodic recertification, reflecting the recognition that continuing competency is vitally important. Given the pace of new research and accumulating evidence for (or against) many practices, periodic reexamination assures the public of a minimum level of competence. IBCLCs are on the cutting edge of health care credentialing, with a level of quality control that other branches are talking of imitating in the years to come. Dread the exam, resent it, even cram for it if you like, but be grateful for its rewards and the global results. You can talk with an IBCLC whom you have never before met, and discover that the two of you share a body of knowledge that differs only in the less significant details. You can refer a mother to an IBCLC on the other side of the world, and be reasonably confident that she will be cared for with concern and competence. The exam works, and works well.

ADHERE TO THE IBLCE CODE OF ETHICS

Our *Code of Ethics* is neither complicated nor difficult to follow, and you need to have a copy of it. You'll find it in its entirety in Appendix A. Most of the code is common sense for any health care professional. A few points have special significance for lactation consultants:

9. *Recognize and exercise professional judgment within the limits of her/his qualifications. This principle includes seeking counsel and making referrals to appropriate providers.*

Coach Smith's Rule 5: Nobody knows everything, including the most experienced LC. It takes self-confidence to say, "I don't know, but I'll try to find out." Ultimately, that willingness can make all the difference. A friend of mine, stymied by an immigrant mother's layers of breastfeeding problems, ultimately drew upon her own background in nutrition, an obstetrician, a pediatrician, a craniosacral therapist, and a neighbor. The contributions of the first four people aren't difficult to figure out. The neighbor was from the mother's country *and* was breastfeeding a child of roughly the same age. My friend arranged a get-together between them to make sure the mother had a "peer support group" of sorts. Appropriate referrals come in all styles!

11. *Provide sufficient information to enable clients to make informed decisions.*

We don't make decisions for mothers. Rather, we enable them to make informed decisions for themselves. One purpose of the information packet that I give to each client who comes for a full consultation is to provide her with information that might not have been covered in the consultation or that she might want to refer to later. We don't have to give all information to mothers orally; it can come in handout or even book form, too. Not long ago, a client of mine opted not to pursue breastfeeding, despite having read "cover to cover" the best breastfeeding book in my lending library. Every unnecessary weaning takes a piece out of my heart, but I can look back and know that I provided the mother with ample information on which to base her decision. Sometimes I feel like a very dim candle in a very great darkness; then I remind myself that my candle is merely information and support. It's up to the mother to provide the flame.

17. *Ensure that professional judgment is not influenced by any commercial considerations.*

This standard is especially important for LCs who sell or lease equipment and products. Work diligently to keep your product judgments free of influence from personal prejudice (and potential income). It's very difficult to profit from the sale or lease of products and not find yourself using them unnecessarily. Also, it's impossible to really know whether you ever do so. Always be aware of the danger, and don't think for a moment that clever little you can outwit the billions of dollars that have been spent over the years figuring out marketing techniques that work. You're not that smart.

I once attended a conference at which LCs complained that a certain product was now being marketed directly to the public, rather than being made available to the public only through lactation consultants. Abruptly, the room became filled for me with turn-of-the-twentieth-century physicians, complaining about formula companies that took their products directly to the consumer: "Only *we* can decide what the consumer needs. This product should be available only through *us*!" The LCs' argument sounded reasonable—but then so did the argument of the doctors who started us on the path to blind health care system reliance on formula company monies.

23. *Present substantiated information and interpret controversial information without personal bias, recognizing that legitimate differences of opinion exist.*

Ours is a young field, and many of our "truths" are being turned upside down. Some of those ridiculous theories you hear from other people will eventually turn out to be right. Keep an open mind, go to conferences when you can, and recognize that the unusual approach taken by a colleague may work well for her and her clients, even if it doesn't work for you. We're interested in the destination with a mother, not the details of the journey. Coach Smith takes a pink baseball cap with her when she speaks at conferences. When her comments are personal opinion, the pink hat goes on. When they are research-based, the hat is off. Eventually some of her hatless statements will be proved wrong, and some of her pink-hat statements will turn out to be right. It's important to know which is which along the way.

24. *Withdraw voluntarily from professional practice if the lactation consultant…has an emotional or mental disability that affects her/his practice in a manner that could harm the client.*

Burnout results, I think, when you labor too long for too little return. That concept means many of us are at risk, and I believe burnout qualifies as a disability that affects our ability to give a client our best. You have an ethical mandate to take breaks when you need them. Some of us document well enough, remember well enough, and have emotional wells deep enough to juggle chronically large case loads; others begin to mix faces and facts when we exceed a certain number of new mothers per week. As you find your personal (and ever-changing) balance point, respect it. Your clients will be glad that you do.

25. *Require and obtain consent to share clinical concerns and information with the physician or other primary health care provider before initiating a consultation.*

Isn't that a surprising mandate to find in our Code of Ethics? Some IBCLCs in private practice don't even realize it's there. Nevertheless, our certifying organization requires us to obtain a client's signature before we begin a consultation. The phrasing of the consent statement is up to us. My own is very simple, and I've put it at the top of my intake form because otherwise I forget to have the mother sign it:

> I understand that a consultation may include a visual and manual examination of my breasts and of my infant's mouth. I give permission for information from this and subsequent consultations to be shared with my child's pediatrician, my own health care providers, my insurance company, and with other breastfeeding specialists as needed to further the understanding of breastfeeding generally or to improve my lactation consultant's knowledge base.

One of my phrases—"and subsequent consultations"—was added belatedly after a client in my neighborhood thought my follow-up visits, which I did free of charge because of our proximity and previous acquaintanceship, were done purely as a neighbor and not as an LC. She was unhappy to learn that I continued to file physician reports on those contacts, and I realized I had given her no way to know for sure whether my visits were being made from neighborly concern or professional obligation. If I had it to do again, I would charge at least a small amount for those visits to keep them clearly professional.

24. *Adhere to those provisions of the International Code of Marketing of Breast-milk Substitutes which pertain to health workers.*

Surprisingly, this point is a recent addition to our *Code of Ethics*. Perhaps it was left out of the original version because it was assumed that we all know a bribe when we see one. Marketing has huge amounts of research behind it to make it both invisible and enticing, however, and it's important for us all to have our boundaries spelled out ahead of time. Read the *Code*, which is summarized in Appendix A, and make it part of your ethical foundation. Formula and baby food companies are no more in business to promote breastfeeding than Ford is in business to promote Chevrolet. It's that simple.

JOIN ILCA

The International Lactation Consultant Association is our professional organization. Join it. Its main publication, the *Journal of Human Lactation*, is one of a tiny handful of professional journals devoted to human lactation, and you need it. Its policies are a major force in deciding the direction of our profession, and you need to participate in the process. ILCA's membership directory offers a great way to locate IBCLCs in other areas, and you need to be able to find them. Its conferences are the ultimate lactation consultant playground, and you deserve—even if it's only once in your career—to play at it.

It's not difficult to spot LCs who don't belong to ILCA. They don't know the leading names in their field. I used to feel I was name-dropping when names like Ruth Lawrence, Jan Riordan, or Peter Hartmann would come up in my get-togethers with LC-wannabes. I'd see their blank faces and feel just a little foolish at how often these names would pop up in my conversation. Later, I realized how difficult it would be to provide an introductory course in, say, psychiatry without mentioning Freud or Jung. Furthermore, I realized that I would absolutely steer clear of any practicing psychiatrist who was unfamiliar with them.

The vast majority of us entered the LC profession by gathering information on our own, not by taking structured university classes. We sought to gather information and create our own "course" in human lactation. If we gather information so poorly, and add to it so poorly that we don't know the names of our own founders, historians, authors, and researchers, then clearly our knowledge base has major holes. Reading the *Journal of Human Lactation* and participating in ILCA fills in the holes.

If you're not in the ILCA directory, you're invisible in your field. You will practice in isolation, using the same old techniques, oblivious to changes in the profession. Fortunately, if you're not in the directory, you're unlikely to receive referrals from any other IBCLCs. Do yourself, your clients, and your peers a huge favor: Join! ILCA is on the Web at www.ilca.org.

FOLLOW ILCA'S STANDARDS OF PRACTICE

Even if you're not a member of ILCA, if you hold the IBCLC certification you are expected to adhere to ILCA's *Standards of Practice*. The full text appears in Appendix A. A few additional thoughts:

1.1.3 *discuss with the mother and document as appropriate all assessment information*

1.3.1 *implement the plan of care in a manner appropriate to the situation and acceptable to the mother*

One of the things of which I am proudest in our profession is the fact that we work *with* a mother—truly *with* her. When I hear a phrase like "patient noncompliance" in other disciplines, I see a failure of health care. The LC's job is to find a woman's strengths, her abilities, and the directions in which she will not go, and then work within that framework. We could write physician's reports criticizing a woman's lack of literacy, or her unwillingness to consider an antibiotic, or her refusal to feed more often than every three hours. People are not bundles of inadequacies, however, but rather blendings of particular strengths. The LC's job is to find the strengths and work with them. If the plan doesn't work for a mother, it isn't a good plan and needs revision. Very simple.

Unless the issue is a simple matter of improving positioning, a mother and I rarely establish a single plan and stick with it. We nudge it here, tweak it there—always making it a plan tailored for this particular woman at this particular time. What a forgiving way to work! It's a little like being a parent, making mistakes, and knowing that it's all right as long as you keep trying. Your first care plan with a mother may not be perfect, but she can leave her visit with you knowing two important things: (1) she now has a clear direction to head, and (2) you'll stick with her if she wants to change direction.

1.3.5 *provide a written report to the primary health care provider as appropriate, including: assessment information, suggested interventions, instructions provided*

1.4.3 *document and communicate to the primary health care provider(s) as appropriate: evaluation of outcomes, modifications in the plan, follow-up*

Because the necessity for reporting is buried halfway through the *Standards of Practice*, because not everyone has a copy of the *Standards*, and because the requirement isn't discussed much, I suspect many IBCLCs in private practice don't routinely file physician's reports. Oh dear!

At first, I found the reports something of a chore. I now realize that they can serve as a lazy way of filling out case notes after a client leaves—your copy becomes invaluable when your memory fails you. More importantly, the reports keep you absolutely on the same page as the doctor. There are no surprises for either one of you, the physician knows exactly what additional help the mother is getting and why, he or she knows the extent to which the baby is being monitored, and the doctor learns to trust your services. Of course, the report is also your discreet little chance to provide a bit of breastfeeding education to the medical community! Seize this opportunity, and don't give the mother's other health care providers the opportunity to think of you as haphazard or secretive. These reports are a cornerstone of the care we provide.

As allied health professionals, LCs are satellites of the primary mother–baby medical team. What we recommend to a mother and baby needs to end up in their main medical record, which is *not* the file in our own office. We may not like a woman's choice of doctors; all the more reason to file those reports, and educate him or her!

These days, I have fun writing the reports. When I write to a doctor whom I know to be sympathetic, I feel I'm writing to a collaborator. When I write to one who is, well, not particularly friendly to breastfeeding, I enjoy finding a way to write the report that slides in some gentle education without letting on that I know the physician's knowledge base is deficient. I *behave* as if we're collaborators, even if we are not.

All of the writing should be respectful enough that the mother can read it, too. While I don't routinely give her a copy of my reports, I do so if asked, and I always write the report with her reading of it in mind. My reports end, not infrequently, with a sentence something like this: "This mother has been working very hard to get where she is, and deserves a great deal of credit for her efforts." Any mother can feel good reading that statement, and I like to think it reminds the doctor to give her a verbal pat on the back at her next visit. Sometimes it's difficult to phrase my concerns in a way that won't upset the mother if she reads it. That dilemma doesn't happen often, because my usual "take" on a client is that she's working a whole lot harder than I had to with my babies.

How often you file a report on a given client is up to you. Some LCs file a report with every pump rental, more as a means of advertising than out of necessity. I rarely file a report for a phone consultation, for two reasons: if we were able to address the mother's concern by phone it wasn't a major problem, and I would never send a report to someone else without the mother's written permission. While I always file a report for an initial full consultation, I may not report on subsequent visits until something significant changes, either in the plan or in the outcome.

LC reports vary greatly in style, from hospital charting formats to wholly narrative descriptions. It's generally best to keep the report to one page, although some of us probably like a more complete record for our own use. Cover the pertinent information well enough that the doctor can understand it today and you can understand it 10 years from today, and choose a format with which you're comfortable, so that you will *do it*!

With whom, exactly, do you file the report? Most of mine go to the pediatrician, because it's primarily a baby issue. Even if it's thrush, I think of the problem as a baby issue, because the mother's thrush may interfere with her ability to breastfeed the baby. If the referral came from her obstetrician or midwife, the report goes to the obstetrician or midwife. Sometimes the pertinent person changes over the course of a long and complicated problem. In that case, I usually keep sending copies to the original report recipient.

I print out a copy for myself as well. My early reports were written on a computer that I no longer have, in a software program that no longer exists. I have those reports on disk, but I can do little with them except stack them. Much as I love my computer, when it comes to permanence it's hard to beat paper. Keep the reports on file according to the law in your community, which often specifies "until the child reaches the age of majority" (18 years or more).

2.4 provide emotional support for continued breastfeeding in difficult or complicated circumstances

It's embarrassing how often the most important thing I do, for all my education and experience, is simply act as cheerleader. Sometimes I've dug up a splendid bit of information for a mother, or found a unique resource for her, perhaps done some very clever equipment troubleshooting, and what is she most grateful for? The fact that I was always optimistic and caring. When mothers express gratitude for such ordinary support, I confess I feel just a little let down. Of course, LCs have a gift that most of our culture has lost: we know that Breastfeeding Works. The confidence with which we talk with a mother, our ability to scare away the shadows, is often all a mother really needs to manage on her own. We may be able to take the pain away sooner or help her rebuild her milk supply faster, but mostly the mother needs confidence. And here it is in section 2.4—a professional obligation to share with her our confidence in breastfeeding, to cheer her on and tell her what a great job she's doing. Isn't that nice?

2.5 share current evidence-based information and clinical skills with other health care providers

Perhaps part of the reason I enjoy writing physician's reports is that I enjoy sharing information. My family and friends really don't care about the latest thinking in nipple wound healing. But the midwife does! There is deep satisfaction in seeing better care gradually spread through a community because you kept sending articles around and offering those demonstrations.

3.4 assist the mother in maintaining an intact breastfeeding relationship with her child

It can be easy to forget that our goal is not putting human milk into human tummies. Our goal is helping mothers toward happy, successful breastfeeding. Breastfeeding is a relationship, not a product or a technique. Sometimes it's the very last piece to fall into place, leaving mothers overjoyed when it finally does. I worked with a mother in a distant state by e-mail, patching up a relationship that had faltered from oversupply. She called when things were greatly improved to say, "I love you!" Nevertheless, there was still more work to do. We e-mailed back and forth about nursing for any old reason. "Even just to keep him quiet when you're on the phone," I wrote. That was a moment of revelation for her. "It's not that I'm not willing to do it, it's just that it would never, never have occurred to me." A few days later, I got another phone call. "I love my baby!" And then they were fine.

Our job is not really finished until a mother's relationship with her baby is stable. It may have stabilized in a pattern we would not have chosen, or it may have stabilized in a breastfeeding relationship that will continue for years. One of the best ways we can help ensure the latter is to encourage her involvement in a mother-to-mother breastfeeding support group. It is a part of our *Standards of Practice* to support whatever breastfeeding support group exists in our community, and to do our best to establish one if none exists.

Standard 4. Legal Considerations: *IBCLC lactation consultants are obligated to…practice with consideration for clients' rights of privacy and with respect for matters of a confidential nature.*

ILCA's section on legal considerations makes an assumption that I have always liked. It is that, if LCs protect the mother and child, we have adequately protected ourselves. This section does not include a long list of safeguards that IBCLCs can put in place to keep from being sued. Rather, it focuses on the need of the mother for respect, confidentiality, and an understanding of just whose body and whose baby we are dealing with. Childbirth educators and doulas rarely have suits brought against them. That's not because they don't make mistakes, but rather because they offer information, not mandates. They empower their clients rather than seeking to control them. They form a bond with them rather than acting as lawmakers over them. IBCLCs have that same philosophy, and it's reflected in our legal considerations.

KEEP UP-TO-DATE THROUGH CONTINUING EDUCATION

To some extent, your continuing education is taken care of for you, just in the course of maintaining your certification. It is possible to become certified and hang out your shingle for five years only, until your certification expires. This book was not written for the IBCLC who plans that approach, however.

With membership in ILCA, you'll find yourself on mailing lists for delectable conferences in your area and around the country, which makes accumulating credits a simple matter of deciding which sweets from the ongoing candy shop you want to sink your teeth into. If you expect from the start to devote a certain portion of your income to covering conference costs, they'll taste all the sweeter, with no bitter aftertaste. As an ILCA member, you'll also receive the candy catalogue known as the *Journal of Human Lactation*. Two other journals of interest are *Breastfeeding Review* from Australia and *Current Issues in Clinical Lactation* (for addresses, see Appendix B).

It would be difficult to maintain an effective private practice today without e-mail. Any private practice IBCLC with e-mail should have some involvement with Lactnet. This international e-mail user group for breastfeeding specialists represents an immediate window on the world of human lactation. When a situation arises that puzzles you (and those situations will come up much more often than you think), you can get immediate input from around the globe, just by posing your question to this intimate group of nearly 3000 participants. Furthermore, Lactnet's archives allow you to tap into the wisdom of past years (Lactnet was founded in 1995), pulling up any posts that contain your desired key word or phrase.

Those of us lucky enough to work in a real, live group practice do a lot of give and take around the coffee machine. We understand that most of these conversations don't qualify as research-based information, and those of us who use Lactnet as an Internet substitute for such a coffee break need to understand the same thing: Whenever you receive information, consider the source. That said, the opportunity to take a coffee break among so many colleagues is an enormous gift.

Many members of Lactnet never or seldom post anything themselves, preferring to "lurk" when they have the time to do so. Very few of us can keep up continually with its four-or-so daily digests of a dozen-or-so posts each. Nevertheless, it's wonderful to have access to Lactnet when you need it, and dipping into it even occasionally will keep you apprised of events, shifts in thought, new research, and new techniques that you might otherwise never encounter.

LCs who are seriously involved in breastfeeding support already form a scattered subset of this culture; IBCLCs in private practice represent a subset of that subset. Lactnet was originally invented for us and by us; its founders, Kathleen Bruce and Kathleen Auerbach, are private practice IBCLCs. They saw Lactnet as a way of bringing professional dialogue to LCs living many miles from their nearest colleagues. It now includes many others—doctors, nurses, and La Leche League Leaders among them—but the focus remains helping LCs who work in a vacuum to feel supported and connected and to have some ability to confer over puzzling cases. I can look back to when I worked all alone in private practice, the only IBCLC in several counties. But I don't want to revisit those days. Lactnet has improved my skills, lifted my spirits, shortened my "response time" for difficult questions, and brought me laughter and tears and friends. I can't imagine life as an LC without it.

For information on joining Lactnet, see Appendix B.

The pioneers of any new profession are self-taught and peer-taught, and lactation consultants are no exception. Linda Wieser[1] investigated which clinical skills were deemed central to lactation consultant practice, and how these skills were learned. She found that three steps were necessary for training future lactation consultants:

EVALUATE AND MONITOR YOUR CLINICAL SKILLS THROUGH PEER REVIEW

1. Observation of mother–infant dyads and of LCs working with these dyads

2. Practice doing the particular skill with both clients and volunteer subjects

3. Feedback from clients and instructors or more experienced clinicians

The lactation consultant profession is now well into its second decade of development. The early pioneers are now the teachers and mentors for novice LCs. As the study of human lactation becomes more established, more opportunities will arise to work with mentors or to shadow experienced LCs, and to have your skills evaluated by others. If you are a new LC, seek structured learning experiences[2] in your community, and travel to obtain in-person, supervised education in the clinical skills. (See Appendix B for more on learning opportunities.)

If you are a seasoned LC or structured feedback from peers is clearly impossible in your situation, you (and I) have an obligation to take advantage of all opportunities that come our way. If you have a group practice, establish a system for observing one another's consultations at intervals. If other IBCLCs practice in your area, strive to make the same arrangement. If you are the only game in town...well, at least remind yourself regularly of how you would feel if the local neurosurgeon performed in permanent isolation, and keep looking for ways to observe and be observed.

Many of us take the time to visit a fellow IBCLC in another town, if her practice is busy enough that we are fairly sure to see her in action on a prearranged day. You may also be able to shadow a hospital IBCLC. You'll be glad of any such contact that you can manage. Having something with which to compare yourself will help you say, "I know now why I like to do it this way," as well as, "That's something I'd like to try." Even hearing someone else give the same information in a different way gives you new insights into things you thought you already knew.

Feedback from clients[3] is helpful, even though they have no basis for comparison. Just as a new mother may leave a hospital with a nonlatching baby and no instructions on obtaining a pump and yet praise the wonderful breastfeeding help she received there, our clients may be thrilled with our care even when we spend weeks figuring out what we could have spotted immediately. What a client *can* help us evaluate is the effectiveness of our "packaging"—the way we wrap our information, ideas, suggestions, and demonstrations to make them work for her. Are we too stand-offish? Too hands-on? The LC's personal approach is personal indeed, so that what proves effective for one LC may not work for another LC. In this area, your clients may do a better job of evaluating you than another IBCLC could do. A sample client feedback tool appears in Appendix C.

Perhaps the most practical, albeit imperfect, system of peer review is an "e-mail group practice." Not long after Lactnet began, I posted a request for a handful of other LCs who wanted to share a very small, day-to-day forum in which we could ask questions too trivial or too embarrassing to send around the world. Our group includes nine LCs, and our daily exchanges are one of the most valuable things I have gained from Lactnet. A few members of the group work in hospitals, some are in private practice, some have La Leche League backgrounds, some are grandmothers, some are familiar with allergies or craniosacral work or lymph drainage or herbs or certain pump brands. Among the group members, someone is bound to know more than the rest of us about whatever topic comes up. We have learned a great deal from one another, and I know it has improved the quality of care that each of us delivers.

ADVOCATE FOR THE PROFESSION

You advocate for your profession financially when you join ILCA. You act as an advocate even in the simple act of including the initials "IBCLC" in your credentials. There are other important ways for you to promote the profession as well. Those well-reasoned letters to the editor of your paper that you sign as an IBCLC make an impression on the general public. The conversation you have with your seatmate on the plane affects his or her view of lactation consultants. Physician's reports, a contribution of time or materials to World Breastfeeding Week, handouts or a brief talk at a childbirth class, a booth at a local health fair—all of these activities let the public know that LCs exist, have valuable skills, and are an integral part of the health care system.

Some of this advocacy will come easily to you, whereas some of it poses a challenge. Just remember that positive visibility is important for all LCs, and do what you can. For my part, I've perfected the art of not making eye contact on planes. On the other hand, I do try to write a letter to the editor of the local paper whenever a breastfeeding issue arises. If you don't like to write letters, you can make a point of talking to your seatmate the next time you fly somewhere, and we'll balance each other out, with my thanks.

FORM RELATIONSHIPS WITH MOTHER-SUPPORT GROUPS

Step Ten of the Baby-Friendly Hospital Initiative (see Appendix A) states, "Foster the establishment of breastfeeding support groups and refer mothers to them on discharge from the hospital or clinic." It doesn't say, "Foster the establishment of IBCLCs in private practice and refer mothers to them," because there's a far greater need for mother-support groups than there is for LCs. Whenever our egos swell too much, we should remember that much of the time, a moderately well-informed neighbor bearing a casserole can do almost as well as we can, especially if she stays in touch.

All most mothers really need is the confidence that a breastfeeding culture gives them. Because we're woefully lacking in the cultural confidence department, a breastfeeding mini-culture is the next best thing—a group of women who have hurt from, worried over, wondered about, laughed at, and enjoyed their own breastfeeding experiences. The largest, best-organized such group in North America is La Leche League International.

I attended a small La Leche League meeting recently at which I realized our shoes were the perfect metaphor for the mothers who benefit from the organization. I saw a pair of traditional pumps with stockings, a pair of youthful platform shoes with stockings, a pair of black Keds with socks, a pair of army boots with tights, and several casual pairs of running shoes. The meeting began with the same statement I have heard at virtually every LLL meeting I have attended since my first one more than 20 years ago. It always goes something like this: "At this meeting, you'll hear a lot of different ideas and see a lot of different parenting styles. Some of what you see and hear you'll think would work for you and your baby, and some of it you won't. Just take from the meeting whatever feels right to you, and leave the rest." This caveat from an organization that some believe to be fanatic, militant, or judgmental!

Certainly, some LLL Leaders don't have enough information or communication skills to ease a mother's concerns. La Leche League is, after all, a lay volunteer organization whose members have limited time and training. Even so, you can become part of that training and improve your local group.

We're all working toward the same goal—happy, healthy breastfeeding relationships for women. That our routes take slightly different paths doesn't make them oppositional. Indeed, the clients of mine who do the best in the long run are the ones who leave the security of my help for the companionship of La Leche League. How sad if a woman must continue going to a specialist for support in maintaining what has become a perfectly ordinary breastfeeding experience. No, she needs to find other breastfeeding women who share her stage of parenting and whose company she enjoys. La Leche League facilitates that quest for her, often acting as a source from which she can form her own weekly playgroup.

Last year I received a call from a woman who wanted to become a lactation consultant. She had a nursing background, and when I suggested attending La Leche League meetings as a starting point, she said, "Oh, La Leche League. I called a Leader once and she was *terrible*! I'd never call them again." I thought about responding, "Oh, hospitals. I went to one once and the nurse was *terrible*. I'd never go to a hospital again." Perhaps I should have. With an attitude like that, she would have made a dangerous IBCLC. Imagine helping a mother through a difficult initiation of breastfeeding, only to scare her away from that important next stage—the shared enjoyment and support of other mothers.

Of course, mother-to-mother support systems needn't be part of La Leche League. When I have a group of clients who are still too fragile, or perhaps too unaccustomed to recognizing their own needs, to attend a regular La Leche League meeting, I may host a small meeting at my home. Even so, if an established breastfeeding support group exists, you need to use it, not snub it. If you feel it's unusable as it is, you need to be a friendly force for change. Attend the meetings and get to know the leaders. Have lunch together. Offer a series of get-togethers at which you can exchange information. Find some sort of common ground and build on it. Doing so is a fundamental responsibility of any IBCLC.

IBCLCs represent a sturdy series of threads in the safety net under breastfeeding mothers. Adhering to the guidelines set forth by our profession helps us ensure that those threads remain strong. On their own, they are not enough, however. Mother-support groups are another sturdy series of threads, and with our enthusiastic support they can become stronger yet. An informed and positive medical community is yet another part of the safety net, and yet another part that benefits from our input. All of these threads together slowly draw the community at large into the structure of the net. And every mother who enjoys breastfeeding her baby adds her own thread.

The safety net won't be entirely secure in our lifetimes, but the holes will get smaller. That's thanks, in part, to you.

SUMMARY

Direct clinical support of mothers and babies is the core function of the private practice lactation consultant. In addition, we have responsibilities to ourselves, our community, and our profession. These responsibilities are listed in the checklist on this page.

✔ Maintaining IBCLC certification

✔ Keeping up-to-date through continuing education

✔ Adhering to the *Code of Ethics* and *Standards of Practice*

✔ Joining ILCA and local lactation consultant affiliates

✔ Advocating for our profession

✔ Evaluating and monitoring our skills through client and peer review

✔ Forming collaborative relationships with mother-support groups, professionals, and other related sources of breast-feeding help and support in our community

RESPONSIBILITIES OF THE PRIVATE PRACTICE LACTATION CONSULTANT

NOTES

1. Wieser, L. How best to learn clinical lactation skills: A survey of practicing lactation consultants. Masters' thesis through Pacific Oaks College/Lactation Institute, Pasadena, CA, 1991.

2. Kutner, L., and Barger, J. *Clinical Experience in Lactation: A Blueprint for Internship.* Chalfont, PA: Breastfeeding Support Consultants, 1997.

3. Turner, M. R. Twenty questions for the consumer: A quality assurance tool for the lactation consultant. *Journal of Human Lactation* 1996;12(1):50053.

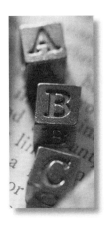

22 Other Aspects of PPLC Work

Linda J. Smith, BSE, FACCE, IBCLC

Providing clinical support services is helping mothers and babies "from the bottom up," at the grassroots level. This work alone can be enormously satisfying and rewarding, encouraging us to constantly sharpen our skills, strengthen our knowledge, and broaden our attitudes for the crucial up-close work we do with mothers and babies.

However, as Kevin Frick stated in his foreword to this book, "The policy process will continue to move ahead whether you take an active role or not." We also need to work "from the top down" if we hope to transform (or return) our culture into a breastfeeding culture. Policies, legislation, legal cases, education, and marketing efforts will be created while we're up to our proverbial elbows in sore nipples. Some of these policy activities will benefit PPLCs, whereas others may not be in our best interest or in the best interest of our clients. Therefore, we all need to carve out time and energy for other aspects of promoting, protecting, and supporting breastfeeding and the lactation consultant profession. This chapter discusses some of these activities, but it certainly does not cover *everything* an individual PPLC might do to achieve worldwide health goals.

"Each one, teach one" was one of ILCA's campaign themes for a time. Educating the general public on the importance of breastfeeding and the role of lactation consultants is an ongoing responsibility. Promotion activities include, but are not limited to, the following:

- Volunteer to discuss breastfeeding with high school "marriage and family" or other appropriate classes.
- Present a lecture to the local Rotary International or Kiwanis club.
- Join the chamber of commerce and advertise your business in chamber forums. (This is also good business!)
- Write letters to local and national newspapers, TV and radio program hosts, and other media outlets.
- Write letters to local, state, and national legislators.
- Join related coalitions and organizations, and bring up the topic of breastfeeding where appropriate (e.g., the local SIDS task force).
- Wear breastfeeding-themed clothing, jewelry, and other items (in appropriate places).

ACTIVITIES THAT PROMOTE BREASTFEEDING: THINK *ADVERTISE BREASTFEEDING*

- Participate in a World Walk for Breastfeeding or some other community-wide activity.

- Coordinate, create, or support World Breastfeeding Week events. These activities could include press releases, displays, open house receptions, and so on. Action Kits for WBW themes are available from WABA (www.waba.org.br), La Leche League International (www.lalecheleague.org), ILCA (www.ilca.org), and other sources.

- Publicize reputable sources of information on breastfeeding, including those listed in the appendices.

ACTIVITIES THAT PROTECT BREASTFEEDING: THINK *LAWS OR POLICIES*

- Testify at governmental hearings on health issues. For example, see my testimony before the Ohio Women's Policy Commission (http://www.bflrc.com/ljs/news/testwprc.htm) and the Greater Miami Valley Breastfeeding Coalition's testimony for the Ohio Department of Health's Title V Maternal and Child Health Block Grant (http://www.ohio-olca.org/news/article/Block%20Grant%202000.htm).

- Research how health policy is made in your community. Find a way to serve on local, statewide, or national committees that influence public policy. For example, Kay Hoover worked closely with other PPLCs to create Philadelphia's city-wide breastfeeding policy. I serve on the U.S. Breastfeeding Committee—for information and the National Agenda, see www.usbreastfeeding.org.

- Make yourself available as an expert witness for breastfeeding mothers and babies involved in divorce, custody, employment, or other civil cases. See "The ABC's of Testifying at a Deposition or at a Trial" in *Core Curriculum for Lactation Consultant Practice*, (pages 492–498) and http://www.lalecheleague.org/LawMain.html.

- Work with local employers to establish work-site lactation programs. Corporate lactation programs are often great business opportunities, and truly a win-win-win situation for the PPLC, mothers and babies, and businesses. See *Business, Babies, and the Bottom Line* by the Washington Business Group on Health.[1]

- Work with professional associations on policy documents. For example, Carol Ryan helped write AWHONN's *Standards and Guidelines for Professional Nursing Practice in the Care of Women and Newborns*, fifth edition (pages 18–19).

- Support UNICEF's *Baby-Friendly Hospital Initiative* (http://www.unicef.org/bfhi or babyfriendlyusa.org) and the *Mother Friendly Childbirth Initiative* (www.motherfriendly.org).

- Work with local hospitals, clinics, health agencies, and school systems to develop appropriate policies for breastfeeding. These institutions may be required to have one or more community representatives on their governing or policy-making committees. For example, I served on a task force charged with developing a family life (sex education) program for all the public schools in our county (kindergarten through twelfth grade). I provided substantial input into the issues of when and how breastfeeding was included in the curriculum and staff training program for the curriculum.

- Participate in a *Code* monitoring project, or work to raise awareness of un-ethical marketing practices of some companies. For example, see the letter on "Gift Packs" in Appendix D that our local coalition prepared for a hos-pital, *Breaking the Rules 2001* from IBFAN, and *Selling Out Mothers and Babies* by NABA.

- Work with insurance companies to establish programs supporting breast-feeding. Some examples of how you might do so appear in *Advancing Women's Health: Health Plans' Innovative Programs in Breastfeeding Promotion* (http://www.4woman.gov/owh/pub/breastfeeding/).

- Stay up-to-date with government policies on breastfeeding. Many U.S. poli-cies are on or available through the Centers for Disease Control and Prevention Web site (www.cdc.gov/breastfeeding).

Roberta Graham de Escobedo writes of her experience with advocacy in Mexico:

Strike While the Iron Is Hot, or Avoiding Sins of Omission

After 71 years of one-party rule, Mexico finally experienced a change of leadership in the person of President Vicente Fox. As President-elect, Mr. Fox encouraged the citizenry to participate in the writing of this new chapter in Mexico's history by offering their sug-gestions, proposals, and ideas. "We want your input," he said over and over in his ad-dresses to the country.

My first corporate lactation program in an assembly plant in the state of Yucatan had been up and running for about 18 months, and four more factories had joined the ranks of companies offering work-site breastfeeding support to their workers. "Why couldn't this model be replicated in other parts of the country?" I asked myself. Wouldn't the new President-elect be interested in a program that would have a positive impact on pro-ductivity in the workplace, and also affect the health and well-being of the country's in-fants and families?

An inner voice kept chanting, "Write to Fox, write to Fox!" I decided to obey after contemplating a scenario in the future where an 80-year-old me was sitting around with friends over steaming cups of coffee, as I recounted how, back when President Fox took office, I really meant to write to him about corporate lactation. To commit a sin of omis-sion, that is to say, doing harm by *not* taking action, seemed an awful price to pay when the risk was so small. After all, if I sent a proposal to the new President-elect the burden would shift to his shoulders, and my conscience would be clear! And so, I faxed Mr. Fox.

Amazingly, *only 20 days later* I received an e-mail response from a person in the tran-sition team involved in the creation of social programs focusing on women's needs. And so began the back and forth of e-mail correspondence between an IBCLC and the tran-sition team of a newly elected president.

After President Fox took office on December 1, 2000, and named his cabinet mem-bers, once again that inner voice took up its chant: "Write to the Secretary of Labor and Welfare!"

In March 2001 I sent a formal proposal to the Secretary of Labor and Welfare ex-plaining how work-site support of breastfeeding would be beneficial to all parties in-volved in the workplace. Mentioning how provision for breastfeeding breaks was already a part of Mexico's Labor Law gave additional credibility to the proposal. All that was lack-ing was a clear plan to make the benefits of the law a reality for Mexico's working women. Corporate lactation was the answer.

The proposal was well received and immediately passed on to the Assistant Secretary of Welfare, who in turn gave instructions to the Office of Gender Equality under his ju-risdiction to integrate the concept of corporate lactation into the administration's three new lines of action promoting women's rights in the workplace. The other two lines of action are concerned with sexual harassment in the workplace and not using pregnancy as a reason for hiring or firing a female employee.

In addition to these actions by the Secretary of Labor and Welfare on a national level, additional attention was recently given to the importance of breastfeeding through the

Secretariat of Social Welfare (similar to the Department of Health and Human Services in the United States).

This secretariat coordinates all the programs whose beneficiaries are those individuals who live in extreme poverty. PROGRESA, the nation?s most important social welfare program, is concerned with three main concepts: education, health, and nutrition. Breastfeeding is intimately related to all three of these concerns, and so I was invited to lead a workshop on breastfeeding in Fall 2001 at several regional meetings held all around the country for the program's community liaisons (women who coordinate the program at the grassroots level in their villages).

These initiatives on a national level, through two different government secretariats, are a direct result of one lone lactation consultant taking advantage of a window of opportunity opened due to a change in political leadership, listening to that inner voice, and taking an action that was really quite small. In this case, faxing a proposal to a newly elected political leader got the ball rolling. The universality and nobility of breastfeeding then took over, working its special magic to effect positive change.

I have witnessed the sincere interest shown by people in government when the topic of breastfeeding is discussed, and I have no doubt that you will be able to make even greater inroads in your own community. Just keep your eyes open, your ear to the ground, your confidence high, and your resolve firm. Any change in local, state, or national leadership is an opportunity waiting to be seized. Carpe diem!

ACTIVITIES THAT SUPPORT BREASTFEEDING: THINK *PREVENT AND SOLVE PROBLEMS*

Of course, your private practice is your primary way of supporting breastfeeding! Here's where you can enhance your standing as part of the health care team.

- Turn your client reports into "teaching reports" sent to the mothers' health care providers in your community. This strategy is a very effective way to both publicize your practice and raise the skill and knowledge of other professionals.

- Maintain and distribute a list of other providers of relevant services or care in your area. This group includes, but is not limited to, breast pump rental and sales outlets, bra suppliers, stores and catalogs where breastfeeding garments are sold, other lactation consultants, hospitals and clinics with lactation support services, WIC clinics with good breastfeeding support and/or peer counselors, and La Leche League and/or other mother-support groups. The list could even include businesses that have made a commitment to being "breastfeeding-friendly."

- Keep up-to-date clinically by

  —Attending conferences and workshops, including ILCA conferences.

  —Reading professional journals, especially the *Journal of Human Lactation*.

  —Searching Medline and other databases for clinically relevant articles.

  —Compiling your own library of books and research articles.

  —Participating in on-line discussion groups for lactation professionals.

  —Arranging for periodic peer review of your practice.

  —Taking or expanding your skills through ancillary training programs (e.g., physical assessent, CPR, oral-motor assessment, cranial-sacral therapy).

  —Seeking further formal education related to breastfeeding (bachelor, masters, and PhD programs are now available—see Appendix B).

— Maintaining membership in professional associations, especially ILCA and local ILCA affiliates.

— Maintaining your IBLCE certification.

• Conduct formal research on pertinent topics, and maintain a list of topics that need more research.

• Present lectures, in-service programs, courses, or seminars to health care professionals. When you are preparing to teach peers and professionals, you'll be even more motivated to thoroughly research the topic you're presenting!

• Create your own policy manual, especially including clinical policies that will be used by all employees and partners/clinicians in your practice.

Wow! That's a lot, and it's only a partial list of possibilities. Obviously, you can't do everything. Pick and choose wisely, and consider the business aspect of everything you do. The bottom line is this: *Work as a team player*. Everyone involved in breastfeeding promotion, protection, and support is working toward the same goals, and the more friends and colleagues we have on our team, the better! This cooperation is what "creating a community safety net" is all about.

SUMMARY

Lactation consultants in private practice primarily provide direct services to breastfeeding families. In addition, and as time allows, participating in activities that promote and protect breastfeeding itself will help strengthen the community safety net for mothers and babies. Likewise, improving clinical skills—both our own and those of other professionals—will help strengthen the network of support for women and children in our society.

NOTES

1. Jacobson, M., Kolarek, M. H., and Newton, M. *Business, Babies, and the Bottom Line: Corporate Innovations and Best Practices in Maternal and Child Health*. Washington, DC: National Business Partnership to Improve Family Health and the Washington Business Group on Health, 1996, www.wbgh.com.

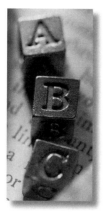

23 Realities of Private Practice

Patricia Lindsey, IBCLC
Pamela Morrison, IBCLC

PATRICIA LINDSEY, IBCLC

I am both a staff lactation consultant for a pediatric office and the owner of a private practice that operates as part of the pediatric office. I was a La Leche League (LLL) Leader for 18 years when I began to think about becoming an International Board Certified Lactation Consultant (IBCLC). First, I contacted a lactation consultant in private practice and asked if I could shadow her for a few days to learn more about the differences between being a LLL Leader and an IBCLC. By the end of the week, I knew that being an IBCLC was what I wanted to do. I also felt I had much to learn, so for the next 18 months I worked as a LC apprentice or intern doing clinical work. I sat for the IBCLE exam in 1996.

While doing my internship with the private practice LC, I met several doctors who referred their patients to that LC's private practice. Some physicians allowed us to do the lactation visit in their office, which is how I met the pediatricians for whom I now work.

HOW MY PRACTICE STARTED

After sitting for the IBCLE exam, but before I even had the results, one of the pediatricians called me at home to ask me about my plans as an IBCLC. He went on to say that he would like me to work in his office, seeing his breastfeeding mothers. I was completely surprised. We met with the office manager and the other pediatrician in the office to hash out the details. I began seeing patients within a few weeks of our first talk. I initially worked only part-time in the office on a contract basis. After a first year filled with overwhelming client satisfaction, I became a salaried employee with benefits.

It was also agreed that I could meet with private patients if any were referred to me. Because the office lacked enough space to have an assessment room or office for lactation, I started out in a pediatrician owner's personal office. The office purchased a recliner for the mothers to sit in while breastfeeding, and I ordered pumps and supplies from Medela as well as a BabyWeigh™ Scale.

The physician owner had been in private practice for about nine years and had one other pediatrician working with him, who became a full partner about six months later. The practice had a large clientele for a two-doctor, one-nurse-practitioner office and was ready for more growth. The caregivers had always encouraged breastfeeding and tried their best to support the breastfeeding mother and baby. When they brought me on board, they began to publicize the fact that they had a lactation consultant on staff to help with breastfeeding. Mostly by word of mouth, they marketed their practice as the breastfeeding friendly pediatric practice and the results were amazing. Within two years of my joining the practice, they had added three doctors and another nurse practitioner to the staff as well as doubled the physical size of the building. A major consideration when building onto the existing building was the needs of the breastfeeding mothers and myself. A nicely sized room was designated as the breastfeeding suite, and I was given my own office for assessments and management of my services. As Jay Gordon, MD, speaking at the 1997 La Leche League International conference in Washington, D.C., noted, "If a pediatric office wants to grow quickly, just have an IBCLC on staff and get the word out and the moms will come." This was surely the case with our office.

I've now been in the pediatric office for more than six years. I work full-time, seeing both the pediatric practice's patients and my private patients. I rent more than 60 pumps as well as sell breast pumps, breastfeeding supplies, and parenting aids. My private practice remains separate from the pediatric office patients so far as the billing and recordkeeping are concerned. I run my pump rentals and retail sales through my private practice.

HOW I OPERATE

As staff lactation consultant for the pediatric practice, mothers and babies are encouraged to see me for four specific lactation visits:

- *First visit: recommended during the first week after birth, and preferably between 3-5 days*. During this visit, I assess the baby's weight and oral anatomy and any breast problems the mother may be experiencing. I observe a breastfeeding session and suggest improvements in comfort, latching-on, attachment, and positioning techniques. At this time, I also answer questions about newborn behaviors. This first visit usually lasts about one hour.

- *Second visit: recommended at weeks 3-6*. During this visit, we discuss any unresolved breastfeeding issues and the introduction of a bottle for either occasional feedings or the mother's return to work. We discuss scheduling, pumping, care, and storage of breast milk.

- *Third visit: recommended at 5-6 months*. This visit focuses on the developmental signs to notice in preparation for starting solid foods. We discuss how to start solids and cup feeding without compromising the mother's milk supply.

- *Fourth visit: the weaning visit*. This visit occurs whenever the mother is ready to wean from the breast to either a bottle or a cup. We discuss how to wean so as to make a gentle transition for the baby, and also how to wean so that the mother will not experience any breast discomfort caused by weaning too quickly.

- *Other visits:* Anytime a concern or problem with breastfeeding or the mother's comfort arises.

Most of our breastfeeding mothers and babies do see me for the first visit, with fewer seeing me for the other visits. The first visit is billed as a sick visit using 779.3 (feeding difficulties of a newborn 28 days or younger). It is usually a level 4 visit because it will take at least 60 minutes. Before I meet with the mother and baby, the mother fills out an intake form with information on her family and her general health, pregnancy, and breastfeeding history as well as a brief history of the baby. During this visit, I do a general assessment of the baby's oral cavity, a naked weigh, and a general assessment of the baby's responsiveness and color. I assess the mother's breast and nipples and then teach optimal latch-on techniques. I observe a feeding and take a test weight before and after the feeding to determine intake. I offer guidance about breastfeeding in the first two weeks of life and a picture of normal newborn behavior. This early intervention usually necessitates only some fine-tuning of latch-on and positioning techniques and suggested care path for sore nipples and/or engorgement.

At the first visit, I see many of the usual breastfeeding challenges that necessitate intervention and/or development of a care path to overcome either a maternal or infant problem. Many times, these issues require follow-up either by phone or another office visit. Referrals are also made to me by the pediatrician or nurse practitioner if the baby's weight gain is not optimal or concerns arise regarding overfeeding, excessive crying, or spitting-up. When a baby is more than 28 days old, the diagnosis code used is 783.3 (feeding difficulties and/or mismanagement of infant to elderly). Follow-up visits or visits in which I spend only about 30 minutes are billed at a level 3.

I chart the assessment information I gathered on my own evaluation and management forms in the baby's chart. Care paths and interventions for improved feedings are also documented here as well. The evaluation and management form is then signed under my signature by the baby's pediatrician. I always include my time spent on the visit in my charting, a necessary step to justify the level of visit billed. Through charting and documentation with physician signature and use of appropriate third-party billing codes, we have enjoyed good results with insurance reimbursement.

PAYMENT FOR SERVICES AND THIRD-PARTY REIMBURSEMENT: PART 1

The American Academy of Pediatrics encourages reimbursement of lactation support in its policy statement on "Breastfeeding and the Use of Human Milk" (*Pediatrics*, vol. 100, No. 6, December 1997, pp. 1035–1039). We did our homework and studied the coding and billing issues. One of our best references for billing for lactation visits in a pediatric office appeared in the *Pediatric Coding Alert* (December 1998, pp. 95–96).

You must consider some special issues when thinking about reimbursement in a physician office. Whether an office is an HMO or PPO in which the physician has a capitated contract instead of a fee-for-service contract can make a big difference in generating revenue to justify paying a salary to a lactation consultant. Capitated contracts pay physicians so much per person per month on the plan. In such a case, the physician gets a set amount per number of persons assigned under the contract, whether those patients visit the office or not. Under this arrangement, the physician profits more when there are fewer office visits. In contrast, physicians who have fee-for-service contracts bill for each office visit and are paid per visit. These offices profit more when there are more office visits, so these practices will be positioned to reap financial benefits from offering the services of a lactation consultant. Why is it important to be a financial benefit to the physician's practice? Because doctors are in business to make money, as well as to serve patients. The bottom line of most businesses is profit.

The ideal physician office in which a lactation consultant can work to generate financial benefit is either a pediatric office or a family practice office. In the pediatric office, all coding must reflect that the infant is the patient. Sore nipples and engorgement become feeding difficulties for the baby so as to code the visit as a baby problem. In a family practice, coding could be for the mother, the baby, or both.

Being on staff in an obstetric office has its shortcomings when it comes to reimbursement. In the insurance world, *bundling*, or *universal billing*, occurs when a flat charge is paid for a complete service. Obstetricians receive a flat fee for prenatal care, delivery, and six weeks postnatal care. They are paid one fee for a vaginal delivery and another fee for a cesarean section, but the six weeks postnatal are included in the flat fee. Thus the lactation consultant could not bill for reimbursement of services under the obstetrician's name during the six-week postnatal period and expect additional payment for those services. As most problems with breastfeeding occur in the first few weeks, having an LC does not provide a financial benefit to the obstetrician's practice.

Other considerations with billing in the pediatric office apply as well. The best reimbursement comes from the baby being seen by only one physician or provider in the same day in the same office. To achieve the best reimbursement, then, the mother would have to bring the baby to the pediatrician for the newborn visit or well-baby checkup on one day and then to the lactation consultant on another day. This scenario is not always ideal.

In our office, we try to determine the most urgent need of the mother–baby pair when the newborn visit is scheduled. We see all our babies at three-to-five days after discharge from the hospital and again at two weeks. If a mother feels the breastfeeding problem is most urgent, she might see me on the first visit out of the hospital and then return to have the baby seen by the pediatrician for the newborn three- to five-day visit on the following day. Alternatively, if the baby is being seen by the pediatrician and he sees that the most important thing is saving the breastfeeding, he will switch the visits and have the mother see me that day and return the following day to see him. Likewise, if I see a four-day-old baby to help with the breastfeeding and the baby is excessively sleepy and glowing like an illuminated pumpkin, I will ask to switch to a physician visit. In this case, I would still work with the mother and baby to achieve an optimal care path to support breastfeeding. We would then bill with modifier 77, which deals with two providers seeing the same patient in the same day in the same office. This modifier doesn't result in consistent reimbursement. Some insurers pay well, whereas others do not pay at all for the second visit. Bottom line—in our office, we do whatever is in the baby's best interest and supports the breastfeeding regardless of reimbursement. Ideally, all physician offices would be equally committed to breastfeeding. Also, because of universal or bundled billing, pediatricians are paid a set fee for their hospital care of the baby whether for two days or four days; for this reason, I do not make rounds at the hospital. No financial benefit arises from my going to the hospital, and the hospitals have their own lactation consultants who can assist the mother during the hospital stay.

My private practice works differently. I do not accept insurance assignment in my private practice. I work strictly on a fee-for-service basis, with payment at the time of service. I do give the patient a receipt for visit.

PAYMENT FOR SERVICES AND THIRD-PARTY REIMBURSEMENT: PART 2

It's a very professional superbill that I developed myself after doing much research on insurance coding and billing. I call my superbill the lactation visit receipt (LVR). For ordering information and to view it, go to http://patlc.com/id41.htm. Along with the LVR, I give the patient instructions on filing for insurance reimbursement. I don't perform insurance assignment because it would necessitate my hiring someone to bill the insurance company, follow up on payment, and then wait three to six months or more for payment. I just don't think it's worth the trouble. I provide a valuable service, and I deserve to be paid in a timely manner. After all, if the choice is seeing me for a lactation visit or using formula, I'm much, much less costly.

MARKETING AND ADVERTISING

I market myself to all the pediatricians, obstetricians, and hospitals without outpatient lactation support services in my area. Marketing is an ongoing necessity to support my practice. If I let several months go by without doing some type of marketing to area physicians, then I start to see a slight decline in my private patients. If your name doesn't surface in physicians' offices often, then they tend to forget about you. In the early years, I would make appointments with the nurse managers of pediatric and obstetric offices. I would take in brochures and business cards, and sometimes cakes or cookies. Today, I don't have time to make these visits. Here are some of the things I do to keep my name out there, instead:

- I'm listed in the phone book.
- I'm listed on the task force breastfeeding resource list that is distributed to all physicians, clinics, and hospitals in the area.
- I take advantage of the Medela mailing at least twice per year. Medela will do two mailings per year to promote your services and pump rental and sales. You furnish the company with a cover letter and the names and addresses of the physicians for the mailing. Medela will also do two mailings per year to promote your services and rentals of its BabyWeigh™ Scale.
- I send out Christmas cards with a special "thank you" note every December.
- Each quarter, I try to do a mailing with business cards and flyers to be placed in new-patient bags (most likely they will go in formula "gift" bags).
- I take advantage of Medela's cooperative advertising reimbursement. I advertise only Medela pump rentals and pump in styles in a local parenting publication. Medela offers reimbursement for the advertising based on my annual lease and purchases from the previous year. Ask your Medela representative for more information or call the company directly.
- I have a Web site, www.PatLC.com. I developed the Web site for a specific reason—not to do Internet sales, but rather to help with my shopping callers. I was getting numerous shopping calls per day. How much is your pump rental? Do you have pump in styles, and what is the price? How much is an office visit? I built the Web site to answer shoppers' questions and to do local advertising. By placing my Web site address on my flyers, business cards, and pager, many mothers will have visited my Web site prior to calling my office. They are then better prepared to either make an appointment or schedule for pump rental or sale. The Web site has saved me tons of time. I built my Web site with very easy-to-use Web site builders software called TrellixWeb.

When I started out six years ago, I had one or two private patients per month. Today, I see one to two private patients per day. I receive almost as many referrals from my former patients as I do from hospitals or physicians. Word of mouth is definitely the most rewarding of referrals, because it reflects your delivery of appreciated services.

I use the pediatric office phone number on my business cards. My private patients are scheduled just as my patients in the pediatric practice are, with one exception. My private patients are informed that I am not a provider on any insurance plan and that my services are provided on a fee-for-service basis at the time of service. I charge a flat fee for first-time patients and a flat fee for follow-up visits. This system keeps matters simple for me. I pay the pediatric office 20 percent of all my private-patient fees to offset the staff support required.

My private patients come into the pediatric office and sign in to see me just as the pediatric practice patients do. Patients are taken to the breastfeeding suite to fill out my consent/financial form and a history form. The breastfeeding suite has two recliners, three other chairs, nursing stools, and pillows. A TV/VCR is available so that mothers can watch either Marshall Klaus's *Talents of the Amazing Newborn* or Johnson & Johnson's *Infant Massage* video, or mothers can read copies of *New Beginnings* while waiting to see me. I try to stick to a schedule, but it's not always possible when working at the individual mother–baby pace. Few mothers become upset about waiting. Occasionally, I have used the breastfeeding suite as an assessment room; I can then go back and forth between the two rooms. At the end of the visit, I fill out the lactation visit receipt with charges and send the mother to the checkout person to pay the bill. My private-patient payments are kept separate, but this system keeps me from having to deal with payments and helps me to move along to the next patient more quickly.

I use the same evaluation and management form with my private patients as with the pediatric practice patients, with one exception: I don't have a physician signature on my private patient forms. This form serves three purposes. First, it represents a medical record of the visit. Second, I fax a copy to the mom and/or baby's physician as a consult report of visit. Third, it serves to justify the charges for the visit and can be requested by the patient's insurance company. For these reasons, it is essential that this form be completed fully with documented time of visit. It is then filed with the consent/financial form as a permanent record. (The consent/financial form also gives consent for release of information concerning the visit to health care providers and insurance companies.)

During all lactation visits, the infant is unclothed and the diaper removed to perform a naked weigh. The infant is then redressed in a diaper only, and a prefeeding weigh is done. The mother sits in a recliner, and any family members sit across from the mother. I do a general assessment of the infant's color and responsiveness and inspect the infant's oral anatomy. I then inspect the mother's nipples and breast for any problems. All information gathered is recorded on the evaluation and management form as well as any intervention or care path. Next, I observe a feeding, providing teaching and instruction for improved feedings. A postfeeding weigh is done at the end of the feeding. I

DOCUMENTATION

discuss key points in the history form, provide an overview of handouts pertaining to this visit, and answer any questions. The visit always ends with my giving the mother a couple of my business cards and reinforcing the importance of calling me with questions and concerns or to discuss changes in the care path.

SUPPLIES AND EQUIPMENT

In the hallway outside my office, there are shelves with pumps, breastfeeding supplies, and a lending library. I sell pumps by Medela, Hollister, and Bailey Medical. I sell baby slings, Happy Baby™ food grinders, and herbs. I also sell most all breastfeeding supplies, including pump parts. I rent Medela Classics and Lactinas™ and Hollister Lact-Es™ and Elites™. I have educated the front-office staff via an in-service program on how to rent pumps and assist mothers with finding parts to pumps. If staff members have a question and I'm not in the building, they page me.

After three years of tracking pumps and billing for pumps in the evenings or on weekends, I obtained part-time help to take over the tracking and billing responsibilities. During the first few years, I used my down time when I had fewer patients to write handouts, track and bill for pumps, and market my business. In the past two years, I've had very little down time.

BUSINESS MANAGEMENT

Setting up a private practice is a business endeavor like any other business. It can be both costly in terms of start-up expenses and risky. I was fortunate to have learned from the pitfalls of other private practice lactation consultants who had gone out of business largely because their bills exceeded their income and/or they mismanaged funds. I also give credit to Kathleen Auerbach and Jan Riordan's *Breastfeeding and Human Lactation*, Chapter 20, "Working Strategies and the Lactation Consultant," for good business advice. In their 1993 edition, they state, "The average length of time LCs are in business before they are no longer putting their profits back into the practice is three years. In some cases, LCs make a profit within two years. The higher the overhead, the longer it takes before earnings exceed the costs of doing business." When I started my private practice, I loaned myself $2000 for furniture, liability insurance, and breastfeeding supplies. My goal was to pay myself back in one year. I was able to pay myself back in six months, but then I left every penny of profit in the bank and did not take an owner's draw for the first two years. It helped that I was drawing a salary from the pediatric practice. Of course, to get my business off to a sound start with a potential of earning a profit, I had to sacrifice my time and endure the lack of pay.

I make sure that all the bills are paid monthly. I keep a reserve fund for paying quarterly sales taxes; quarterly estimated self-employment taxes, yearly liability insurance, continuing education, and yearly association dues. I make sure that my running balance exceeds all outstanding bills, such as my pump leases, which are billed 30 days in arrears, as well as enough to ship all my pumps back if I suddenly had to close my practice. My business always comes before my being paid a salary from the private practice. I have never had a carryover of pump lease fees and have always paid for all inventories at the time of purchase. For me, this is just good business; I have to take care of the business first for it to have the potential to take care of me.

It's important to have both short-term and long-term goals when setting up a private practice. My short-term goals were for the business to stand on its own, to show steady growth, to be known for my integrity, and to be recognized as a valuable professional allied health care specialist in my community. My long-term goals are to grow to a size that I can hire an LC to work with me and offer prospective LCs clinical opportunities.

I have enjoyed steady growth, with the number of private patients nearly doubling each year. I'm now at a point of mothers telling me that their obstetricians referred them as well as their pediatricians, hospitals, and friends. The pediatric office in which I work just hired a new doctor. When he was introduced to me, he said, "I've heard a lot about you." I smiled and said, "I hope the doctors said good things about me." He said, "Oh no, not from the doctors here. My wife and I were at a school function, and it seemed as if all the mothers with babies said you were their lactation consultant." He was most impressed with the fact that the mothers went to different pediatricians around the city and were referred to me by these doctors. For me, this result represents the best of success—having high patient satisfaction and the respect of the medical community.

LESSONS LEARNED

So far, it might sound as if I have a little piece of heaven. Of course, there are also drawbacks and downsides:

- By my own choice, I'm on call 24 hours a day, 7 days a week, 365 days a year. From my years with La Leche League, I feel strongly that an LC must be available to her patients at all times—after all formula is. When I go to a conference, take a few days off, or go on vacation, I have no one to triage my phone calls or see my mothers. Therefore, my pager and my cell phone go where I go, and I triage even when I'm on vacation. We do have one hospital that offers outpatient lactation, to which I refer mothers who need immediate help.

- In the beginning of my practice, I did lots of follow-up calls. These experiences were as valuable to me as to the patients. Without follow-up, I don't know how you would know if the care path was helpful and how you would grow in knowledge of practice. As my practice became busier, I couldn't call to follow up on every patient. There just aren't enough hours in a day. Today, my consent form states that it is the responsibility of the patient to call me to discuss progress, continued problems, and changes in care paths. I also stress this point in the visit. Every patient receives my business card with my office phone, pager number, Web site address, and e-mail address. I actively do follow-up only on those patients with whom I'm most concerned.

- Because I have only part-time help, the phone often goes to voicemail and I call patients or perspective patients back when I get a chance. I inform my patients that I don't answer the phone or return calls when I'm with a patient unless it's an emergency; otherwise, they can expect a return call in the late afternoon or early evening.

- Another consideration of being self-employed is the extra taxes you have to pay. When hired by an employer, the employee pays only half the Social Security tax and the employer pays the other half. Not so when you are self-employed: The self-employed individual pays both shares. The first year my husband and I filed our income tax return after I started my private practice, we had to pay several thousand dollars in income tax. My husband said, "You have an expensive hobby." The following year, I spoke with an accountant and started paying quarterly self-employment taxes. I also set up a SEP-IRA to help reduce the amount of taxes I would owe each year. I would advise anyone setting up a small business to speak with an accountant or take a small business course at a community college. Also, you must keep records and receipts of everything.

Are you beginning to figure out that I put in a lot of hours in exchange for a very modest income? I can't measure my success in dollars earned per hour. That's not why I work as an LC. Yes, getting paid is important. It helps keep my husband happier about my working so much. I feel what I do is a sort of ministry in helping mothers learn to love their babies (Titus 2:3–4). I have a passion for mothers, babies, and families. I also feel that I'm a pioneer in the field of lactation consulting. I'm helping to build a reputation for the importance of good lactation help. Perhaps someday in the future, a standard in pediatric care will be to have an LC on staff in every pediatric setting. Pioneers often make sacrifices to pave the future for others in their field. I sacrifice my time, but it's truly my labor of love.

RECOMMENDATIONS

Not everyone will enjoy the good fortune that I had, when physicians knocked on my door and asked me to become part of their practice. I would like to share a few ideas that you might want to consider in proposing a lactation position to a physician:

- Look for a pediatric or family practice office that is breastfeeding-friendly and (ideally) has enough physical space for you to operate in the office.
- Choose a practice that only has fee-for-service insurance reimbursement contracts.
- List the advantages of having an LC on staff:
  1. Revenue for lactation visits
  2. Marketing to bring in parents who choose to breastfeed and wish to have optimal help available
  3. Savings in terms of physician and staff time (They don't have to spend time discussing feeding problems or answering breastfeeding questions, as these are referred to you for office visits or triage.)
  4. Client appreciation (New parents feel that their physician is supporting them in their choice to breastfeed when they are offered reliable help.)
- Keep your proposal flexible. You might suggest initially being a contract employee as opposed to a salaried employee. Don't go in with a fixed proposal; have options.
  1. You might ask to do a 60- or 90-day trial of your services asking for 50–60 percent of revenues that you generate.
  2. If office space is available, you might ask for use of that space to set up private practice in exchange for seeing a certain number of the practice's patients per month or a percentage of revenue for its patients. State explicitly the advantages of your having a private practice in the office.

3. When private clients come into the physician's office to see you, it show-cases the practice. Your clients may change care providers to come to this office because it is viewed as breastfeeding-supportive.

4. Your private clients will share with their friends their impressions of the office in which you work. Again, this is good marketing for the practice.

- Think of the first 60-90 days of working in the physician office as showing what you can do for the practice, and then renegotiate at the end of the 60- to 90-day period. You are proving your worth. During this period, you must keep good records of the time involved in visits and triage time. If at the end of the trail period, the physician is not willing to give you what you feel you are worth, consider your options:

1. Is there another practice that you might approach?

2. You might continue with this practice, but keep it on a limited time con-tract with renegotiations in another three to six months.

3. Remember it takes time to establish your value and to build a clientele. Be patient.

- Start out little and build as your business grows. If you feel you need to add breast pumps and supplies, start with the bare necessities and then expand slowly as your business grows.

- Know some things about the physician's practice to which you plan to offer your services so as to make a fair offer. Don't expect a small practice with only one to five newborns per month to be able to offer more than what you will bring to the practice. (The practice in which I work averages at least one newborn per day.)

- Are you quitting a job with an established income and a benefits package? If so, you are unlikely to match the income or benefits of the job you are quitting for some time. I once talked with a RN/IBCLC who was an LC at a lactation hospital outpatient clinic and was interested in quitting the hos-pital and working with a group of pediatricians. I suggested that she ask for the lowest amount she need to continue to support her family. The pedia-tricians turned her down because she wanted more than they felt they could justify for her services. Yet, she would have hurt her family and her-self to have asked for less.

- Keep in mind that pediatricians and family practice doctors are generally at the lowest end of income scale for physicians. Before proposing a salary, know what the physicians pay their nurses. Do they have RNs or just LPNs or MAs? What do they pay their nurses? Some LCs think that they should make as much as a nurse practitioner; I disagree. On an average day, a good nurse practitioner could see 20-25 patients, generating about $1500-2000. On my best day, I can see 7-8 breastfeeding dyads and generate about $300-500; on average, I see 3-4 pediatric office patients per day. Most LCs feel they need to ask for more than a nurse, but physicians may not see mat-ters in the same way. Remember, physicians are in business to make money, and they have to consider their overhead.

- If you take a job with a physician office, when the parents thank you for your help, tell them to thank the physicians because they determine whether your services will continue to be part of their practice. *This is very important.* One of my pediatric practice mothers told the physician owner,

"I don't know what you pay Pat, but it's not enough. She is awesome." Make sure you save "thank you" notes and share them with management.

- Bottom line: Be willing to negotiate, be willing to prove yourself and your skills, and be patient.

If you would like to visit my office and/or the pediatric office for which I work, you can visit www.patlc.com or www.pedsplus.com. You may even share our Web sites with the physician to whom you offer your proposal. Whatever type of practice you decide to set up, I wish you success.

PAMELA MORRISON, IBCLC

I have worked in private practice in Zimbabwe for the last 11 years. I suspect that I have the most wonderful job in the world—working as the only lactation consultant in a country where breastfeeding is the cultural norm.

I HAD A DREAM...

Late in 1989, two lactation consultants came to Zimbabwe to present at a landmark workshop for senior Ministry of Health and hospital staff, which was to mark the beginning of an aggressive and effective national breastfeeding-promotion campaign. One of them told me about her "dream job" as a lactation consultant in Europe. Although it had never been done before, and the IBCLC profession, still in its infancy, was completely unknown, it seemed that there might be a gap that could be filled by an inexperienced, but enthusiastic, pioneer. My vision was to address the discrepancy that existed in infant feeding practices between the ordinary African woman, for whom *not* to breastfeed is unthinkable, and the comparatively small, but hugely influential population of socially and economically advantaged mothers, the trend-setters of tomorrow, who enjoyed the luxury of access to private health care but tended to experience so many problems with breastfeeding.

The IBLCE Exam Board accepted me as a candidate and proved incredibly helpful as I commenced trying to set up the exam in Harare, not knowing if I would be the only African candidate for 1990. Obtaining study and exam materials was something of a nightmare. My first order of books was lost en route from the United States. Then, with only days to go before the exam, the Customs Department seized the exam booklets and slides, demanding an exhorbitant amount of duty before they would release what they viewed as "educational materials." The exam itself went off smoothly until the clinical portion, when it was discovered that the young man working the projector had loaded many of the slides upside down or sideways, identifiable in one case only by the direction of the drip milk tracking along the screen. I and my co-candidate, who had arrived unexpectedly at the eleventh hour from Mauritius, were thoroughly unnerved by being asked to leave five minutes into the afternoon session, while the proctors conferred, the slides were reloaded, and everyone hoped for the best!

PLANNING

Where to Start?

The success of my practice has exceeded my wildest dreams, although "floundering around in the dark" is the only way to describe how I set about starting up my practice and becoming known. There were no precedents. I knew of no other LC in private practice, and very little literature was available at that time to guide me. Clarifying how I could work within the health care system and taking care of legal and financial matters seemed to be the most important first steps. Next, it would be necessary to decide which services I wanted to offer and where I wanted to work.

My Office

I converted a small room in my home in Harare into an office, with a desk, couch, filing cabinet, baby scale, sterilizer, and shelves for reference books, pumps, and other equipment. I bought pillows, linens, towels, wipes, and bowls, feeding cups, and spoons. I gave careful thought to developing the forms I would need to keep track of my would-be clients' details, breastfeeding histories, and follow-ups. I also developed some tear-off care plans for common breastfeeding difficulties, and information sheets on various topics, printed in different colors, to use as handouts. In addition to office consults, I had decided to offer home and hospital visits. I therefore needed a bag large enough to hold supplies, and small enough to carry easily. I have since obtained my own computer, which I would recommend to any would-be private practice LC as an absolutely essential item. (See Chapter 12.)

Legal Requirements

Clutching my new IBLCE certificate, I made an appointment with the Registrar of the Health Professions Council, only to be told "you haven't got a snowball's chance in hell of being registered with us." Nevertheless, he confirmed that I was free to practice. I spoke to a lawyer about legal implications and engaged an accountant. I was lucky enough to find a female insurance broker who became fascinated by my plans and managed to talk an insurer into providing me with professional liability insurance. She even obtained a no-claims bonus for me at the beginning of my second year, when it became apparent that the practice of lactation consulting did not constitute a major risk.

Being Available

Being reachable posed something of a problem in those early days. Zimbabwe's phone system is reputedly one of the worst in the world. I shared a party line with nine other subscribers, some of whom would leave their phones off the hook, clogging up the line for days. In the rainy season, the whole line might go dead for a week at a time. There was no chance of obtaining a direct line as the waiting list was several years long. I persuaded some friends, a husband and wife who ran a home business, to act as my answering service. If my phone went "off," I would collect my messages two or three times each day and find some way to get back to my waiting clients. The husband became quite good, over the years, at soothing distraught mothers and offering basic breastfeeding tips until I could get back to them. Finally, I managed to persuade a sympathetic technician to take pity on my mother–baby clients and speed up my application. The luxury of having my own direct phone line still has not palled. Nowadays the availability of cell-phone networks in Zimbabwe makes everything easier still.

Reimbursement

My husband developed a computerized invoicing system for me. Even so, the question of how to charge clients for consultations was problematic, because I was used to working as a volunteer. I decided to charge slightly less than a physiotherapist, to charge strictly by time, and to invoice each client at the successful resolution of her problem, on the rationale that a client would be more inclined to keep following up with me if she didn't need to pay cash for every consultation. This system has worked well. I often worked with a single mother–baby dyad over several months, hiring out or selling equipment to them, and only invoicing at the end of the problem. Unexpectedly encouraging was the extremely low rate of bad debts—only two in the first eight years of my practice—which I took as an indication of my clients' level of satisfaction.

The changing economic climate has demanded that I rethink this method of reimbursement and change to a mostly cash basis to remain financially viable. For the LC who wishes to expand a new practice in a strong economy, however, I would still recommend invoicing.

Breastfeeding Aids and Devices

The lactation consultant in a developing country may have access to minimal breastfeeding aids and devices. For instance, I have never seen a hospital-grade double electric pump! Nevertheless, the absence of too much gadgetry can be an advantage. Most of the mothers with whom I work do not have pumps, so I teach hand-expression; with practice, they become very proficient at this technique. Nevertheless, I have found that my success in resolving very severe lactation and breastfeeding difficulties has been enhanced by working to access two items that I now consider absolutely essential: simple but effective manual, cylinder-style breast pumps, and nipple shields. Sometimes it has been necessary to be very persuasive to explain the urgency of these needs to businessmen, to be inventive in finding outside alternative sources of supply, and to plan and budget for these items far in advance so as to cope with delays in ordering, delivery, hold-ups in the customs department, and fluctuations in currency values due to scarce foreign exchange.

Marketing

Once everything else was in place, it was time to let my target audience know that the services of a lactation consultant were available in Harare. Because I wished to be seen as a "professional," I made a conscious decision to follow the example of the other professions in this part of the world, where doctors, health care providers, lawyers, and accountants neither advertise nor actively market their services.

I restrained myself to writing formal letters on my new letterhead to introduce myself and my skills to the best-known obstetricians, pediatricians, and general practitioners (family doctors) in Harare. I followed up my introductory letters by making appointments to meet each one in person, taking little stacks of business cards in the hope that they would hand them out to their patients. None of the doctors had ever heard of a lactation consultant before (their receptionists always said, "A what?"). Consequently, I had no idea how the doctors would react, and I was quite nervous. I described how I hoped to assist mothers with routine and special-circumstance lactation and breast-feeding, asking if they supported breastfeeding (who could say no?), or if they had any special recommendations about how I should work with their patients. I hoped that this meeting would provide them with opportunities to express concerns at the outset, and let them know that I would be careful. My questions elicited a surprising range of answers and allowed me to learn more about each doctor and the way he or she liked to work.

I did not expect the exceptional level of courtesy, interest, and even outright wild enthusiasm with which I was received, often ahead of a waiting room full of patients ("This is a *fantastic* idea!"). I was especially nervous when three of Harare's finest obstetricians wanted to meet me all at once. Unknown to me, however, one of them served on the board of the best private hospital in Harare, and offered to speak to the matron about the possibility of my obtaining visiting privileges. The matron made it clear that I was not to upset her nursing staff, but was otherwise happy to allow me to offer lactation consultations in her hospital.

My Clients

My first client was referred by an acquaintance, and I made a home visit to consult with the mother of a three-week-old breastfed baby with "colic." This experience was quickly followed by a few referrals from some of the doctors I had recently visited. Suddenly, there I was, a lactation consultant in private practice!

I keep a log book recording who I see, and when, also noting the reason, time taken, items of equipment provided, fee, and date paid. In 11 years I have been privileged to work with nearly 3000 mothers and babies, each one unique and fascinating, and many in situations that have proved extremely challenging and demanding. My clients come from all racial and ethnic groups—mostly European mothers of many nationalities, but with a sprinkling of Indian and Colored mothers, and a growing number of sophisticated African women who increasingly experience the same kind and range of breastfeeding difficulties traditionally experienced by their American and European counterparts. Many of my clients come from neighboring countries such as Zambia, Malawi, Mozambique, Botswana, South Africa, Angola, and Mauritius to give birth in the good private hospitals in Zimbabwe. They are often highly motivated to breastfeed because of the primitive conditions and paucity of health care in their countries of residence. I also see many expatriate and diplomatic wives, from all over the globe, each with their own special traditions and expectations.

In Zimbabwe, there is almost 100 percent initiation of breastfeeding, and 39 percent of mothers are still exclusively breastfeeding at four months. Most African mothers in Zimbabwe breastfeed for nearly two years. One becomes aware of practices and trends over time. Where many marginally motivated European women from the middle-income suburbs and farmers' wives used to abandon breastfeeding as they left the hospital, this group will now often breastfeed for at least the first six weeks before giving up. In that time, some of them get "hooked," generating a ripple effect of longer breastfeeding for a whole group of their friends. An increasing number of my clients are exclusively breastfeeding until six months, and many more are breastfeeding well into the second year of life.

The youngest baby I have worked with has been one hour old; the oldest was a six-year-old tandem-nursing with his younger brother. I work with many mothers of twins, and I have even helped one set of triplets. Unbelievably, one of my clients realized that she was pregnant only when she went into labor. I work with first-time mothers of 16, and another mother aged 42. I assist mothers to breastfeed babies with down syndrome, cleft lip/palate, or other congenital abnormalities. African traditional beliefs about babies who cannot breastfeed make these situations especially difficult for the mother, and thus for the LC. The personal risk of working in an environment where 30 percent to 40 percent of all pregnant women test positive for HIV infections on anonymous sentinel surveillance testing also creates its own difficulties and need for self-care and caution.

It has been a special challenge to work with mothers from countries where breastfeeding rates are very low. Some of these women have been somewhat disconcerted to discover that the concept of infant feeding choice is unknown in Zimbabwe's hospitals, because every mother is expected to initiate breastfeeding and enjoy 24-hour rooming-in, and because formula simply is not available for healthy babies. It has been especially rewarding to find that many of these mothers have gone on to breastfeed for long periods, admitting that had they been "at home" they would never have enjoyed this wonderful experience.

Referrals

Referrals can be generated from several sources. First, the doctors of your mother–baby clients can be one of your best resources for referrals and information. One of the most important and fulfilling aspects of working as a lactation consultant in private practice is the development of respectful working relationships with members of the medical profession in your community. The lone lactation consultant working in private practice would be wise to nurture good relationships with her clients' obstetricians, pediatricians, and general practitioners. After several years, I realized that some doctors referred clients to me even without having met me first, which is especially pleasing, because it means that my reputation alone has been enough! Being responsible and professional in reporting to doctors, backing up your care plans with up-to-date citations and references, and sharing interesting items of new research with them will enhance your reputation and increase their trust in your abilities

Second, you can receive referrals from hospital nursing staff. Zimbabwe's strong breastfeeding policy, and the fact that our pediatricians strongly support breastfeeding for all babies, create conditions where hospital nursing staff are, for the most part, already very experienced in assisting mothers to breastfeed. The solo private practice LC in a developing country may find that she is referred clients by nursing staff themselves in three general situations:

- In the extremely difficult situations where the nurses themselves have already exhausted their expertise

- When the hospital is short-staffed (e.g., on weekends or public holidays)

- Where staff perceive that a mother is reluctant to breastfeed and they hope that you persuade her, which can make for some challenging and tricky situations

Third, and probably most importantly, new clients come following word of mouth from former clients. Always remember that each mother you help has the potential to become your ambassador, with the power to influence the number of referrals you receive many years into the future, as she will tell her relations, friends, and doctors about your work.

My clients' initial contact form includes space to record "Referred by...." It can be really fulfilling to hear a new client tell you she was referred by "Oh, everyone! The sister at the clinic, my pediatrician, my sister-in-law who you helped to breastfeed four years ago, and my friend with a two-month-old." Furthermore, you may find that mothers will come back to you with their second or third babies—even if the breastfeeding outcome with their first baby was not what you had hoped.

Logistics

The private practice LC can offer consultations in several different settings. There are benefits and disadvantages to each.

Office Consults

Working from an office in my home serves me and my clients very well. I can save hours of traveling time by having clients come to me and, depending on my workload, I sometimes do so. I also have all the equipment and information materials I might possibly need close at hand.

One disadvantage can be that bored siblings of the nursing baby may race through my office pulling everything off shelves, which both the mother and I find distracting! Another can be that friends or relations may drop a client off and then abandon her with me long past the time that our consultation has ended, so that I am more or less "stuck" with her until she is retrieved. A third problem arises when clients pop in unexpectedly to drop off books, pay bills, or just to show me their beautiful babies. I find it acutely unprofessional, on a day that I anticipated was going to be quiet, to be caught in my caftan and bare feet at 10:30 A.M.! I am lucky to have an excellent male cook/housekeeper in my employ so that I am never alone and thus have no qualms about inviting strangers into my home, but I would imagine that this could be a risk for some LCs.

Home Visits

The private practice LC is able to offer one service that perhaps no one else provides—the chance for a mother to receive tailor-made breastfeeding assistance in the comfort and safety of her own home. Offering this unique service brings both benefits and risks for the LC. The benefits are that you may get more work by offering home visits and can make a more realistic assessment of a mother's individual circumstances and level of support when you see what happens in her home. The disadvantages are that you will use time and fuel to travel to many different locations, leaving you less time to see more clients. You also need to carry with you all equipment, forms, and reference materials that you might conceivably need.

Hospital Visits

The solo LC may have an opportunity to make hospital visits by virtue of the fact that she may possess additional expertise or skills that are needed in especially difficult breastfeeding situations. Nevertheless, you, as the LC, run the risk of aggravating professional jealousy from the midwives employed by the hospital every time you walk through the door. I especially enjoy doing consultations in hospitals. Approximately 25–30 percent of my work takes place in several of Zimbabwe's private hospitals, and occasionally I visit at municipal clinics and government hospitals. I am very careful to appear to be and practice as just one member of the "team." I have learned that, when I am referred to a client by the staff themselves, the case will be one of those "last resort" things, because they will already have done whatever they can to resolve the difficulty themselves. I always make sure to chat to the sister-in-charge, or to the nurse looking after my new client on my way in, listening carefully to the sister's assessment of "the problem." On my way out, I let whoever is responsible know what I thought and what I suggested, thanking them for their help. After several years of hospital visiting, I was asked to write up my consultation briefly in the patient's notes so that everyone could be clear about what I had seen and what I had suggested to resolve the difficulty. This invitation stopped me from feeling like a ghost (wafting in and out of the hospitals with no record of my visit). Now I take a special notepad and carbon paper in my tote bag so that I can copy what I wrote up in the hospital notes, and then staple it to my own consultation form when I return to my home office.

Clients first seen in the hospital are mother–baby pairs from 1 to 72 hours postpartum. They are usually experiencing latching difficulties, delayed lactogenesis, or may be reluctant to initiate breastfeeding. Sometimes mothers from out of town just want to get off to a really good start before they go home to an isolated farm with little help to breastfeed. Mothers with uncomplicated vaginal deliveries are usually discharged after about 48 hours, whereas mothers with cesarean sections or those from far away often stay longer. The pediatricians will not usually discharge a baby until he is breastfeeding well, although often I am used as a backup: "You can go home if Pam says it's okay." I am always conscious of the huge responsibility in these cases, and I especially enjoy the continuity of being able to assist a mother right from the beginning in the hospital and then following up after hospital discharge.

Hospital Practices

In our hospitals, mothers are not expected to exercise a choice about infant feeding; formula is never provided for full-term healthy babies, and all mothers are expected to breastfeed. Thus the baby whose mother, for whatever reason, really does not want to breastfeed is quickly identified, and staff may call on me in the hope that I can change the mother's mind. This scenario represents a very challenging situation as the mother may state verbally that she wants to breastfeed but her actions frequently prevent it from taking place. The baby's nutrition must be protected, and the hospital staff, obstetrician, and pediatrician share the expectation that the LC (whose job, after all, is to promote breastfeeding) can fix it! I have worked with mothers who in effect may starve the baby until they can take him home and feed him formula. One pediatrician told me, in a resigned tone, that he knows that these mothers have formula waiting in the car!

Things are no easier for the more assertive mother. I have known a matron in charge of a postnatal ward who dropped everything to obtain clearance from the obstetrician and pediatrician to discharge a mother and twins when it became obvious that the mother intended to bottle-feed her babies in the hospital. The matron stated categorically that she was not having "that" going on on her ward, and arranged for them to go home within the hour!

Conversely, I have also worked with a mother of a large baby, who was highly motivated to breastfeed, but who produced no colostrum and whose milk simply never "came in." The baby was discharged home at six days, having lost 16 percent of his birth weight, yet the pediatrician had been unconcerned. It was obvious that this baby needed urgent formula supplementation once he came home and I was able to follow up until the mother came to terms with the fact that she was one of the rare and tiny percentage of mothers who did not lactate.

Another common reason for hospital consults is to assist initiation of lactation, and eventual breastfeeding, for preterm babies in neonatal units (NNUs). The smallest babies with whom I have worked were twins born at 25 weeks gestation, survivors of a triplet pregnancy, who were finally discharged home from the neonatal unit, exclusively breastfed at 100 days of age.

Our NNUs may be fairly unique in that formula is used only minimally, on a case-by-case basis, in tiny amounts for the first 24–48 hours, for babies who are well enough to be fed, but whose mothers are not yet producing sufficient expressed breast milk. Often, these tiny preterm babies will be on an I.V. drip for several days. The pediatricians will then call for mother's milk, and the babies will go straight on to expressed breast milk via nasogastric tube. I may be called to see the mothers of the smaller babies when they want to start expressing their milk, if the milk supply appears to dip below the baby's needs, and again to assist with positioning when direct breastfeeding begins.

Bottles and pacifiers are never used or even seen in our NNUs, "gifts" of formula are not permitted by law, and any formula used is charged to the mother's account. Preterm babies are fed the mother's own milk as it comes (with no manipulation of fat content), every two or three hours depending on their weight. The tiny babies sometimes receive supplementary vitamin D, and human milk fortifiers are unknown. The baby who has reached 31–33 weeks gestational age and is well enough will be put to the breast for practice breastfeeds. During a changeover period, the baby may do some breastfeeding combined with top-ups of expressed breast milk via nasogastric tube or by cup/spoon. Eventually, babies will be discharged at 1800 g, fully breastfed. Babies who have reached this weight but are not yet breastfeeding stay in the hospital until they are. I see many of these cases, because everyone wants to go home. Working in such a baby-friendly atmosphere is a real joy, with everyone (mothers, nursing staff, pediatricians) working toward the same goal—effective breastfeeding for these tiny, at-risk babies. Having the opportunity to facilitate and be a part of the success when these babies grow and thrive on mother's milk alone is a thrill that never palls.

Security and Other Issues for the Isolated LC

Risks to your personal safety or politically driven constraints may need to be factored in as you decide whether to offer consultations outside your own office environment. Escalating levels of poverty and unemployment in recent years have caused security to become an important issue in Harare; some of my clients may live in mini-fortresses with security guards, electric fences, and locked gates, and therefore gaining entry (and exit) is sometimes difficult. After having a couple of frightening experiences, I learned to say no to requests for home visits in certain areas. I also decline outside consultations when the initial phone contact just doesn't "feel right," and I no longer go out after dark. Recently, incidents of armed robbery and kidnapping on the roads, even in broad daylight, are on the increase in Zimbabwe. Now that I have a cell phone, I don't go out without it; it increases my sense of security if I can phone home to let my cook (my right-hand man!) or my family know where I am. I also often phone ahead to clients to ask them to open their gates promptly, as waiting at a locked gate is a known risk factor for carjacking.

Political tension has also led to work sick-outs, strikes, riots, and demonstrations in and around Harare. I have learned to look out for rioters or truckloads of armed riot police, and to do fast U-turns. The irony is that the worse the unrest, the more your clients need your help to breastfeed their babies!

During our worst fuel shortages, I rearranged my time, plugging my laptop into the cigarette lighter in my car so that I could read my e-mail while sitting in fuel queues, which often lasted five to six hours starting at 4 A.M. I also limited home or hospital visits to times and places where I could easily combine them with collecting my boys from school. I was once persuaded by a desperate father to make a hospital visit in exchange for a full tank of fuel, to our mutual benefit. Allowing a total stranger to drive away in my car seemed a little risky, but after all, he had trusted me with his baby!

Teamwork

There is a special challenge in working to meet your client's need to initiate or preserve lactation or breastfeeding, while simultaneously working amicably with hospital policies, and with what your client's obstetrician and pediatrician have ordered. Sometimes other health professionals are involved as well; at different times I have had to work with a cardiologist, a neurologist, a psychiatrist, psychologists, orthopedic and plastic surgeons, an orthodontist, physiotherapists, dentists, anaesthetists and intensive care unit specialists (for mother or baby), some or all of whom have an interest in an aspect of the mother's or baby's health that can compete with lactation or breastfeeding. The lactation consultant who is able to work as a member of a team, with the mother's and baby's best health outcome as the main goal, will be rewarded by being treated as a professional

Typical Day

I enjoy the flexibility of being able to choose my own working hours, enabling me to work around my family's needs. I usually see two to four mothers per day, and I also provide phone consults and make follow-up calls. The volume of work is very up and down, and nearly always unpredictable. One day is quiet, then on other days everyone seems to need you at once. For instance, I had no work at all on Friday, I made two hospital visits on Saturday, and received one call at 7:30 P.M. from an out-of-town mother on Sunday. I am almost never booked up much in advance, and this Monday morning my diary showed an absolutely blank day. As often happens, today turned out to be one of *those* days and my morning went like this:

6:23 A.M. Call from a grandmother of a four-day-old baby at home, requesting a home visit for the mother, arranged for 11 A.M. The mother was a former client, seen with her last baby five years ago.

6:40 A.M. Download e-mail. Of special interest is a message from someone in Australia about an upcoming Codex meeting in Berlin, commenting on whether labeling of weaning foods should state from four or six months, and an astute message from an LC in the United States on the "HIV and breast-feeding" list. I leave the Lactnet messages to read later, when I have more time.

7:15 A.M. Follow-up call from a mother of another four-day-old, seen in the hospital on Saturday for a latching difficulty (tongue-sucking). The mother wants to let me know that the baby is now breastfeeding for 20 minutes at a time every 2 1/2 hours, and now she is afraid of getting sore nipples. We have a long discussion about this success, and ways to avoid/treat nipple pain.

8:00 A.M. Call from an African mother who attended my last antenatal class. The baby is six days old. The mother has one engorged breast and the nipple is ungraspable. We discuss whether the mother is able to hand-express milk (taught at the class), but she is undecided about whether she would prefer a breast pump. I suggest that this issue needs to be resolved promptly (drainage by manual expression and use of cabbage leaves) and offer an office consult later in the day if she is not managing. She will get back to me.

8:30 A.M. Call from sister-in-charge of the postnatal ward at the largest private clinic. She requests a hospital visit for one of the patients. When I speak to the mother, I find out that she is very young (only 16, white Zimbabwean by the accent). Her baby boy is one day old and a healthy 3270 g, but is not latching to the breast easily. I ascertain that she would prefer to bottle-feed. Oh dear. I advise her that the hospital will not provide formula, discuss the cost of for-mula feeding, suggest that she consider breastfeeding for now, take her pedi-atrician's advice (I know he will recommend *breastfeeding*), and get back to me if she would like me to make a hospital consult to show her how to re-solve the latching difficulty.

9:15 A.M. Call from an out-of-town mother. Her exclusively breastfed three-week-old is gaining weight well, but feeding for short times at short intervals. The mother has formed unrealistic expectations and has been trying to "struc-ture" her baby's sleep/feed intervals in accordance with guidelines set out in a popular (detachment-parenting) baby-care book. She is a highly organized, intelligent mother, so we discuss recent research on breast milk synthesis and gastric emptying times, and she is reassured.

10:00 A.M. Call from a second-time mother of another three-week-old. The baby is gaining well, spitting up, has a blocked nose, writhes around, and seems uncomfortable. We explore possible sensitivity to bovine proteins in-gested by the mother and what to expect.

11:00 A.M. Home consult arranged earlier in the day. Third baby, three days old, somewhat jaundiced, sleeping long periods, and having difficulty latching in cradle hold, has a receding upper gum and a high palate. The mother has moderate breast engorgement. We review how to use her own pump and latch techniques in football hold. The baby sucks well, so I suggest the fol-lowing: breast compression during nursing to increase intake, feed 50 ml EBM every three hours if the baby is not alert enough to breastfeed, see pediatri-cian if the jaundice spreads to the baby's arms and palms.

FINDING SUPPORT AS AN ISOLATED LACTATION CONSULTANT

Keeping Abreast

One of the most difficult problems of being an isolated LC is obtaining access to good, up-to-date information on lactation and breastfeeding. Having no one to ask means that you will need to be able to access written information. This effort has two aspects:

• Knowing which reference materials are really worthwhile to obtain

• Knowing where to locate information on a particular topic again when you need it, once you know you've read it somewhere!

Publications written especially for the lactation community, such as the *Journal of Human Lactation*, *Breastfeeding Review*, *Breastfeeding Abstracts*, and *ALCA Galaxy*, as well as the annual reading list for the IBLCE exam are all good sources of information. Obtaining these materials has been a particular challenge for me, because Zimbabwe's foreign exchange regulations limit how many and what kind of books and subscriptions I can order, and the value of our dollar and the cost of postage render them prohibitively expensive. LC friends and colleagues overseas have often overwhelmed me with their generosity in sending me their older editions of vital materials when they update their own libraries, and my own budget places a high priority on obtaining books and journals.

While studying for the IBLCE exam in 1989, I soon became overwhelmed by the vast quantity of information on lactation and breastfeeding that was available even then, realizing that I would never be able to remember it all! My husband suggested a way of keeping track of information by topic, which I have used ever since. I obtained tickler boxes and stacks of cards and jotted down information by subject (which was also a great way of studying), noting where to find it in my reference books. I filed the cards alphabetically so that I could easily look up the topic again. I call this set of little boxes, marked "A-E," "F-O," and "P-Z," my "brain" because I couldn't do without it! If I want information for a mother with a nipple bleb, I can look up "bleb" (also cross-referenced under "nipple blister") and find a good description in *Breastfeeding Review*, July 1991, pages 118-119. There is more in *Breastfeeding Matters*, page 161, *The Breastfeeding Answer Book*, page 174, and *Breastfeeding and Human Lactation*, page 387. Whenever I receive a new journal, I note information of interest in my "brain" so that it is continually updated. This system saves me hours of time whenever I encounter a rare problem that I know I've read about somewhere (but where?) or whenever I want references from the literature to share with a doctor.

Keeping Notes

One of your best assets will be your own experience. A lone LC does not enjoy the luxury of being able to discuss case histories with colleagues, but as your number of clients grows you can learn from your own experience, as carefully recorded in your own notes. Keeping full, comprehensive notes of anatomy, history, care plans, and outcomes can provide you with an opportunity to see what works and what doesn't, can force you to think through each situation carefully, and provides an easy-to-follow record of each client's progress. I open a folder for each client, starting with initial contact and initial lactation consultation forms, and drop notes of each subsequent contact, and any reports, into the file as they occur. My archive system allows me to pull a client's file months later, for the same baby, or even several years later when she comes back again with a third baby, which provides me with anticipatory guidance when working with the client again.

I also have a box file marked "Case Histories" where I record details of very unusual or difficult situations, including the client's name and the dates when I worked with her. Thus I can look up the whole file if necessary. Case histories are filed alphabetically by subject (e.g., "abcess," "imperforate anus," "laryngomalacia," or "rabies").

Developing a Support Network

One of the biggest challenges of working as an isolated LC is the loneliness of not having a colleague who speaks your language and not having any way of measuring the success of your practice. Thus finding ways to maintain contact with other lactation consultants, albeit at long distance, can be vital to ensure your own support, to keep abreast of current trends, and to keep up-to-date with what is happening in the wider world. Being an ILCA member will be helpful. Many countries have ILCA affiliate groups, and joining the one nearest to you can help to keep you in touch. Many ILCA affiliates run a sister program whereby a group may "adopt" a lone LC. I will be forever grateful to the U.S. group that adopted me, helping me financially by paying my ILCA subscriptions when doing so was so difficult from Zimbabwe, writing and sending me their newsletters and personal notes, and allowing me in the first lonely years of my practice to write them long letters picking their collective brains!

As an extremely isolated LC, the single biggest change for me occurred when I discovered e-mail. After working for several years alone, and feeling as if I was blind, my LC life and outlook were completely revamped by finding Lactnet, an e-mail list of more than 2000 lactation professionals from all over the world. I subsequently had the opportunity to join an e-mail list for lactation consultants in private practice. E-mail has been a lifeline for me, enabling me to keep in constant contact with colleagues and professional friends, to learn so much, to contribute to professional journals and international debates on breastfeeding issues, and to participate in the international breastfeeding arena, even at this distance.

Mentoring and Professional Networking Relationships

It is also advisable to try and form a mentor relationship with a local pediatrician and an obstetrician, whereby you can ask for education and information on medical matters that you suspect may affect lactation and breastfeeding. In return, these health professionals may ask you questions on behalf of their patients. I sometimes gladly see my friendly pediatrician's government hospital patients at no charge for two reasons. First, it is a way of expressing my gratitude for his help to me. Second, the breastfeeding problems are always extremely severe, and the babies very wasted and sick, and I find them especially challenging and rewarding to help.

Emergencies

The LC in private practice is likely, sooner or later, to find herself in the middle of an emergency situation by virtue of the fact that the mother–baby dyads she sees will have left the hospital but may not have sought medical advice for a health problem as yet. Your assessment of a mother's or baby's ability to breastfeed can reveal an urgent need for additional medical care. Furthermore, the LC who spends an hour or more in the company of a mother–baby pair may be in a position to observe a problem that a quick doctor's visit may not have picked up. I have been the first person to know that an 11-day-old baby was 30 percent below birth weight, and that a preterm baby remained 20 percent below birth weight at one month of age. I have urgently referred back to their pediatricians babies with undiagnosed imperforate anus and undiagnosed congenital heart defects, and an extremely jaundiced eight-day-old whose total serum bilirubin was shown to be 28 mg/dL. A baby in my office once had convulsions that a family doctor had attributed to "colic" on the basis of the mother's description; the baby was subsequently found on CT scan to have fairly severe brain damage. A lone LC does not have the luxury of conferring with colleagues about these worrying situations. At times like these, it is vital to know how you can reach your clients' doctors in an emergency. For your own protection, ensure that you are covered by insurance, and as soon as possible afterward make extremely detailed notes of what you observed, what you suggested, what was done, and to whom you referred the client.

Outreach

A unique opportunity exists for the lone LC to increase her own range of experience and enhance her visibility by assisting general breastfeeding promotion efforts in her community and even on a national scale. If you are the only lactation professional in your area or country, consider offering your services to people or organizations that might need them. Even though you may not get paid, a gift of your time and talents to promote breastfeeding can make you more widely known and often brings unexpected bonuses. I have had the opportunity to help set national policy on breastfeeding by serving on Zimbabwe's national multisectoral committee for nearly a decade.

I have also had the very rewarding experience of contributing to the Baby Friendly Hospital Initiative (BFHI) in my country as a trainer/facilitator at BFHI workshops for health care staff, as a BFHI assessor in government and municipal hospitals, of which Zimbabwe now has 46, and finally as a member of the national BFHI Task Force. BFHI assessments have provided some heartwarming and uniquely African experiences:

- Interviewing new mothers and realizing that none of them knew what teats and pacifiers were

- Being able to award a 100 percent score to a male laboratory technician who clutched his white coat to his chest to give a perfect example of manual expression of breast milk

- Having the chance late one night to observe a newborn baby girl crawl up her mother's abdomen and self-attach to the breast while an overworked midwife had to choose between assisting with the first breastfeed or searching frantically for mislaid sutures

- Being able to slip in an extra assessment for a crestfallen male security guard, missed in random sampling, who had been through all the training and was dying to show off all his breastfeeding knowledge "in case the mothers need help with breastfeeding while they are waiting in the queue at the gate"

Possibly the greatest highlight, however, was teaching staff at the hospital where my own babies had been born 20 years ago how to be "baby-friendly" and then assessing them later to make sure!

It has also been extremely satisfying to officially monitor industry violations of the International Code of Marketing of Breastmilk Substitutes. I was also able to provide input toward, and haggle with industry over, the provisions of national legislation that was finally passed through parliament to implement the Code.

I have blatantly "pushed" breastfeeding by offering talks to high-school students, on the rationale that within five to ten years these young men and women will be parents. These events have been immensely fulfilling for me. The most challenging questions I have ever been asked have come from these young people. I have also been the guest of a dozen radio or TV talk shows and phone-in programs to share my fascination with the subject of lactation and breastfeeding; these appearances, too, are really fun to do.

Special Interests

A phone call from a distraught mother six years ago sparked my current special interest in the ongoing international debate on the thorny issue of whether HIV-infected mothers should breastfeed. In turn, this interest led to a related issue—the question of human rights and breastfeeding. Work on these issues resulted in publication of several articles and letters and subsequent invitations to participate at meetings and conferences in countries as far away as Australia and Brazil, where I have met some of the finest minds in the lactation world.

Politics

Being a member of a minority racial group in Africa requires showing sensitivity to local cultural practices and traditions, some of which are beneficial to breastfeeding and some of which are detrimental. The LC who wishes to give a little of her time to breastfeeding advocacy work will eventually become aware of the political alliances and hierarchies found in her community or country. It requires a certain degree of skill, and something of an instinct for self-preservation, to work in and around the very sensitive areas that often include a hidden agenda. I have found that the best way to skirt this professional minefield is to keep my focus firmly on what I am working to achieve— namely, to help the *individual* mother breastfeed her baby for as long as possible. As far as I am able, I make it clear that I am working toward this end and that I will work with anyone else who shares the same goal.

When working in a country or area where there is war, conflict, or civil unrest, it becomes very obvious that the needs of mothers and babies cut across all racial, ethnic, and political boundaries. Recently, my clients have included the wives and sisters of individuals whose names may have appeared prominently in negative press reports. I have also helped the victims—for instance, the farmer's wife who thought she had lost her milk the day after she had been given two hours to pack all her worldly possessions into two suitcases and flee for her life with her baby, as well as others whose homes are surrounded by "invaders" or whose residences have been actually seized. These mothers experience identical difficulties in breastfeeding, and the background of politics, lawlessness, and mayhem is of no consequence as I work with *this* mother and *this* baby to help them breastfeed.

Avoiding Burnout

The lone LC, by virtue of her isolation and lack of support, is at risk for burnout in any situation involving stress or distress. Perhaps the baby of one of your clients dies, you are overextending yourself by taking on too much, or you must deal with stressful situations within your own family. It is important to know whether continuing to see mothers when you are distressed affects the quality of the assistance you provide, and to act accordingly. I find that I completely forget about my own stresses the minute I start taking a client's details, instead becoming caught up in the fascination of finding out what the mother needs to be able to breastfeed her baby. For me, time spent during a consult is almost like a personal emotional holiday. One exception occurred recently when my son was charged with a serious crime after a car accident. Justice prevailed and he was eventually acquitted, but I was such a basketcase that I knew I would have to avoid consulting whenever he had to appear in court.

When you are the *only* LC around, it is difficult to say "no" when too many people need the assistance and skills that only *you* can provide, or when you are trying to work on many outreach projects while still keeping your private practice going. I have learned that I can comfortably see no more than four clients in one day if I am working on other things as well, although I can just squeeze in eight if nothing else is scheduled. If I am attending all-day workshops, I sometimes arrange to see clients very early or very late in the day; this schedule can be so exhausting that I can't do it for more than two days in a row, however. If you are also writing articles or critiquing others' work and trying to meet too many simultaneous deadlines, it is tempting to work until late at night and become very tired. Having fallen prey to a mystery "virus" that nearly killed me two years ago after I had stayed up until the early hours of the morning for several months running, and having been prostrated for six weeks as a result, I have learned to pace myself, to stop when I become tired, to be choosy about the tasks I take on, and to deliberately schedule time for family, friends, relaxation, and just "smelling the roses."

EVALUATION

Summary: Reviewing What It Takes

The solo LC in an isolated setting, while facing many constraints and difficulties for which no easy solutions exist, has the opportunity to work as creatively and imaginatively as she wishes, to put her unique stamp on whatever she achieves, and to succeed by her own efforts alone. There is almost no end to the opportunities for the LC who is prepared to do the following:

- Invest the time and energy to give each client 100 percent
- Plan carefully
- Do the paperwork and keep up-to-date
- Nurture her sources of referral
- Give a little time to outreach in her community and/or internationally

The Realization of a Dream

I had a dream of working professionally in private practice to help more mothers breastfeed, and for longer periods of time. I dreamed of doing something that I love, and being paid to do so. My dream has come true beyond my wildest imagination, and the realization of it has turned out to be a stepping stone to an even wider world.

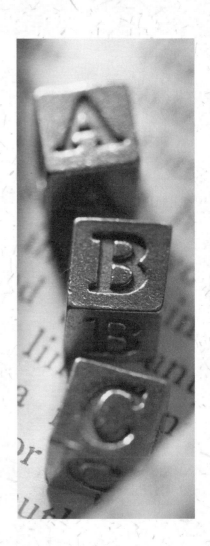

Professional Documents

Code of Ethics
Standards of Practice for Lactation Consultants
Scope of Practice and Education Guidelines
Innocenti Declaration
WHO Code Summary: *The International Code of Marketing of Breast-Milk Substitutes*

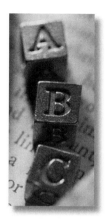

Code of Ethics

International Board of Lactation Consultant Examiners

PREAMBLE

It is in the best interests of the profession of lactation consultants and the public it serves that there be a Code of Ethics to provide guidance to lactation consultants in their professional practice and conduct. These ethical principles guide the profession and outline commitments and obligations of the lactation consultant to self, client, colleague, society, and the profession.

The purpose of the International Board of Lactation Consultant Examiners (IBLCE) is to assist in the protection of the health, safety, and welfare of the public by establishing and enforcing qualifications of certification and for issuing voluntary credentials to individuals who have attained those qualifications. The IBLCE has adopted this Code to apply to all individuals who hold the credential of International Board Certified Lactation Consultant (IBCLC).

PRINCIPLES OF ETHICAL PRACTICE

The International Board Certified Lactation Consultant shall act in a manner that safeguards the interests of individual clients, justifies public trust in her/his competence, and enhances the reputation of the profession.

The International Board Certified Lactation Consultant is personally accountable for her/his practice and, in the exercise of professional accountability, must:

1. Provide professional services with objectivity and with respect for the unique needs and values of individuals.

2. Avoid discrimination against other individuals on the basis of race, creed, religion, gender, sexual orientation, age, and national origin.

3. Fulfill professional commitments in good faith.

4. Conduct herself/himself with honesty, integrity, and fairness.

5. Remain free of conflict of interest while fulfilling the objectives and maintaining the integrity of the lactation consultant profession.

6. Maintain confidentiality.

7. Base her/his practice on scientific principles, current research, and information.

8. Take responsibility and accept accountability for personal competence in practice.

9. Recognize and exercise professional judgment within the limits of her/his qualifications. This principle includes seeking counsel and making referrals to appropriate providers.

10. Inform the public and colleagues of her/his services by using factual information. An International Board Certified Lactation Consultant will not advertise in a false or misleading manner.

11. Provide sufficient information to enable clients to make informed decisions.

12. Provide information about appropriate products in a manner that is neither false nor misleading

13. Permit use of her/his name for the purpose of certifying that lactation consultant services have been rendered only if she/he provided those services.

14. Present professional qualifications and credentials accurately, using IBCLC only when certification is current and authorized by the IBLCE, and complying with all requirements when seeking initial or continued certification from the IBLCE. The lactation consultant is subject to disciplinary action for aiding another person in violating any IBLCE requirements or aiding another person in representing herself/himself as an IBCLC when she/he is not.

15. Report to an appropriate person or authority when it appears that the health or safety of colleagues is at risk, as such circumstances may compromise standards of practice and care.

16. Refuse any gift, favor, or hospitality from patients or clients currently in her/his care that might be interpreted as seeking to exert influence to obtain preferential consideration.

17. Disclose any financial or other conflicts of interest in relevant organizations providing goods or services. Ensure that professional judgment is not influenced by any commercial considerations.

18. Present substantiated information and interpret controversial information without personal bias, recognizing that legitimate differences of opinion exist.

19. Withdraw voluntarily from professional practice if the lactation consultant has engaged in any substance abuse that could affect her/his practice; has been adjudged by a court to be mentally incompetent; or has an emotional or mental disability that affects her/his practice in a manner that could harm the client.

20. Obtain maternal consent to photograph, audiotape, or videotape a mother and/or her infant(s) for educational or professional purposes.

21. Submit to disciplinary action under the following circumstance: If convicted of a crime under the laws of the practitioner's country which is a felony or a misdemeanor, an essential element of which is dishonesty, and which is related to the practice of lactation consulting; if disciplined by a state, province, or other local government and at least one of the grounds for the discipline is the same or substantially equivalent to these principles; if committed an act of misfeasance or malfeasance which is directly related to the practice of the profession as determined by a court of competent jurisdiction, a licensing board, or an agency of a governmental

body; or if violated a Principle set forth in the Code of Ethics for International Board Certified Lactation Consultants which was in force at the time of the violation.

22. Accept the obligation to protect society and the profession by upholding the Code of Ethics for International Board Certified Lactation Consultants and by reporting alleged violations of the Code through the defined review process of the IBLCE.

23. Require and obtain consent to share clinical concerns and information with the physician or other primary health care provider before initiating a consultation.

24. IBCLCs must adhere to those provisions of the International Code of Marketing of Breast-Milk Substitutes that pertain to health workers.

TO LODGE A COMPLAINT

IBCLCs shall act in a manner that justifies public trust in their competence, enhances the reputation of the profession, and safeguards the interests of individual clients.

To protect the credential and to assure responsible practice by its certificants, the IBLCE depends on IBCLCs, members of the coordinating and supervising health professions, employers, and the public to report incidents which may require action by the IBLCE Discipline Committee.

Only signed, written complaints will be considered. Anonymous complaints will be discarded. The IBLCE will become involved only in matters that can be factually determined, and will provide the accused party with every opportunity to respond in a professional and legally defensible manner.

Complaints that appear to fit the scope of the Discipline Committee's responsibilities should be sent to the:

Chair of the Discipline Committee
IBLCE
7309 Arlington Blvd., Suite 300
Falls Church, VA 22042-3215 USA

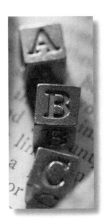

Standards of Practice for IBCLC Lactation Consultants

International Lactation Consultant Association

PREFACE

T his text is the second edition of Standards of Practice for IBCLC Lactation Consultants published by the International Lactation Consultant Association (ILCA).

ILCA recognizes the certification conferred by the International Board of Lactation Consultant Examiners (IBLCE) as the professional credential for lactation consultants. All individuals representing themselves as IBCLC lactation consultants should adhere to these Standards of Practice and the Code of Ethics for International Board Certified Lactation Consultants in any and all interactions with clients, clients' families, and other health care professionals.

INTRODUCTION

Q uality practice and service constitute the core of a profession's responsibility to the public. Standards of practice have been defined as stated measures or levels of quality that serve as models for the conduct and evaluation of practice. Standards promote consistency by encouraging a common systematic approach. They also are sufficiently specific in content to meet the demands of daily practice. These standards are presented as a recommended framework for the development of policies and protocols, educational programs, and quality improvement efforts. They are intended for use in diverse settings, institutions, and cultural contexts.

STANDARD 1.
CLINICAL PRACTICE

T he clinical practice of the IBCLC lactation consultant focuses on providing lactation care and clinical management. This is best accomplished within the framework of systematic problem solving in collaboration with other members of the health care team and the client. IBCLC lactation consultants are responsible for decisions and actions undertaken as a part of their professional role, including the:

- assessment, planning, intervention, and evaluation of care in a variety of situations
- prevention of problems
- complete, accurate, and timely documentation of care
- communication and collaboration with other health care professionals

1.1 Assessment

1.1.1 Obtain and document an appropriate history of the breastfeeding mother and child.

1.1.2 Systematically collect objective and subjective information

1.1.3 Discuss with the mother and document as appropriate all assessment information

1.2 Plan

1.2.1 Analyze assessment information to identify concerns and/or problems

1.2.2 Develop a plan of care based on identified concerns or problems

1.2.3 Arrange for follow-up evaluation

1.3 Implementation

1.3.1 Implement the plan of care in a manner appropriate to the situation and acceptable to the mother

1.3.2 Exercise principles of safety and universal precautions

1.3.3 Demonstrate procedures, techniques, equipment, and devices

1.3.4 Provide appropriate instruction

1.3.5 Provide a written report to the primary health care provider as appropriate, including:

- Assessment information
- Suggested interventions
- Instructions provided

1.3.6 Facilitate referral to other health professionals, community services, and support groups as needed

1.4 Evaluation

1.4.1 Evaluate outcomes of planned interventions

1.4 2 Modify the plan based on the evaluation of outcomes

1.4.3 Document and communicate to the primary health care provider(s) as appropriate:

- Evaluation of outcomes
- Modifications in the plan
- Follow-up

STANDARD 2. BREASTFEEDING EDUCATION AND COUNSELING

Breastfeeding education and counseling are integral parts of the care provided by the lactation consultant.

2.1 Provide education to parents and families to encourage informed decision making about infant and child feeding

2.2 Provide anticipatory teaching to:

- promote ideal breastfeeding practices
- minimize the potential for breastfeeding problems or complications

2.4 Provide emotional support for continued breastfeeding in difficult or complicated circumstances

2.5 Share current, evidence-based information and clinical skills with other health care providers

The IBCLC lactation consultant has a responsibility to maintain professional conduct and to practice in an ethical manner and is accountable for professional actions and legal responsibilities.

STANDARD 3. PROFESSIONAL RESPONSIBILITIES

3.1 Adhere to these Standards of Practice and the IBCLE Code of Ethics.

3.2 Practice within the scope of the International Code of Marketing of Breast-Milk Substitutes and subsequent relevant resolutions, and maintain an awareness of conflict of interest when/if profiting from the rental or sale of breastfeeding equipment.

3.3 Act as an advocate for breastfeeding women, infants, and children.

3.4 Assist the mother in maintaining an intact breastfeeding relationship with her child.

3.5 Use breastfeeding equipment and devices appropriately by:

- Refraining from unnecessary or excessive use.
- Discussing the risks and benefits of recommended use.
- Evaluating safety and effectiveness.
- Assuring cleanliness and good operating condition.

3.6 Maintain and expand knowledge and skills for lactation consultant practice by participating in continuing education.

3.7 Undertake periodic and systematic appraisal for evaluation of one's clinical practice.

3.8 Support and promote well-designed research in human lactation and breastfeeding and base clinical practice, whenever possible, on such research.

IBCLC lactation consultants are obligated to practice within the laws of the geopolitical region and setting in which they work. They must practice with consideration for clients' rights of privacy and with respect for matters of a confidential nature.

STANDARD 4. LEGAL CONSIDERATIONS

4.1 Work within the policies and procedures of the institution where employed, or if self-employed, have identifiable policies and procedures to follow.

4.2 Clearly state applicable fees prior to providing care.

4.3 Obtain informed consent from all clients prior to:

- Assessing or intervening
- Reporting relevant information to the primary health care provider or other health care professional(s)
- Taking photographs for any purpose
- Seeking publication of information associated with the consultation

4.4 Protect client confidentiality at all times.

4.5 Maintain records according to legal practices within the work setting.

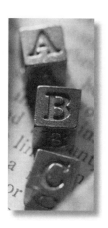

The International Board Certified Lactation Consultant: Scope of Practice and Education Guidelines

International Lactation Consultant Association

INTRODUCTION

The purpose of this document is to inform consumers, health care professionals, employers, health care policy makers, third party payors, educators, and students regarding the basic knowledge, skills, and competencies of an International Board Certified Lactation Consultant.[1] It also serves as the framework for evaluation and accreditation of International Board Certified Lactation Consultant education programs.

ROLE DEFINITION

The International Board Certified Lactation Consultant is a health care professional whose scope of practice encompasses working collaboratively with primary care providers to assure appropriate clinical/practical management of breastfeeding and lactation in order to protect, promote, and support breastfeeding. Such practice includes providing education, counseling, and clinical/practical management to allow breastfeeding to be seen as the expected way in which healthy newborns are to be fed, as well as to prevent and solve breastfeeding problems. Education efforts extend to the community as well as to breastfeeding families and health care colleagues.

The role of the International Board Certified Lactation Consultant is dynamic and changes as the theory and practice of breastfeeding support and lactation management evolve to incorporate research findings and to adapt to (trends) societal needs. Practice is based on the principles outlined in this document, on the *Standards of Practice for IBCLC Lactation Consultants,* and on the *International Board Certified Lactation Consultant Examiners (IBLCE) Code of Ethics.*

CERTIFICATION

Lactation consultants who are certified by the IBLCE have the professional responsibility to maintain the IBLCE credential. Certification is evidence that the individual has achieved and does maintain the knowledge, skills, and wisdom required for the provision of competent breastfeeding care and services. International Board Certified Lactation Consultants are accountable for the outcomes of their practice and are responsible for complying with the laws within their practice jurisdictions.

FRAMEWORK FOR EDUCATION AND PRACTICE

The theoretical framework for International Board Certified Lactation Consultant education derives from the health, biological, and social sciences. Clinical/practical preparation involves acquiring the knowledge, judg-

266

ment, and skills necessary to provide optimal, safe care for the breastfeeding mother and child. Acceptable clinical/practical practice and educational curricula are based on a foundation of fundamental principles, professional responsibilities, core knowledge, and competencies.

FUNDAMENTAL PRINCIPLES

- Breastfeeding is a normal physiologic and developmental process for the majority of mothers and infants.
- Breastfeeding promotes optimal child health as well as optimal maternal health and is a vital component of public health policy.
- Every child has the right to receive human milk, and every woman has the right to breastfeed her child unless there is a medical contraindication.
- Every woman has the right to receive accurate, evidence-based information, support, and clinical/practical management for herself and her child.
- Mothers and infants have the right to receive, when needed, skilled assistance and clinical/practical management to breastfeed effectively.

PROFESSIONAL RESPONSIBILITIES

International Board Certified Lactation Consultants have a professional responsibility to:

- Recognize that breastfeeding provides a foundation for optimal health outcomes and nurturing behaviors.
- Strive to support women to make informed decisions and take responsibility for their own well-being and that of their children.
- Work in respectful partnership with women and their chosen support systems.
- Advocate for the health and well-being of children by providing information about infant needs to guide mothers in informed decision-making about infant and child feeding.
- Integrate observation, knowledge, and intuition in assessing mothers and children and in developing breastfeeding management strategies.
- Demonstrate clinical/practical competency, professional accountability, and legal responsibility.
- Facilitate the collaborative care of the mother and infant.
- Critically evaluate and incorporate research findings to provide and maintain evidenced-based practice.
- Participate in self-evaluation, peer review, continuing education, and other activities to ensure quality practice.
- Engage in professional conduct and practice in an ethical manner.
- Promote and protect breastfeeding through community outreach.
- Stay informed about the national and international issues and trends in maternal-newborn care and women's health.

CORE KNOWLEDGE OUTLINE (SUBJECT AREAS FROM THE IBLCE EXAMINATION BLUEPRINT)

A. Anatomy

    Mother

        General

        Breast and nipple (specific to lactation)

Infant

   General

   Head

     Oral

   Neck and shoulders

   Gastrointestinal

B. Physiology and Endocrinology

  Mother

   General maternal hormones

   Milk synthesis and production

   Fertility/family planning

   Induced lactation and re-lactation

  Infant

   General infant hormones

   Neuro-endocrine-gut reactions

   Sucking, swallowing, and breathing

   Digestion

   Elimination

C. Nutrition and Biochemistry

  Mother

   Principles of nutrition for women of childbearing age

   Weight loss and gain

   Cultural diet issues/ritual foods during post partum period

   Milk composition

   Effect of maternal diet on milk composition

  Infant

   Guidelines for infant feeding

   Comparison between human milk and artificial feeding products

   Complementary and supplementary foods

   Food sensitivities

   Weaning/introduction of solids

D. Immunology and Infectious Disease

  Protective properties of human milk

   Immune system factors

    Cells, antibodies, and other immunoglobulins in human milk

   Non-antibody factors—lactoferrin, bifidus factor, enzymes, hormones, growth factors, oligosaccharides, etc.

  Decreased risk of infections and some chronic illnesses

   Etiology

   Manifestations

   Prevention

   Management

Decreased risk of allergies

Etiology

Manifestations

Prevention

Management

E. Pathology

Maternal

Labor and birth complications

Breast problems

Engorgement

Sore nipples

Yeast infections

Mastitis/abscesses

Plugged ducts

Insufficient glandular development

Breast surgery

Breast implants

Breast cancer

Acute illnesses

Chronic illnesses

Physical disabilities

Infant

Birth trauma

Inability to coordinate breathing/sucking/swallowing

Respiratory distress

Sucking problems

Swallowing difficulty

Preterm birth

Hyperbilirubinemia

Slow weight gain

Failure to thrive

Congenital anomalies/birth defects

Acute illnesses

Chronic illnesses

Oral pathology

Neurological impairment

F. Pharmacology and Toxicology

Pharmacology

Role of lactation consultant

Resources

Pharmacokinetics

Effects of drugs and substances commonly used during lactation

Over-the-counter medications

Alcohol

Tobacco

Management of lactation during drug therapy

Contraindications for breastfeeding

Pharmacologic family planning

Galactogogues/milk suppressants

Recreational/street drugs

Complementary therapies

　　Herbs

　　Homeopathic remedies

　　Acupuncture

　　Other

Toxicology

　　Environmental pollutants

G. Psychology, Sociology, and Anthropology

Adult learning

Counseling skills

Mother issues

　　Incorporating breastfeeding into ones lifestyle

　　Breastfeeding outside the home

　　Maternal empowerment

　　Employment

　　Post partum depression/psychosis

　　Domestic violence/sexual abuse

Parenting role

　　Mother-infant relationship

　　Father-infant relationship

　　Sibling-infant relationships

　　Other family roles

　　Single parenting

　　Adolescent parenting

Alternative family styles

Cultural beliefs and practices

Support systems

H. Growth Parameters and Developmental Milestones

Social, adaptive, psychosocial, and physical assessment of the child

　　Prenatal growth

　　Feeding cues

　　Infant needs and temperament

　　Feeding patterns and normal growth curves throughout breastfeeding

Developmental milestones of the early years

   Small and large motor development

   Cognitive development

   Markers of developmental delays

Developmental issues throughout breastfeeding

   Feeding and sleeping patterns

   Breastfeeding toddler

   Tandem breastfeeding

   Weaning

I. Interpretation of Research

Critical reading and interpretation

   Study design

   Human rights issues

   Results

Application to lactation consultant practice

Lactation measurement tools

Research terminology

Basic statistics

Data collection for research purposes

J. Ethical and Legal Issues

Medical-legal responsibilities

   Standards of Practice for IBCLC Lactation Consultants and other pertinent documents

   IBLCE Code of Ethics and other pertinent documents

   Evidence-based Guidelines for Breastfeeding Management During the First Fourteen Days

   Confidentiality

   Informed consent

   Referrals

   Charting and report writing

Ethical practice

   Remaining current

   Interdisciplinary relationships

   Neglect, maternal/infant abuse cases

   Expert witness role

   Rental and sale of equipment

   Evaluating practice

K. Breastfeeding Equipment and Technology

Identification of breastfeeding devices and equipment

   Appropriate use of breastfeeding equipment

   Alternatives to high technology solutions

Milk collection, storage, and use

Donor milk banking

  L. Techniques

    Breastfeeding techniques

      Positioning

      Latching on

      Feeding management skills

      Evaluating effectiveness of milk transfer

    Typical feeding patterns

    Multiple birth infants

    Manual expression

  M. Public Health

    Community education

    Health promotion activities

    Workplace issues

    IBCLC lactation consultant as change agent

    Creating and implementing protocols

    International Code of Marketing of Breast-Milk Substitutes and other resolutions

    The Innocenti Declaration

    The Baby Friendly Hospital Initiative

    Affecting public policy

    Nutrition programs providing for vulnerable populations

    International Labor Organization (ILO) recommendations

INTERNATIONAL BOARD CERTIFIED LACTATION CONSULTANT COMPETENCIES

The International Board Certified Lactation Consultant demonstrates multiple competencies. It is essential that the International Board Certified Lactation Consultant:

- think critically and reflectively in order to affect the clinical/practical management of the mother-baby dyad.
- sustain an evidence-based practice.
- collaborate effectively with the client and in multidisciplinary health care teams.
- continually update knowledge and skills.
- maintain awareness of the need to promote breastfeeding.

Practice Guidelines

I. Client Care Competencies

In order to provide appropriate care, a systematic process of assessment, management, and evaluation is used by the lactation consultant to:

1. Obtain an appropriate breastfeeding history for the mother and child.

2. Perform a comprehensive breastfeeding assessment of the mother-infant dyad.

3. Evaluate all assessment data to develop a plan of care that is both appropriate for specific problems and acceptable to the client.

4. Function as a member of the interdisciplinary health care team by collaborative systematic problem solving. Effectively coordinate breastfeeding care by providing written reports of consultations and making appropriate referrals to other health care providers and community service/support resources.

5. Identify the need for and provide client teaching and anticipatory guidance appropriate to the client's age, developmental status, (dis)ability, culture, religion, ethnicity, and support system.

6. Evaluate results of management using accepted outcome criteria; revise the plan accordingly, and consult and/or refer when needed.

7. Maintain comprehensive client records.

8. Provide safe care and understand the principles of universal precautions.

II. Lactation Consultant-Client Relationship Competencies

In order to establish a collaborative and supportive relationship with the client, the International Board Certified Lactation Consultant:

1. Promotes client autonomy, dignity, and self-determination by providing care that is non-judgmental and sensitive to client needs.

2. Establishes a partnership with the client to provide individualized optimal care consistent with the client's health belief system, and facilitates informed decision-making and self-care.

3. Acknowledges personal values and cultural differences and recognizes their impact on the provider/client relationship.

4. Uses effective communication and counseling skills.

5. Provides a physically safe and confidential environment for care.

6. Offers comfort and emotional support to clients and their families.

7. Functions as an advocate for the mother and child within the family.

8. Advocates for the mother and child within the health care system.

III. Health Education and Counseling Competencies

In order to plan, develop, coordinate, and provide appropriate breastfeeding education and counseling in response to the needs of clients, including breastfeeding families, health care professionals, and the community, the International Board Certified Lactation Consultant:

1. Provides information that meets client needs, promotes informed choice, and is appropriate to culture, language, and literacy.

2. Uses adult learning principles when providing educational experiences for clients.

3. Shares current evidence-based information.

4. Evaluates teaching strategies and effectiveness.

5. Demonstrates techniques and appropriate use of equipment according to the needs of the client.

6. Works collaboratively with others providing support and assistance, i.e., paraprofessionals, volunteers with community breastfeeding support groups, peer counselors, etc.

IV. Professional Role Competencies

In order to contribute to the practice of lactation consulting and the advancement of the profession, the International Board Certified Lactation Consultant:

1. Maintains IBLCE certification.

2. Adheres to these Guidelines, the *ILCA Standards of Practice for IBCLC Lactation Consultants*, and the *IBLCE Code of Ethics*.

3. Practices within the scope of the *International Code of Marketing of Breast-Milk Substitutes* and subsequent relevant resolutions.

4. Works within the policies and procedures of the institution where employed, or if self-employed, has identifiable policies and procedures, including informing clients about fees, obtaining informed consent, protecting confidentiality, and maintaining appropriate client records.

5. Uses breastfeeding equipment in an appropriate manner, including discussing benefits and risks, assuring cleanliness, and maintaining an awareness of conflict of interest when/if profiting from the rental or sale of breastfeeding equipment.

6. Maintains and expands knowledge and skills for lactation consultant practice by participating in continuing education programs and professional development activities in addition to reading current literature.

7. Evaluates own practice periodically and systematically in order to strive for improvement of care.

8. Supports and promotes well-designed research in human lactation and breastfeeding and bases clinical/practical practice on such research whenever possible.

9. Serves as a role model, preceptor, and mentor to other lactation consultants and students.

10. Seeks information about ethical, legal, and political issues regarding client advocacy and health care.

11. Participates in legislative and institutional policy-making activities related to breastfeeding.

12. Acts as an advocate for breastfeeding women, infants, and children in the community (including the media), the workplace, and within the health care system.

13. Interprets and promotes the role of the International Board Certified Lactation Consultant to consumers, other health care professionals, and the community.

14. Develops, uses, and maintains collaborative relationships with health care professionals to strengthen the role of the International Board Certified Lactation Consultant.

15. Maintains membership and participates in ILCA and local affiliate, if available.

Education Guidelines

Philosophy and Objectives

An International Board Certified Lactation Consultant education program is based upon a clearly articulated philosophy of what constitutes quality care for the breastfeeding mother-child dyad and the role of the lactation consultant in the provision of that care. An International Board Certified Lactation Consultant education program emphasizes individualized family care, client autonomy with informed decision-making, and optimal health care through a collaborative, supportive relationship with clients and primary care providers. In order to provide care, support, and services for breastfeeding families, practitioners must be able to clearly define both the necessary services and the role of the International Board Certified Lactation Consultant as the service provider.

The first objective of an International Board Certified Lactation Consultant education program is to prepare an individual for entry-level practice with emphasis on clinical/practical support and the management of normal breastfeeding and lactation. A secondary objective may be to provide continuing education opportunities for practicing International Board Certified Lactation Consultants. Such education is based upon understanding the interrelationship of many academic subject areas including: maternal and infant anatomy; physiology and endocrinology; nutrition and biochemistry; pathology; psychology, sociology, and anthropology; public health; normal growth and development; ethics and law; and evidence-based management principles. The body of scientific knowledge that forms the basis for the field of breastfeeding and human lactation results from a comprehension of the interrelationships between these subject areas and their impact on the care of a mother-infant dyad.

ILCA believes that the profession of lactation consulting is responsible for setting and maintaining the standards for the educational preparation of International Board Certified Lactation Consultants. ILCA further believes that professional education is a lifelong endeavor. The expanding body of knowledge of human lactation and breastfeeding, coupled with corresponding changes in health care and society, presents a continuing challenge to International Board Certified Lactation Consultant educators and creates a mandate for ongoing review of educational processes and outcomes.

II. Program Organization

Evaluation of any International Board Certified Lactation Consultant education programs is based on the following criteria:

1. The program has defined goals, measurable objectives, and adequate resources, in addition to appropriate curriculum, program design, and faculty.

2. The faculty of an International Board Certified Lactation Consultant program will offer expertise in breastfeeding and human lactation. It is also desirable that they be multidisciplinary and, where appropriate, culturally diverse. To serve as both mentors and role models, the majority of the faculty will possess current IBLCE credentials and maintain their competence through regular clinical/practical practice. The academic director of the program will be a recertified International Board Certified Lactation Consultant prepared at the master level of formal education or equivalent experience.

3. Clinical/practical preceptors are qualified by education and experience in the management of the breastfeeding mother and child. They are also competent in clinical/practical instruction. The use of experienced IBCLC practitioners as preceptors is preferred, whenever possible. A faculty/student ratio of no greater than 1:10 for supervised clinical/practical practice or a preceptor/student ratio of no greater than 1:2 is recommended.

4. The International Board Certified Lactation Consultant education program has clear admission criteria that may include specific content courses recommended by IBLCE for eligibility for certification.

Beginning in the exam year 2003, an applicant for the IBLCE exam must document background or completion of courses in anatomy & physiology, sociology, psychology or counseling, child development, nutrition, and medical terminology. A degree (including diploma RN) in one of the licensed health care professions is sufficient documentation. Applicants with other academic backgrounds will need to provide specific documentation. Additionally, all applicants will need to provide evidence of a minimum of 45 documented clock hours of education in lactation, reflecting the exam content outline, in the three years immediately preceding the exam.

Qualified applicants are admitted without regard to gender, race, disability, marital status, ethnic origin, creed, age, or sexual orientation. Selection and admission criteria are established by the sponsoring institution and its lactation consultant education faculty. Programs encourage enrollment and retention of students from culturally diverse populations.

5. Adequate classroom and clinical/practical teaching facilities, administrative support, and teaching aids are designated for the program. Students have access to adequate library resources. Technology support is sufficient to maintain distance learning programs, where offered.

6. Student records and program data are maintained in a manner that ensures confidentiality, retrievability and permanence. Transcripts are available upon student request.

III. Program Curriculum

Evaluation of an International Board Certified Lactation Consultant education program curriculum is based on the following criteria:

1. Curriculum content prepares students to meet standards of practice and prepares students in total or in part to be eligible for international certification.

2. Teaching strategies are based on currently accepted theories and principles of adult education.

3. The curriculum content includes the fundamental principles, professional responsibilities, core knowledge, and competencies, as outlined in this document under *Framework for Education and Practice*, pages 266–274.

IV. Program Evaluation

Assessment of International Board Certified Lactation Consultant education programs is based on the following criteria:

1. The program employs a variety of evaluation strategies to measure student achievement of IBCLC lactation consultant competencies. These strategies may include written tests and reports; observation of the student in the classroom, laboratory, and clinical/practical settings; conferences with the faculty and/or clinical/practical mentors; peer review and self-assessments.

2. Evaluation is ongoing, and students review their progress regularly with a faculty mentor.

3. There are written policies regarding expected levels of achievement, probation, dismissal, and withdrawal. These policies include expectations for mentor/preceptorship and any time limits for completion of the program.

4. A formal student grievance procedure exists.

5. There is a regular, formal evaluation of the total educational program. Evaluation is an integral part of the planning process and allows for timely revisions. Formative and summative evaluations are suggested and could include the following: program philosophy and goals, curriculum objectives and content, clinical/practical settings and experience, student-to-faculty ratios, faculty and clinical/practical mentor/preceptor performance, and student outcomes.

6. Surveys are conducted on both a short- and long-term basis to assess the impact of the program on career development and role satisfaction, as well as the impact of the graduates on the provision of breastfeeding/human lactation support and services. Sources of data and feedback to the program may include the following: students, preceptors, faculty, graduates, employers, funding sources, clients, and records of certification examination performance.

Accreditation is a voluntary external review process. It recognizes lactation consultant education programs that have achieved a level of quality that deserves the confidence of the student consumer and the public. Accreditation often is used as a criterion in decision-making by funding organizations, state regulatory bodies, employers, third party payors, student loan/scholarship granting agencies, and potential students. Because accreditation status is reviewed periodically, it encourages continuous self-study and improvement. This document outlines the basic knowledge, skills, and competencies of a practitioner and provides the basis for evaluation and approval of International Board Certified Lactation Consultant education programs by an official accreditation body.

ACKNOWLEDGEMENTS

The Professional Education Council of the International Lactation Consultant Association acknowledges the assistance of the Association of Women's Health, Obstetric and Neonatal Nurses (AWHONN) and the National Association of Nurse Practitioners in Reproductive Health (NANPRH). Their jointly prepared document, The Women's Health Nurse Practitioner: Guidelines for Practice and Education served as a general model of clear, unified guidelines for practice and education. The Professional Education Council also thanks the North Carolina Nurses Association for their helpful discussion of multiple competencies in their North Carolina Nurses Association Position Paper, Registered Nurse Education in the 21st Century.

NOTES

1 Note: The International Lactation Consultant Association (ILCA) recognizes the International Board Certified Lactation Consultant (IBLCE) credential as the appropriate certification for lactation consultants.

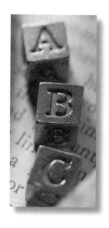

Innocenti Declaration

On the Protection, Promotion and Support of Breastfeeding

RECOGNISING THAT:

Breastfeeding is a unique process that:

- Provides ideal nutrition for infants and contributes to their healthy growth and development

- Reduces incidence and severity of infectious diseases, thereby lowering infant morbidity and mortality

- Contributes to women's health by reducing the risk of breast and ovarian cancer, and by increasing the spacing between pregnancies

- Provides social and economic benefits to the family and the nation

- Provides most women with a sense of satisfaction when successfully carried out and that

Recent Research has found that:

- these benefits increase with increased exclusiveness of breastfeeding during the first six months of life, and thereafter with increased duration of breastfeeding with complementary foods, and

- programme intervention can result in positive changes in breastfeeding behaviour

WE THEREFORE DECLARE THAT:

As a global goal for optimal maternal and child health and nutrition, all women should be enabled to practise exclusive breastfeeding and all infants should be fed exclusively on breastmilk from birth to 4-6 months of age.[1] Thereafter, children should continue to be breastfed, while receiving appropriate and adequate complementary foods, for up to two years of age or beyond. This child-feeding ideal is to be achieved by creating an appropriate environment of awareness and support so that women can breastfeed in this manner.

Attainment of this goal requires, in many countries, the reinforcement of a "breastfeeding culture" and its vigorous defence against incursions of a "bottle-feeding culture." This requires commitment and advocacy for social mobilization, utilizing to the full the prestige and authority of acknowledged leaders of society in all walks of life.

Efforts should be made to increase women's confidence in their ability to breastfeed. Such empowerment involves the removal of constraints and influences that manipulate perceptions and behaviour towards breastfeeding, often by subtle and indirect means. This requires sensitivity, continued vigilance, and a responsive and comprehensive communications strategy involving all media and addressed to all levels of society. Furthermore, obstacles to breastfeeding within the health system, the workplace, and the community must be eliminated.

Measures should be taken to ensure that women are adequately nourished for their optimal health and that of their families. Furthermore, ensuring that all women also have access to family planning information and services allows them to sustain breastfeeding and avoid shortened birth intervals that may compromise their health and nutritional status, and that of their children.

All governments should develop national breastfeeding policies and set appropriate national targets for the 1990s. They should establish a national system for monitoring the attainment of their targets, and they should develop indicators such as the prevalence of exclusively breastfed infants at discharge from maternity services, and the prevalence of exclusively breastfed infants at four months of age.

National authorities are further urged to integrate their breastfeeding policies into their overall health and development policies. In so doing they should reinforce all actions that protect, promote, and support breastfeeding within complementary programmes such as prenatal and perinatal care, nutrition, family planning services, and prevention and treatment of common maternal and childhood diseases. All healthcare staff should be trained in the skills necessary to implement these breastfeeding policies.

OPERATIONAL TARGETS

All governments by the year 1995 should have:

- Appointed a national breastfeeding coordinator of appropriate authority, and established a multisectoral national breastfeeding committee composed of representatives from relevant government departments, non-governmental organizations, and health professional associations;

- Ensured that every facility providing maternity services fully practises all ten of the Ten Steps to Successful Breastfeeding set out in the joint WHO/UNICEF statement "Protecting, promoting and supporting breastfeeding: the special role of maternity services;"

- Taken action to give effect to the principles and aim of all Articles of the International Code of Marketing of Breast-Milk Substitutes and subsequent relevant World Health Assembly resolutions in their entirety; and

- Enacted imaginative legislation protecting the breastfeeding rights of working women and established means for its enforcement.

WE ALSO CALL UPON INTERNATIONAL ORGANIZATIONS TO:

- Draw up action strategies for protecting, promoting and supporting breastfeeding, including global monitoring and evaluation of their strategies;

- Support national situation analyses and surveys and the development of national goals and targets for action; and

- Encourage and support national authorities in planning, implementing, monitoring and evaluating their breastfeeding policies.

The Innocenti Declaration was produced and adopted by participants at the WHO/UNICEF policymakers' meeting on "Breastfeeding in the 1990s: A Global Initiative," co-sponsored by the United States Agency for International Development (A.I.D.) and the Swedish International Development Authority (SIDA), held at the Spedale degli Innocenti, Florence, Italy, on 30 July–1 August 1990. The Declaration reflects the content of the original background document for the meeting and the views expressed in group and plenary sessions.

Further information may be obtained from UNICEF, Nutrition Cluster (H-8F), 3 United Nations Plaza, New York, NY 10017.

NOTES

1. Subsequent to the signing of the Innocenti Declaration in 1990, the World Health Organization has clarified the optimal duration of exclusive breastfeeding with the following language: "To achieve optimal growth, development and health, infants should be exclusively breastfed for the first six months of life. Thereafter, to meet their evolving nutritional requirements, infants should receive nutritionally adequate and safe complementary foods while breastfeeding continues for up to two years of age or beyond."

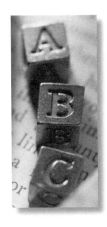

WHO Code Summary

The International Code of Marketing of Breast-Milk Substitutes

World Health Organization

The Code seeks to encourage and protect breastfeeding and to control incorrect marketing practices used to sell products for artificial feeding.

The Code applies to: artificial milks for babies; other products used to feed babies, especially when they are marketed for use in a feeding bottle; feeding bottles and teats.

Provisions:

1. No advertising of these products to the public.

2. No free samples to mothers. (Includes "gift" bags)

3. No promotion of products in health care facilities. (Includes providing free or low-cost supplies of formula and related products to hospitals).

4. No company mothercraft nurses to advise mothers.

5. No gifts or personal samples to health workers. (Includes pens, pads, coffee cups, etc.)

6. No words or pictures idealizing artificial feeding, including pictures of infants, on the labels of the products.

7. Information to health workers should be scientific and factual.

8. All information on artificial feeding, including the labels, should explain the benefits of breastfeeding, and the costs and hazards associated with artificial feeding.

9. Unsuitable products, such as sweetened condensed milk, should not be promoted for babies.

10. All products should be of a high quality and take account of the climatic and storage conditions of the country where they are used.

Notes: The Code was adopted by the World Health Assembly in 1981 following a vote in which 118 Member States were in favor, one was against (the USA) and three abstained (Argentina, Japan and Korea). In 1994 the USA was party to the adoption of World Health Assembly Resolution 47.5, which reaffirms support for the resolution that adopted the Code. The USA is thus now deemed to support the Code.

The Code is primarily aimed at governments and companies. Governments are expected to use the Code as a "minimum requirement" and implement it "in its entirety," either as a law or as a voluntary measure. Companies are called upon, "independent of any . . . measures taken for implementation" of the Code to "ensure that their conduct at every level conform" to the provisions of the Code. (IBFAN)

For more information, ILCA publishes a monograph on the Code implementation and interpretation, which was originally published in the *Journal of Human Lactation*.

Adapted from *Protecting Infant Health: A Health Workers' Guide to the International Code of Marketing of Breastmilk Substitutes* published by the International Organization of Consumers Union and the International Baby Food Action Network (IBFAN), 1987.

Internet site: http://www.who.org
http://www.infactcanada.ca/whocode/codeview.htm

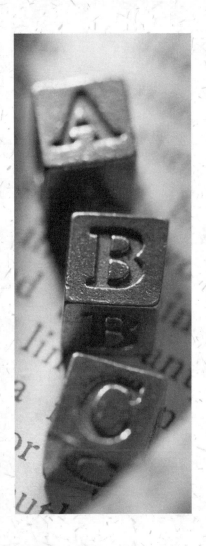

Educational Resources

Resources for Professional Education
IBCLE Suggested Reading List
Reference Book List
Shadowing/Observation Guidelines
Interview Questions for Lactation Consultant Candidates
Development of Professional Lactation Education
Guidelines for Evaluating Educational Materials

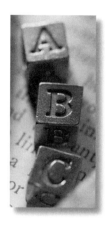

Resources for Professional Education

International Lactation Consultant Association (ILCA)
1500 Sunday Drive, Suite 102
Raleigh, NC 27607
Phone: (919) 787-5181; fax: (919) 787-4916
Internet: www.ILCA.org

ILCA's *Guide to Selecting a Course or Program*,
http://www.ilca.org/courseguide.html
ILCA's *Directory of Lactation Management Courses*,
http://www.ilca.org/courses.html
LactNews (private site; lists conferences and educational programs),
www.lactnews.com

Union Institute, www.tui.edu
Pacific Oaks College/Lactation Institute, www.pacificoaks.edu

International Board of Lactation Consultant Examiners (IBLCE)
7309 Arlington Blvd., Suite 300
Falls Church, VA 22042-3215
Phone: (703) 560-7330; fax: (703) 560-7332
Internet: www.IBLCE.org
E-mail: iblce@iblce.org

La Leche League International
1400 N. Meacham Rd., P.O. Box 4079
Schaumburg, IL 60168-4079
Phone: (847) 519-7730; fax: (847) 519-0035
Internet: www.lalecheleague.org

Research Sites
PubMed, http://www.ncbi.nlm.nih.gov/PubMed
NewJour, http://gort.ucsd.edu/newjour
Free Medical Journals site, www.freemedicaljournals.com

IBLCE Suggested Reading List

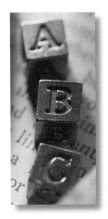

International Board of Lactation Consultant Examiners

The Suggested Reading List is neither all-inclusive, nor does it cover all exam items. The IBLCE recommends that candidates become familiar with a wide range of literature, scientific studies, and journals, including materials published outside their own countries. Additionally, it is useful to review good basic texts on child development, neonatology, prematurity, research methodology, and statistics, as well as mother-support literature that covers breastfeeding management in a range of situations.

BOOKS AND SERIES

The letters in parentheses after a title in the alphabetical listing refer to Disciplines in the Exam Blueprint that are well covered in that book or series. General lactation texts and practical breastfeeding management texts do not have discipline reference numbers after them, as they cover a broad spectrum of topics.

Asterisks indicate materials on this list that may be ordered from LLLI (*) or NMAA (**). The addresses for ordering are at the end of this list.

General Lactation Texts:

International Lactation Consultant Association. *Core Curriculum for Lactation Consultant Practice.* Walker, M. (ed). Sudbury, MA: Jones and Bartlett Publishers, 2001.

Lawrence, Ruth. *Breastfeeding: A Guide for the Medical Profession*, Fifth Edition. St. Louis, MO: CV Mosby, 1999 edition.*

Riordan, J., and K. Auerbach. *Breastfeeding and Human Lactation*, Second Edition. Sudbury, MA: Jones and Bartlett Publishers, 1999.

Practical Breastfeeding Management Texts:

Biancuzzo, M. *Breastfeeding the Newborn: Clinical Strategies for Nurses.* St. Louis, Mosby, 1999.

Brodribb, W. *Breastfeeding Management in Australia: A Reference and Study Guide.* Nunawading, Australia: Nursing Mothers' Association of Australia, 1997 rev. ed. **

Henschel, Dora, and Sally Inch. *Breastfeeding: A Guide for Midwives.* Cheshire, England: Books for Midwives Press, 1996.

Lauwers, J., and D. Shinskie. *Counseling the Nursing Mother.* Sudbury, MA: Jones and Bartlett Publishers, 2000.

Mohrbacher, N., and J. Stock. *The Breastfeeding Answer Book*. Schaumburg, IL: La Leche League International, 1997. *

The Royal College of Midwives. *Successful Breastfeeding: A Practical Guide for Mothers and Midwives and Others Supporting Breastfeeding Mothers*. London; Melbourne; New York: Churchill Livingstone, 1991 ed.

Alphabetical Listing of Books, Series, and Publications:

AAP *Birth to Five Years*, Shelov S (ed), 2nd edition, 2001, AAP [J]

Auerbach, K. and J. Riordan. *Clinical Lactation: A Visual Guide*. Sudbury, MA: Jones and Bartlett Publishers, 2000.

Bornmann, P., *Legal Chap in ILCA's Core Curriculum*. [J]

Hale, Thomas. *Medications and Mothers' Milk*. Amarillo, TX: Thomas Hale, updated annually. [F]

Hoover, K. and B. Wilson-Clay. *The Breastfeeding Atlas*. Austin, TX: LactNews Press, 1999.

Human Relations Enrichment Workbook. Schaumburg, IL: La Leche League International, 1994. [Counseling skills workbook geared toward breastfeeding counselors.] [G] *

ILCA, *Scope of Practice for Lactation Consultants*, 2001. [J]

Merewood A./Phillip BL, *Breastfeeding Conditions and Diseases*. Pharmasoft Publications 2001. [J]

National Academy of Sciences, Institute of Medicine. *Nutrition During Pregnancy and Lactation: An Implementation Guide*. Washington, DC: National Academy Press, 1992. [C] *

Polit, D.F., & B.P. Hungler. *Nursing Research: Principles and Methods*. Philadelphia: Lippencott, 1995. [I]

Roberts, Kathryn and Beverly Taylor. *Nursing Research Processes: An Australian Perspective*. 102 Dodds Street, South Melbourne VIC, 3205 Australia, 1998. [I]

Scott, J. *Ethical Chap in ILCA 's Core Curriculum* [J]

Standards of Practice for Lactation Consultants. Chicago, IL: International Lactation Consultant Association (ILCA), 1995. [M]

Stuart-Macadam, P., and Kathryn Dettwyler, ed. *Breastfeeding: Biocultural Perspectives*. Hawthorne, NY: Aldine de Grnyer, 1995. [G]

Topics in Breastfeeding. Nursing Mothers' Association of Australia, Lactation Resource Centre. [mostly B, C, E, G, K, and I] **

WHO. *International Code of Marketing of Breastmilk Substitutes*. Geneva: WHO, 1981 [M]

WHO/UNICEF Statement. *Protecting, Promoting and Supporting Breastfeeding: The Special Role of Maternity Services*. Geneva, Switzerland: WHO, 1989. [Translated into 22 languages, including German, Italian, French, and Spanish.] [M]

JOURNALS, NEWSLETTERS, AND LITERATURE REVIEW

ABM News and Views. Quarterly newsletter. Available by subscription from the Academy of Breastfeeding Medicine, PO Box 81323, San Diego, CA 92138-1323. Telephone: (877) 836-9947, Fax: (619)295-0056, email: abm@bfmed.org, website: www.bfmed.org

Breastfeeding Abstracts. Quarterly annotated summary of new breastfeeding research. Available by subscription from LLLI. *

Breastfeeding Review. Semi-annual journal. Available by subscription from NMAA. **

Journal of Human Lactation. Quarterly journal. Available by membership in International Lactation Consultant Association (ILCA), 1500 Sunday Drive #102, Raleigh NC 27607-5163 USA. Telephone: 1 (919) 787-5181, Fax: 1 (919) 787-4916, e-mail: ilca@erols.com.

*   LLLI: La Leche League International, 1400 North Meacham Rd., Schaumburg, IL 60173-4840 USA. Telephone: 1 (847) 519-7730, Fax: 1 (847) 519-0035

** NMAA: Nursing Mothers Association of Australia, PO Box 4000, Glen Iris VIC 3146 AUS-TRALIA. From outside Australia: Phone +(61-3) 9885 0855, Fax +(61-3) 9885 0866, email: nursingm@nmsa.asn.au

U.S. National Library of Medicine (NLM) offers its MEDLINE database of more than 8.8 million references to articles published in 3800 biomedical journals free of charge on the World Wide Web. Access PubMed or Internet Grateful Med through http://www.nim.nih.gov/

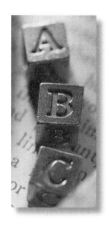

Reference Book List

Compiled by Linda J. Smith, BSE, FACCE, IBCLC, February 2002

Akre J, ed. *Infant Feeding, The Physiological Basis*. Bulletin of the World Health Organization Supplement to Vol. 67 (1989). Geneva: World Health Organization, 1991.

Als H. *Manual for the Naturalistic Observation of Newborn Behavior (Preterm and Fullterm Infants)*. Copyright H. Als, 1981; 1984 revision. The Children's Hospital, Boston, MA 02115. Unpublished manuscript, available from author.

Als H, Lester BM, Tronick E, and Brazelton TB. Manual for the assessment of preterm infants' behavior (AFPB). In Fitzgerald JE, Lester BM, Jogman MW, eds. *Theory and Research in Behavioral Pediatrics, Vol. 1.* New York: Plenum, 1982.

Amir L, Hoover K, and Mulford C. *Candidaisis and Breastfeeding*. Lactation Consultant Series, Unit 18. Garden City Park, NJ: Avery Publishing Group, 1995.

Apple RD. *Mothers and Medicine: A Social History of Infant Feeding 1890–1950*. Madison, WI: University of Wisconsin Press, 1987.

Arms A. *Immaculate Deception II*. Berkeley, CA: Celestial Arts, 1996.

Arnold LDW, ed. *Recommendations for Collection, Storage, and Handling of a Mother's Milk for Her Own Infant in the Hospital Setting*. Sandwich, MA: Human Milk Banking Association of North America, 1993, and subsequent editions.

Arnold LDW. *The Role of Donor Milk in the Reduction of Infant Mortality and Morbidity: A Child Survival Issue*. Sandwich, MA: Health Education Associates, 1996.

Arnold LDW and Tully MR, eds. *Guidelines for the Establishment and Operation of a Donor Human Milk Bank*. Sandwich, MA: Human Milk Banking Association of North America, 1994, and subsequent editions.

Auerbach KG. *Breastfeeding Techniques and Devices*. Lactation Consultant Series, Unit 17. Garden City Park, NJ: Avery Publishing Group, 1987.

Auerbach KG. *Maternal Employment and Breastfeeding*. Lactation Consultant Series Unit 6. Wayne, NJ: Avery Publishing Group, 1987.

Bar-Yam N. *The Right to Breast: Breastfeeding and Human Rights*. Sandwich, MA: Health Education Associates, 2000.

Baumgarner NJ. *Mothering Your Nursing Toddler*, 3rd revised ed. Schaumburg IL: La Leche League International, 2000.

Baumslag N and Michels D. *Milk, Money and Madness*. Westport, CT: Bergin and Garvey, 1995.

Bergman DA, ed. *Practice Parameters from the American Academy of Pediatrics: A Compilation of Evidence-Based Guidelines for Pediatric Practice*. Elk Grove Village, IL: American Academy of Pediatrics, 1997.

Bertelsen C and Auerbach KG. *Nutrition and Breastfeeding: The Cultural Connection*. Lactation Consultant Series Unit 11. Wayne, NJ: Avery Publishing Group, 1987.

Biancuzzo M. *Breastfeeding the Newborn: Clinical Strategies for Nurses*. St. Louis: Mosby, 1999.

Bing E and Colman L. *Laughter and Tears: The Emotional Life of New Mothers*. New York: Henry Holt, 1997.

Black RF, Jarman L, and Simpson J. *Lactation Specialist Self-Study Modules #1–4*. Sudbury, MA: Jones and Bartlett, 1998.

Blum BL. *Psychological Aspects of Pregnancy, Birth and Bonding*. New York: Human Sciences Press, 1980.

Bocar DL and Moore K. *Acquiring the Parental Role: A Theoretical Perspective*. Lactation Consultant Series, Unit 16. Wayne, NJ: Avery Publishing Group, 1987.

Bonica JJ. *Obstetric Analgesia and Anesthesia*. Amsterdam: World Federation of Societies of Anaesthesiologists, 1980.

Bornmann PG. *Legal Considerations and the Lactation Consultant—U.S.A.* Lactation Consultant Series, Unit 3. Wayne, NJ: Avery Publishing Group, 1986.

Brackbill Y, Rice J, and Young D. *Birth Trap: The Legal Low-Down on High-Tech Obstetrics*. St Louis: C.V. Mosby.

Breaking the Rules, Stretching the Rules 2001: Evidence of Violations of the International Code of Marketing of Breastmilk Substitutes and Subsequent Resolutions. Penang, Malaysia: IBFAN, 2001.

Breastfeeding Advocacy Kit. Weston, MA: NABA, 1997.

Briggs GG, Freeman RK, and Yaffe SJ. *Drugs in Pregnancy and Lactation*, 5th ed. Baltimore: Williams and Wilkins, 1998.

Brodzinsky DM, Gormly AV, and Ambron SR. *Lifespan Human Development*, 3rd ed. New York: Holt, Rinehart and Winston, 1986.

Cadwell AL. *Collaboration and Motivation*. Sandwich, MA: Health Education Associates, 1999.

Cadwell AL and Turner-Maffei C. *Toward Evidence-Based Breastfeeding Practice*. Sandwich, MA: Health Education Associates, 2000.

Cadwell K. *Growing the Breastfeeding Friendly Community*. Sandwich, MA: Health Education Associates, 1996.

Cadwell K and Turner-Maffei C. *Concerns about Infant Formula*. Sandwich, MA: Health Education Associates, 2000.

Cadwell K, Turner-Maffei C, O'Connor B, and Blair A. *Maternal and Infant Assessment for Breastfeeding and Human Lactation*. Sudbury MA: Jones and Bartlett, 2002.

Care in Normal Birth: A Practical Guide. Geneva: World Health Organization Technical Working Group, 1996.

Chamberlain D. *The Mind of Your Newborn Baby*. Berkeley, CA: North Atlantic Books, 1998.

Code of Ethics. Falls Church, VA: International Board of Lactation Consultant Examiners, 1996.

Cohen, NW. *Open Season: A Survival Guide for Natural Childbirth and VBAC in the 90s*. New York: Bergin & Garvey, 1991.

Davis M. *The Lactation Consultant's Clinical Practice Manual*. Dayton, OH: Bright Future Lactation Resource Centre, 1998. www.bflrc.com.

Davis-Floyd, R. *Birth as an American Rite of Passage*. Berkeley: University of California Press, 1992.

Desmarais L and Browne S. *Inadequate Weight Gain in Breastfeeding Infants: Assessments and Resolution*. Lactation Consultant Series, Unit 8. Schaumburg, IL: La Leche League International, 1990.

Dunham C. *Mamatoto: A Celebration of Birth*. New York: Penguin Books, 1991.

Ehrenreich B and English D. *Complaints and Disorders: The Sexual Politics of Sickness*. New York: Feminist Press, 1973.

Ehrenreich B and English D. *For Her Own Good*. Garden City, NY: Anchor Books, 1979.

Ehrenreich B and English D. *Witches, Midwives and Nurses*. Out of print.

Engelking C and Page-Lieberman J. *Maternal Diabetes and Diabetes in Young Children: Their Relationship to Breastfeeding*. Lactation Consultant Series, Unit 5. Wayne, NJ: Avery Publishing Group, 1986.

An Evaluation of Infant Growth. Geneva: World Health Organization Nutrition Unit, 1994.

Evidence for the Ten Steps to Successful Breastfeeding. Geneva: World Health Organization Division of Child Health and Development, 1998.

Evidence-Based Guidelines for Breastfeeding Management During the First Fourteen Days. Raleigh, NC: International Lactation Consultant Association, 1999.

Fildes V. *Breasts, Bottles and Babies: A History of Infant Feeding*. Edinburgh: Edinburgh University Press, 1986.

Fildes V. *Wet Nursing: A History from Antiquity to the Present*. New York: Basil Blackwell, 1988.

Fox I. *Being There: The Benefits of a Stay-at-Home Parent*. Hauppauge, NY: Barron's Educational Series, 1996.

Frantz K. *Breastfeeding Product Guide and Supplement*. Sunland, CA: Geddes Productions, 1999.

Gabay M and Wolfe SM. *Unnecessary Cesarean Sections: Curing a National Epidemic*. Washington, DC: Public Citizen Action Group, 1994.

Gardiner J, Lauwers J, Woessner C, and Bernard B. *Relationships and Roles: The Lactation Consultant and Lay Breastfeeding Groups*. Lactation Consultant Series, Unit 7. Wayne, NJ: Avery Publishing Group, 1986.

Goer H. *Obstetric Myths versus Research Realities: A Guide to the Medical Literature*. Westport, CT: Bergin and Garvey, 1995.

Goer H. *The Thinking Woman's Guide to a Better Birth*. New York: Perigree Books by Berkley Publishing Group of Penguin Putnam, 1999.

Granju KA and Kennedy B. *Attachment Parenting*. New York: Pocket Books, 1999.

Griest D, Chesney MR, and Miner K. *The Lactation Consultant as an Allied Health Worker*. Lactation Consultant Series, Unit 4. Wayne, NJ: Avery Publishing Group, 1986.

Gromada KK. *Mothering Multiples*. Schaumburg, IL: La Leche League International, 1999.

Hale T. *Clinical Therapy in Breastfeeding Patients*. Amarillo, TX: Pharmasoft Publishing, 1999.

Hale T. *Medications and Mothers' Milk*. Amarillo, TX: Pharmasoft Publishing, 2000.

Handley R. *Homeopathy for Women*. London: Harper Collins, 1993.

Hauth JC and Gerald BN. Merenstein, eds. *Guidelines for Perinatal Care*, 4th ed. Elk Grove Village, IL: American Academy of Pediatrics, and Washington, DC: American College of Obstetricians and Gynecologists, 1997.

Heller S. *The Vital Touch*. New York: Henry Holt, 1997.

Herforth DT. *Counseling Grieving Families*. Lactation Consultant Series, Unit 12. Wayne, NJ: Avery Publishing Group, 1986.

Herzfeld J. *Sense and Sensibility in Childbirth*. New York: W. W. Norton, 1985.

Huggins K and Ziedrich L. *The Nursing Mother's Guide to Weaning*. Boston: Harvard Common Press, 1994.

Human Relations Enrichment Workbook, 3rd ed. Schaumburg, IL: La Leche League International, 1994.

Hypoglycemia of the Newborn: Review of the Literature. World Health Organization, 1997.

Inch S. Antenatal preparation for breastfeeding. In *Effective Care in Pregnancy and Childbirth, Vol 1: Pregnancy.* Oxford: Oxford University Press, 1989.

Institute of Medicine (Subcommittee on Nutrition During Lactation, Food and Nutrition Board). *Nutrition During Lactation.* Washington, DC: National Academy of Sciences, 1991.

Institute of Medicine. *Nutrition During Pregnancy.* Washington, DC: National Academy of Sciences, 1991.

Jensen RG. *Handbook of Milk Composition.* San Diego: Academic Press, 1995.

Karen R. *Becoming Attached.* New York: Oxford University Press, 1998.

Kitzinger S. *Becoming a Grandmother.* New York: Fireside Books, 1996.

Kitzinger S. *The Complete Book of Pregnancy and Childbirth.* New York: Alfred A. Knopf, 1989.

Klaus MH and Kennell JH. *Maternal–Infant Bonding.* St. Louis: C.V. Mosby, 1976.

Klaus MH and Kennell JH. *Parent–Infant Bonding*, 2nd ed. St. Louis: C.V. Mosby, 1982.

Klaus MH, Kennell JH, and Klaus PH. *Bonding: Building the Foundations of Secure Attachment and Independence.* St. Louis: Mosby, 1995.

Klaus MH, Kennell JH, and Klaus PH. *Mothering the Mother.* Reading, MA: Addison-Wesley, 1993.

Klaus MH and Klaus PH. *Your Amazing Newborn.* Reading, MA: Perseus Books, 1998.

Kleinman RE, ed. *Pediatric Nutrition Handbook*, 4th ed. Elk Grove Village, IL: American Academy of Pediatrics, 1998.

Knoben JE and Anderson PO. *Handbook of Clinical Drug Data*, 6th ed. Hamilton: Drug Intelligence Publications, 1988.

Korte D and Scaer R. *A Good Birth, a Safe Birth*, 3rd revised ed. Boston: Harvard Common Press, 1992.

Lang S. *Breastfeeding Special Care Babies.* London: Balliere Tindall/WB Saunders, 1997.

Lauwers J and Shinskie D. *Counseling the Nursing Mother*, 3rd ed. Sudbury, MA: Jones and Bartlett, 2000.

Lawrence R. *A Review of the Medical Benefits and Contraindications to Breastfeeding in the United States* (Maternal and Child Health Technical Information Bulletin). Arlington, VA: National Center for Education in Maternal and Child Health, October 1997.

Lawrence RA and Lawrence RM. *Breastfeeding, A Guide for the Medical Profession*, 5th ed. St. Louis: Mosby, 1999.

Lee N. *Benefits of Breastfeeding and Their Economic Impact.* Sandwich, MA: Health Education Associates, 2000.

Lee N and Kellogg-Spadt S. *Sexuality and Human Lactation.* Sandwich, MA: Health Education Associates, 2000.

Love SM. *Dr. Susan Love's Breast Book*, 3rd ed. Reading, MA: Addison-Wesley, 2000.

Marmet C and Shell E. *Lactation Forms: A Guide to Lactation Consultant Charting.* Encino, CA: Lactation Institute, 1989.

McIntyre A. *The Complete Woman's Herbal.* New York: Henry Holt, 1995.

Merewood A and Philip BL. *Breastfeeding: Conditions and Diseases, A Reference Guide.* Amarillo, TX: Pharmasoft Publishing, 2001.

Minchin M. *Breastfeeding Matters*, 4th revised ed. St. Kilda, Australia: Alma Publications, 1998.

Mitford, J. *The American Way of Birth.* New York: Penguin Books, 1992.

Montagu A. *Touching: The Human Significance of the Skin*, 3rd ed. New York: Harper and Row, 1986.

Moore KL and Persaud TVN. *Before We Are Born: Essentials of Embryology and Birth Defects*, 4th ed. Philadelphia: W. B. Saunders, 1993.

Morbacher N and Stock J. *The Breastfeeding Answer Book, Revised Edition*. Schaumburg, IL: La Leche League International, 1997.

Mother-Friendly Childbirth Initiative Consensus Document. Washington, DC: Coalition for Improving Maternity Services, 1996. www.motherfriendly.org.

Neville MC and Neifert MR. *Lactation: Physiology, Nutrition and Breastfeeding*. New York: Plenum Press, 1983.

Newton N. *Maternal Emotions*. New York: Paul E. Hoeber, 1955.

Nichols FH and Zwelling E. *Maternal-Newborn Nursing: Theory and Practice*. Philadelphia: W. B. Saunders, 1997.

Oakley, A. *The Captured Womb: A History of the Medical Care of Pregnant Women*. Oxford: Basil Blackwell, 1984.

Odent, M. *The Nature of Birth and Breastfeeding*. Westport, CT: Bergin and Garvey, 1992.

Olds SB, London ML, and Ladewig PW. *Maternal-Newborn Nursing: A Family-Centered Approach*. Redwood City, CA: Addison-Wesley Nursing, 1992.

Osofsky, JD. *Handbook of Infant Development*. New York: John Wiley & Sons, 1987.

Palmer G. *The Politics of Breastfeeding*, 2nd ed. London: Pandora Press, 1993.

Panuthos, C. *Transformation Through Birth*. New York: Bergin & Garvey, 1984.

Parker D and Williams N. *Teens and Breastfeeding*. Schaumburg, IL: La Leche League International, 2000.

Peter G, ed. *1997 Red Book: Report of the Committee on Infectious Diseases*, 24th ed. Elk Grove Village, IL: American Academy of Pediatrics, 1997.

Popper BK. *The Hospitalized Nursing Baby*. Lactation Consultant Series II, Unit 1. Schaumburg, IL: La Leche League International, 1998.

Position Paper on Infant Feeding. Raleigh, NC: International Lactation Consultant Association, 1994.

Powell DE and Stelling CB. *The Diagnosis and Detection of Breast Disease*. St. Louis: Mosby–Year Book, 1994.

Price J. *Motherhood: What It Does to Your Mind*. London: Pandora Books, 1988.

Protecting, Promoting and Supporting Breastfeeding: The Special Role of Maternity Services. A Joint WHO/UNICEF Statement. Geneva: World Health Organization Nutrition Unit, 1989.

Pryor K and Pryor G. *Nursing Your Baby*. New York: Pocket Books, 1991.

Relactation: Review of Experience and Recommendations for Practice. Geneva: World Health Organization, 1998.

Riordan J and Auerbach KG. *Breastfeeding and Human Lactation*, 2nd ed. Sudbury, MA: Jones and Bartlett, 1999.

Riordan J and Riordan S. *The Effect of Labor Epidurals on Breastfeeding*. Schaumburg, IL: La Leche League International, 2000.

Royal College of Midwives. *Successful Breastfeeding*, 2nd ed. London and New York: Churchill Livingstone, 1991.

Satir V. *The New Peoplemaking*. Mountain View, CA: Science and Behavior Books, 1988.

Satter E. *Child of Mine: Feeding with Love and Good Sense*. Palo Alto, CA: Bull Publishing, 1983.

Satter E. *How to Get Your Kid to Eat... But Not Too Much*. Palo Alto, CA: Bull Publishing, 1987.

Savage F. *Helping Mothers to Breastfeed*. Nairobi, Kenya: African Medical and Research Foundation, 1994.

Sears W and Sears M. *The Baby Book: Everything You Need to Know About Your Baby from Birth to Age Two*. Boston: Little, Brown, 1993.

Small MF. *Our Babies, Ourselves: How Biology and Culture Shape the Way We Parent*. New York: Random House, 1998.

Smith LJ. *Coach's Notebook: Games and Strategies for Lactation Education*. Sudbury, MA: Jones and Bartlett, 2002.

Smith LJ. *Comprehensive Lactation Consultant Exam Review*. Sudbury, MA: Jones and Bartlett, 2001.

Snyder JB. *Variation in Infant Palatal Structure and Breastfeeding* (master's thesis). Pasadena, CA: Pacific Oaks College, 1995.

Standards of Practice for Lactation Consultants. Raleigh, NC: International Lactation Consultant Association, 1999.

Stark Y. *Human Nipples: Function and Anatomical Variations in Relationship to Breastfeeding* (master's thesis). Pasadena, CA: Pacific Oaks College, 1994.

Stillerman E. *Mother Massage*. New York: Dell Publishing, 1992.

Stuart-Macadam P and Dettwyler KA. *Breastfeeding: Biocultural Perspectives*. New York: Aldine De Gruyter, 1995.

Sutherland A and Auerback KG. *Relactation and Induced Lactation*. Lactation Consultant Series, Unit 1. Wayne, NJ: Avery Publishing Group, 1985.

Taylor MM. *Transcultural Aspects of Breastfeeding—USA*. Lactation Consultant Series, Unit 2. Wayne, NJ: Avery Publishing Group, 1985.

Thoman EB and Browder S. *Born Dancing: How Intuitive Parents Understand Their Baby's Unspoken Language and Natural Rhythms*. New York: Harper and Row, 1987.

Ullman D and Cummings S. *Everybody's Guide to Homeopathic Medicines*. New York: Jeremy P. Tarcher/Perigree Books, 1991.

U.S. Breastfeeding Committee. *Protecting, Promoting, Supporting Breastfeeding in the United States: A National Agenda*. Raleigh, NC: United States Breastfeeding Committee, 2001.

U.S. Department of Health and Human Services. *HHS Blueprint for Action on Breastfeeding*. Washington, DC: U.S. Department of Health and Human Services, Office of Women's Health, 2000.

Van Esterik P and Menon L. *Being Mother-Friendly: A Practical Guide for Working Women and Breastfeeding*. Penang, Malaysia: World Alliance for Breastfeeding Action, 1996.

Van Esterik, P. *Beyond the Breast-Bottle Controversy*. New Brunswick, NJ: Rutgers University Press, 1989.

Van Esterik P. *Women, Work, and Breastfeeding*. North York, Ontario: York University Press, 1994.

Varney, H. *Varney's Midwifery*, 3rd ed. Sudbury, MA: Jones and Bartlett, 1997.

Walker, M. *Core Curriculum for Lactation Consultant Practice*. Sudbury, MA: Jones and Bartlett, 2002.

Walker M. *Mastitis in Lactating Women*. Lactation Consultant Series II, Unit 2. Schaumburg, IL: La Leche League International, 1999.

Walker, M, ed. *Selling Out Mothers and Babies: Marketing of Breastmilk Substitutes in the USA*. Weston, MA: National Alliance for Breastfeeding Advocacy, 2001.

Waring M. *If Women Counted: A New Feminist Economics*. San Francisco: Harper & Row, 1998.

Weed S. *Wise Woman Herbal: The Childbearing Year*. New York: Ash Tree Publishing, 1996.

Weimer J. *The Economic Benefits of Breastfeeding: A Review and Analysis. Food Assistance and Nutrition Research Report No. 13*. Washington, DC: Food and Rural Economics Division, Economic Research Service, U.S. Department of Agriculture, 2001.

Wertz RW and Wertz DC. *Lying-in: A History of Childbirth in America*. New York: Shocken Books, 1979.

West D. *Defining Your Own Success: Breastfeeding after Breast Reduction Surgery*. Schaumburg, IL: La Leche League International, 2001.

Whaley LF and Wong DL. *Nursing Care of Infants and Children*, 4th ed. St. Louis: Mosby–Year Book, 1991.

White E. *The Association Between Breastfeeding, Higher IQ, and Better Visual Functioning*. Sandwich, MA: Health Education Associates, 1996.

Williams-Arnold LD. *Human Milk Storage for Healthy Infants and Children*. Sandwich, MA: Health Education Associates, 2000.

Winnicott DW. *Babies and Their Mothers*. Reading, MA: Addison-Wesley, 1987.

Wolf LS and Glass RP. *Feeding and Swallowing Disorders in Infancy*. San Antonio: Therapy Skill Builders, 1992.

The Womanly Art of Breastfeeding, 6th revised ed. Schaumburg, IL: La Leche League International, 1997.

Worthington-Roberts B and Williams SR. *Nutrition in Pregnancy and Lactation*, 5th ed. St. Louis: Mosby, 1993.

Young EWD. *Alpha and Omega: Ethics at the Frontier of Life and Death*. Reading, MA: Addison-Wesley, 1989.

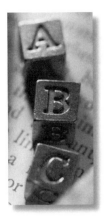

Shadowing/Observation Guidelines

Linda J. Smith, BSE, FACCE, IBCLC

1. Seek permission from the facility, LC, and client being observed, or the La Leche League Leader. Remember, the facility or LC may welcome you but the mother may feel uncomfortable with your presence.

2. Obey any local protocols (e.g., wearing scrubs). Do not observe on a day when you are ill in any way.

3. You are an observer, not a participant in the care of the mother/client. Seek permission from the mother to observe, introduce yourself, and say "thank you." At a La Leche League meeting, you are a guest. The Leader is in charge.

4. Take copious notes on what you've observed. Arrange with the observed party to spend time after the observation period or meeting to talk and ask questions.

5. Be respectful of the IBCLC or La Leche League Leader when asking questions. If you've observed something with which you disagree, tactfully and privately request information on the LC's or Leader's rationale. It is easy to offend someone if you have an attitude that you know better than the LC or Leader. You may be surprised to find out that the LC's or Leader's actions or information was most appropriate for that circumstance regardless of what the books say or what your previous experience dictates.

6. Always thank the client being observed for her willingness to allow you into her "space."

7. Restrain yourself from exhibiting tell-tale negative body language, in the presence of both your hostess and the client. Always be courteous, patient, and kind.

8. Thank the LC or La Leche League Leader in person and again with a note. Let her know how she facilitated your education and describe the positive things that you experienced and saw.

9. If problems arise during the observation, discuss them with your faculty mentor.

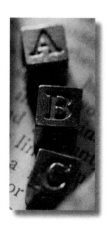

Interview Questions for Lactation Consultant Candidates

Linda J. Smith, BSE, FACCE, IBCLC
Diane Wiessinger, MS, IBCLC

FROM LINDA SMITH

N *ote:* The interview questions are in *italics*. Responses are categorized as "poor" or "good." Someone knowledgeable in breastfeeding management should be on the interview team! I would appreciate receiving feedback regarding how these questions were used.

Place yourself where you feel you fit on this self-assessment tool (or use the IBLCE exam grid) that addresses normal breastfeeding situations and management of problems, and academic areas related to lactation consultant practice. Why did you place yourself where you did?

Poor response: Limited experience with normal situations. Limited experience with problem management.

Good response: Broad range of experiences with normal situations and problems.

Describe how the World Health Organization's International Code of Marketing of Breastmilk Substitutes would apply to our setting.

Poor response: No knowledge. Treats the *Code* as applicable only in other countries. Sees no problem with formula company money used for breastfeeding promotion or education.

Good response: Clearly describes inappropriate advertising, gifts to health workers, and so on. Mentions some of the criteria for educational materials. Bonus for a candidate who praises and understands the *10 Steps to Successful Breastfeeding* and/or the *Baby Friendly Hospital Initiative*.

Tell us some of the risks of bottlefeeding/infant formula/artificial feeding products to the mother and baby.

Poor response: Reluctance to discuss the downside of not breastfeeding for fear of making mother who does not breastfeed "feel guilty." Emotional statements that are alarmist and not based in research.

Good response: Any factual information on health risks in general, alterations of oral responses, separation of mother and baby, sanitation issues, effects on fertility, and so on.

Describe the relationship between breastfeeding and fertility.

Poor response: Breastfeeding isn't a contraceptive.

Good response: Explanation of the Lactation Amenorrhea Method (LAM). Exclusive breastfeeding in the first six months, as long as the mother is amenorrheic, provides 98 percent protection against ovulation. The mother must be nursing at least 60 minutes per day, and go no longer than six hours between nursings. Once menstruation begins, the mother is assumed to be fertile but may not actually ovulate for several months.

What is your position on weaning?

Poor response: Specific length of time to breastfeed, especially if 12 months or less. Saying that "nursing longer than (any age)" is inappropriate in any way. First discussing any drawbacks of extended breastfeeding. Mother-led weaning at any age.

Good response: Baby-led weaning, preferably past 12 months. No solids before six months. Encouragement to nurse past 12 months. No drawbacks mentioned. Some benefits of long nursing mentioned.

Comment on the pros and cons of combining breastfeeding and bottle-feeding in the first three months.

Poor response: Including only the advantages of this approach without discussing the risks of nipple confusion or preference, exposure to nonhuman proteins, and the resultant risk of allergies. Stressing the need for the father's involvement in feeding. Stressing the ease of using formula when back at work instead of collecting breast milk.

Good response: Discussing the health benefits of exclusive breastfeeding and the drawbacks of introducing any nonhuman proteins prior to gut closure, around six months. Discussing the importance of mother–baby togetherness, and the importance of using breast milk when the mother is separated from the baby. Discussing nipple confusion or preference.

What factors are most important in teaching mothers how to start breastfeeding?

Poor response: No knowledge of latch-on and positioning. Discussing supply and demand only, without including the risks of pacifiers and bottles, or reading baby cues for starting and ending feeds. Schedules for feeding. Limiting time at breast.

Good response: Including correct positioning and deep grasp of the areola. Stressing enough time at the breast (minimum of 140 minutes, or 8–12 times per 24 hours). No limits to time at breast. Stressing importance of nursing early, within the first hour after birth, and rooming-in. Feeding on cue, day and night.

What are the practices that most negatively affect the mother's milk supply?

Poor response: Emphasizing the mother's diet or fluid intake. No warnings about the hazards of bottles and pacifiers, or limiting time at breast. Encouraging the baby to sleep through the night or limiting night nursings. Overemphasis on let-down reflex.

Good response: Milk retention for any reason. Limiting time at breast for any reason. Nipple shields, other sucking objects. Discussing autocoine feedback, hormonal influences, ineffective suck by baby, interfering relatives, oral contraceptive use.

What is a common breastfeeding pattern in a nine-month-old?

Poor response: Exclusive breastfeeding. Pressure to wean baby. No idea whatsoever. No knowledge of developmental characteristics of this age baby (separation anxiety, teething, night waking).

Good response: Separation anxiety in baby. Decreased daytime nursing except at naps, bedtime; increased nighttime waking and nursing. Playfulness at breast. Attempts to bite. "Gymnastic" nursing.

If you have only one 10-minute opportunity to discuss breastfeeding with a pregnant woman, what would you do?

Poor response: Bombard her with facts. Preach the benefits. Hand her literature without talking to her. Tell her someone will do it later.

Good response: Listen to her. Stress the following: (1) it's good for you and your baby; (2) it's comfortable and easy to do; and (3) we know how to help you breastfeed.

Describe the effect of the mother's fluid and nutritional status on her milk volume and milk composition.

Poor response: Lengthy discussion of the ideal diet or required or forbidden foods. Emphasis on increased fluid intake.

Good response: No significant effects on volume or composition. Diet and fluids are important for the general health of all postpartum women. Other factors are more important to milk volume. Composition is essentially stable.

How would you discuss breastfeeding with a pregnant woman who is allergic to cow's milk and smokes a pack of cigarettes a day?

Poor response: Discuss benefits only. Discourage her because she smokes.

Good response: Find out her desires. Gently help her reduce smoking. Include benefits to the baby because of its protection against allergy and the increased protection against illnesses caused by secondhand smoke. (Extra credit if the candidate discusses the risk of using cow's milk-based formulas.)

Discuss how you would prioritize the dispensing of breast pumps if your supply of pumps is limited.

Poor response: No intimate knowledge of how pumps can be used in the management of problems. No knowledge of differences between pumps.

Good response: Specific knowledge of pump use in prematurity, maternal illness, mothers returning to work, and mothers at risk of weaning for any reason. Knowledge of other sources of pumps in the community and sources of third-party reimbursement.

Describe three situations in which you would refer a mother to another professional, and describe why and to whom you would refer her.

Poor response: No referrals out. Referral for basic technical issues that an LC should be able to handle.

Good response: Referral to MD for drug questions and infections. Referral to a dietitian for a mother with diabetes. Referral to La Leche League for support of toddler nursing.

If you could design a perfect prenatal and postpartum breastfeeding program, what would it include?

Poor response: Outpatient only. Prenatal education only. Teaching of benefits only; promotion only without knowledgable clinical support. In-hospital visits by outpatient staff without involving the hospital in a coordinated progam. No system of early (first two weeks) follow-up. No medical coordination. No assurance of steady administrative backing, including funding. Use of materials from formula companies.

Good response: Written policies. Continuum of care, preferably with consistent care from one provider. Layered system of providers, including peer counselors/peer support groups and LLL, tangent staff with additional training in breastfeeding management, and IBCLCs. Smooth flow of referrals between agencies and professionals. Sufficient equipment, supportive paperwork, medical backing, and secure funding. Multicultural health workers and educational materials. Absence of funding or materials from formula companies.

FROM DIANE WIESSINGER

If I ran a private practice LC agency (if such a thing existed), I might ask the following questions of applicants:

Have you nursed any children yourself? For how long?

Some might object to the question, saying it isn't necessary for a cardiologist to have experienced heart trouble to do his or her job well. But breastfeeding, like childbirth, tumbled rather accidentally into the medical arena. In the past it involved a culture-wide woman-to-woman sharing; I hope it will return, with rare exceptions, to that same low-intervention sharing of sound cultural wisdom. Some excellent IBCLCs have never breastfed; I'm sure they see themselves as being at somewhat of a disadvantage. How long you nursed is relevant in that the woman whose children weaned at one year or 18 months is inclined to set those figures at the peak of her normal curve. The best figures we have, at the moment, suggest a normal "weaning window" of 2 1/2 to 7 years, with the occasional outlier. It's important that we either have personal experience with that range or have come to respect and promote it, especially in private practice, where, unlike in hospital jobs, we get calls for help from mothers of 2 1/2-year-olds and older.

If you had to choose between exclusively bottle-feeding your child using only human milk and exclusively breastfeeding your child using only formula, which would you choose?

There is no correct answer to this question, but if you leap immediately to bottle-feeding human milk, you aren't giving nearly enough weight to the importance of the *process*. Too many IBCLCs are happy to support a woman in bottle-feeding expressed milk before exhausting all reasonable options for helping her establish a breastfeeding relationship. We are not breast *milk* specialists; we are breast*feeding* specialists. We have a formalized obligation to support that relationship. Perhaps the correct answer to this question is an agonized, "Oh dear, I'll have to think that one over carefully!"

What is the best pump company? Brand of formula? Type of nursing pillow? Way to supplement a non-nursing baby?

Like the preceding question, these are all very complicated questions. The right answer to any one of them is either a long answer or a very short one—"That depends."

How will you deal with situations that seem to be beyond you?

The IBCLC in private practice needs to have in place—and continue to develop—a network of human resources for dealing with difficult cases. Lactnet, local referrals to breastfeeding and other specialists, personal contacts—these are all important, much more often than we think at first.

What if the mother doesn't want to breastfeed?

This question deserves a short answer. After you have provided her—in whatever way is comfortable and comprehensible to her—with adequate information, you help her in the direction of her choice.

Will you refer mothers to any organization after they "graduate" from your services?

The IBCLC who scorns La Leche League or any other mother-to-mother support group is missing the point badly and needs to catch up. According to the World Health Organization, mothers involved in such groups tend to breastfeed longer, and with greater exclusivity in the early months.[1] Just as importantly, studies would be unlikely to point so consistently in this direction if the mothers were not also nursing with greater satisfaction and confidence. Any volunteer-run group is bound to fall short in one area or another—perhaps its leaders need more help with their counseling skills, or perhaps they could benefit enormously from an occasional in-service program on new information. These are reasons to be involved with the groups, not to ignore them!

What if you don't like the baby?

I would hope that your answer would be, "I can't imagine a baby I wouldn't like."

NOTES

1. World Health Organization. *Evidence for the Ten Steps to Successful Breastfeeding.* WHO/CHD/98.9, Geneva, 1998.

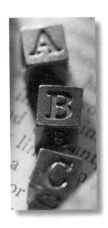

Development of Professional Lactation Education

Linda J. Smith, BSE, FACCE, IBCLC

E ffective professional breastfeeding support in the United States has dual roots in medical education and mother-to-mother support.

1903: An International Congress of Obstetricians observed the Budin clinic in Paris dispensing processed cow's milk to mothers for feeding their infants. The Congress asserted that pediatricians and clinics were encouraging artificial feeding at the expense of breastfeeding.

1920s: Articles on increased mortality and cognitive compromise associated with artificial feeding began appearing in medical literature. For example, Hoefer and Hardy reported that breastfed babies walked more than two months earlier than artificially fed babies; none of the babies with IQs exceeding 130 were artificially fed. (Hoefer, C., and Hardy, M. C. Later development of breastfed and artificially fed infants. *Journal of the American Medical Association* 1929; 92: 615.)

1921: Julius Parker Sedgwick, MD, wanted to "prove on a large scale his contention that the vast majority of mothers could nurse their babies, provided only that they had the enthusiastic and informed cooperation of their own physicians." "He made up his mind that more time (in medical school) should be given to observing and studying this natural function, and less to the study of artificial feeding and formula making." He designed a demonstration project through the Breastfeeding Investigation Bureau of the Department of Pediatrics, University of Minnesota, and the Minneapolis municipal health department. The results: "More than nine-tenths of the babies born in Minneapolis over a test period were kept on natural feeding for their first month; and over three-fourths of them were still nursing at the end of nine months!" (quoted in Richardson, pp. 18–21). (Sedgwick, J. P., and Fleischner. Breastfeeding in the reduction of infant mortality. *American Journal of Public Health* 1921; 11: 153–157.)

Soon after, Dr. Florence McKay and the Brooklyn Pediatric Society replicated the Minneapolis study in Nassau County, New York. "Pediatric and obstetric advisors to the state Health Department...took over the project as part of the curriculum for the plan of postgraduate medical education just then being started." Their conclusion: "Breastfeeding could never again be considered a regional matter; it was a matter of medical education and lay instruction." The results of the Nassau County project "showed how almost universal is its applicability, when a concerted effort is exerted by a community organized to put it across" (quoted in Richardson, pp. 24–26). (McKay, F.

Infant mortality in relation to breastfeeding. *New York State Journal of Medicine* 1924; 24: 433–438.)

1940: Dr. Edith Jackson began the Rooming-In Project in New Haven, Connecticut. Dr. Jackson introduced rooming-in, encouraged mother-to-mother discussions in the maternity ward, and trained medical students in this philosophy.

1953: Frank Richardson, MD, published *The Nursing Mother.* "To every mother who really wants to nurse her baby, this book is dedicated by a doctor who honestly believes that she can." Dr. Richardson described Sedgwick and McKay's work in detail, including Sedgwick's pamphlet that contained "essentials for successful breastfeeding: 1. Conviction on the part of the doctor as to its desirability; 2. Conviction on the part of the mother as to her ability to succeed; 3. Stimulation of the breasts at regular intervals; 4. Complete emptying of the breasts, by the baby, or by manual expression, after each feeding; 5. Patience and perseverance." Sedgwick also listed the "causes of failure from insufficient milk: failure to empty breasts, poor nipples, poor nursing by baby, fatigue, irregular nursing, poor diet, and state of mind of nursing mother" (p. 22).

1953: Barnes, B. F., Lethin, A. N., Jackson, E. B., et al. Management of breastfeeding. *Journal of the American Medical Association* 1953; 151: 192. This article is one of the few published in a medical journal to address the *management* of breastfeeding and not simply the benefits. It appeared 20 years after Sedgwick and McKay published the results of their projects.

1956: Seven mothers in the Chicago area founded what became La Leche League International (LLLI). Dr. Jackson and Dr. Richardson served on LLLI's Professional Advisory Board. The core principle of this organization's effectiveness is mother-to-mother support.

1958: LLLI published the first edition of *The Womanly Art of Breastfeeding.*

1961: Other mother-support groups and breastfeeding groups affiliated with childbirth education associations are formed, including Nursing Mothers Council in Philadelphia and similar groups in Boston and around the United States. Similar associations in other countries emerged, notably in the Scandinavian countries and Australia. Trained volunteer "counselors" became a central focus of organized breastfeeding support groups.

1963: Karen Pryor wrote *Nursing Your Baby.*

1964: LLLI's first convention was held. Although 75 people were expected, 450 attended.

1970: Mavis Gunther, MD, published *Infant Feeding.* Dr. Gunther carefully studied the baby's position at breast, which was the first published examination of the "mechanics" of breastfeeding.

1973–1975: LLLI's first Physician's Seminar on Breastfeeding was held. LLLI announced the establishment of the Paul György Annual Award for the best original paper on breastfeeding submitted by a student enrolled in a medical school. The first papers were submitted in 1975. The momentum began to build toward effective lactation education of health care providers.

1977: Audrey Naylor, M.D., DrPH, and Ruth Wester, RN, C.P.N.P., started the San Diego Lactation Program at University of California, San Diego, which was incorporated as Wellstart International in 1985.

1979: Chele Marmet and Ellen Shell founded the Lactation Institute in Los Angeles, CA.

1980: Ruth Lawrence, MD, published *Breastfeeding, A Guide for the Medical Profession*. Edith Tibbets and Johanna Goldfarb, MD, published *Breastfeeding Handbook, A Practical Reference for Physicians, Nurses, and Other Health Professionals*.

1981: Edward Cerutti, M.D., and Sarah Danner, R.N., C.P.N.P., C.N.M., opened the Lactation Clinic in Cleveland, OH.

1982: LLLI made a commitment to foster the development of a mid-level counselor with more formalized training and a credentialing examination, partly to bridge the gap between physicians and mother-support groups. This effort led to the formation of the International Board of Lactation Consultant Examiners (IBLCE) in 1985. The UCLA Extension Lactation Educator course began in California. Wellstart's international training program began, in cooperation with the U.S. Agency for International Development.

1983: *A Practical Guide to Breastfeeding* was written by Jan Riordan, RN. *Counseling the Nursing Mother* was published, which developed from the experiences of breastfeeding counselors in CEA of Greater Philadelphia. *Lactation: Physiology, Nutrition and Breastfeeding* was written by Margaret Neville, PhD, and Marianne Neifert, MD.

LLLI began a program to train outreach workers to work in public health settings with minority and low-income women, which evolved into the Breastfeeding Peer Counseling Program. Most peer counseling programs in the United States today are modeled on or directly use the LLLI program guidelines. Several other courses emerged, supporting the movement toward making education in breastfeeding and lactation management more widely available.

1984: The U.S. Surgeon General convened a "Workshop on Breastfeeding and Human Lactation," which started a decade of renewed interest in breastfeeding. Professional education was one of six core areas to be addressed for breastfeeding to become the "community norm."

1985: The International Board of Lactation Consultant Examiners (IBLCE) began operations. IBLCE is an independent corporation and not part of either La Leche League or the International Lactation Consultant Association. Its Board of Directors has delegates from medical societies, LLLI, ILCA, and international breastfeeding organizations. The exam combines scientific facts with practical breastfeeding management principles.

1985: The International Lactation Consultant Association (ILCA) was formed as an association for professional lactation consultants. Its Board of Directors includes individuals with highly diverse backgrounds, practice settings, and nationalities.

1993: ILCA convened the first Lactation Education/Course Director's Meeting to begin development of international standards for professional lactation management education.

1995: ILCA published *Standards of Practice for Lactation Consultants*. IBLCE published *Code of Ethics for IBCLC Lactation Consultants*.

1999: ILCA formalized the Professional Education Council, which grew out of the Lactation Course Directors meetings.

2001: ILCA published *Core Curriculum for Lactation Consultant Practice*, edited by Marsha Walker, and *Scope of Practice and Educational Guidelines*. It also established the International Lactation Education Accreditation Council.

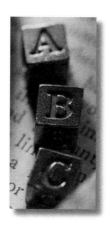

Guidelines for Evaluating Educational Materials[1]

Linda J. Smith, BSE, FACCE, IBCLC

Materials for breastfeeding education or promotion should *include* factors that are necessary for breastfeeding success, and *exclude* factors that contribute to breastfeeding failure or are irrelevant to lactation success. The proportion of space for a topic should correspond to its relative importance to the breastfeeding relationship.

SECTION I: TOPICS THAT SHOULD BE INCLUDED TO FOSTER SUCCESS

Maternal factors that are necessary for successful breastfeeding are:

A. Motivation, founded in

    1. A belief in the superiority of human milk, and

    2. A belief in her own ability to breastfeed.

B. Trust in herself and her baby to find loving ways of interacting.

C. Commitment, including persistence and a tenaciousness of purpose.

D. Access to skilled, knowledgeable, and timely help that prevents and solves technical problems related to lactation.

E. Access to support systems, including clinical settings, that foster the mother–baby interactions necessary for successful breastfeeding.

Statements, photographs, images, and ideas that support any of these factors are supportive of breastfeeding. Most mothers know that "breast is best," but need instruction and support to make it a reality. *Listing advantages does not assure success; mothers need accurate and complete information on the process.*

The five central messages of **"why breastfeed"** are:

1. Human milk is species-specific nourishment for the baby.

2. Human milk produces optimal growth and development.

3. Human milk provides substantial protection from illness.

4. Lactation is beneficial to the mother's health.

5. Breastfeeding biologically supports a special mother–baby relationship.

The five central concepts of **"how to breastfeed"** are:

1. Nurse soon and often, within the first hour after birth.

2. All sucking should be at the breast; the length and frequency of feedings are determined by the baby.

3. Position the baby so nursing is comfortable and milk transfer is maximized.

4. Watch the baby's urine and stool output for assurance of supply.

5. Problems have solutions. Help is available.

Understanding the primary causes of lactation failure helps prioritize the information presented to mothers. In order of frequency, the causes of breastfeeding failure are:

A. Perceived or actual milk insufficiency, caused by inappropriate feeding practices rooted in:

   1. Lack of understanding of the process of lactation.

   2. Lack of knowledge of infant behavior.

B. Pain during breastfeeding, caused by:

   1. Nipple trauma from inappropriate technique or practices.

   2. Breast pain from inappropriate technique.

   3. Nipple or breast pain from pathological organisms.

C. Lack of support or undermining the decision, from:

   1. Family and friends.

   2. Health professionals.

   3. Employers and school administrators.

The five central **causes of problems** in the first six weeks are:

1. *Too few nursing sessions per day.* A normal pattern is 8–12 sessions per day; more are fine. Watch the baby for hunger cues.

2. *Nursings too short, ended by the mother.* Session length should be unrestricted. Let the baby end the session.

3. *Overuse of pacifiers and bottles.* Nipple confusion can lead to breast refusal. Use of supplements decreases milk supply.

4. *Poor attachment, causing nipple pain and low milk transfer.* Breastfeeding should never hurt the mother. Any pain associated with breastfeeding should be investigated.

5. *Blaming breastfeeding for normal newborns' need for closeness, cuddling, holding, and so on. All* babies need frequent feeding, carrying, and comforting.

SECTION II: CAUSES OF BREASTFEEDING FAILURE

Any statement, photograph, image, or product that undermines the mother's belief in the superiority of her milk, her trust in her ability to make milk, her need for breastfeeding to be comfortable and pleasant, or her need for support from society undermines breastfeeding. *Errors are italicized*; *the most serious errors are also underlined*.

SECTION III: COMMON ERRORS IN EDUCATIONAL MATERIALS

Errors in Content of Narration and Written Text

See also Auerbach, Kathleen. Beyond the issue of accuracy: Evaluating patient education materials for breastfeeding mothers. *Journal of Human Lactation* 1988; 4: 108–110.

Errors in Presenting Lactation Physiology

1. <u>*Hinting that milk supply may be inadequate, fixed, or unchangeable*</u>.
   "Not enough milk" is the most common cause of breastfeeding failure. True milk insufficiency is exceedingly rare. Establishing, maintaining, and increasing the milk supply is usually quite easy.

2. <u>*Restricting the length of nursings by:*</u>
   - *Emphasizing the removal of the baby from the breast.*
   - *Establishing rules for feeding length.*

   The baby should determine the end of feedings, not the mother; the baby will stop swallowing and release the breast when finished. Arbitrary rules for feeding length interfere with the balance of nutrients that change dynamically during the course of the feeding and with total milk volume consumed by the baby.

3. <u>*Making strict rules for the number or frequency of nursing sessions*</u>, *especially without stressing the need for watching the baby for hunger and satiety cues.*
   No restrictions should be placed on the number or frequency of nursing sessions. Normal demand-fed infants consume irregular quantities of milk at irregular intervals from each breast according to their own needs. An average minimum number of sessions may be suggested, but not a maximum.

4. <u>*Failing to discuss the risks of pacifiers, bottles, and supplements to an adequate milk supply*</u>.
   The use of bottles, pacifiers, and supplements is a primary cause of lactation failure and early weaning. Other sucking objects may disrupt the oral response. Giving other fluids results in milk retention in the breast, which suppresses further milk production.

5. *Recommending elaborate prenatal "nipple preparation" routines.*
   Except for correcting severely retracted nipples, prenatal preparation has not been shown to be beneficial. Excessive manipulation or rough treatment can cause premature labor contractions and tissue damage.

Errors in Presenting Biochemistry and Immunology

6. <u>*Implying the equivalence of human milk and infant formula*</u>.
   Implying equivalence disregards species specificity and reduces human milk to a combination of carbohydrates, proteins, and fat. Nutrients from other species or vegetable sources differ substantially from human nutrients. Implying equivalence also disregards the presence of protective proteins and cellular components in human milk that are absent in all prepared formulas. See also #18.

7. <u>*Suggesting that mother must eat a perfect diet, eat a restricted diet, or follow a pure lifestyle to breastfeed safely*</u>.
   Human milk volume and composition are essentially unaffected by the mother's diet. Most medications are compatible with breastfeeding. If the "safety" or "purity" of mother's milk is brought up, the issue of risks and safety of alternatives must likewise be discussed. Overemphasis on an ideal maternal diet can be interpreted as requiring the mother to be a martyr to breastfeed. While good nutrition is important for general health, maternal diet has minimal effects on lactation success.

8. _Minimizing the benefits of human milk and the process of lactation_.

   Human milk protects the baby's health in many ways; lactation protects the mother's health in several ways. Failure to breastfeed has both short- and long-term health implications.

Errors in Presenting Psychosocial Factors

9. _Implying that the mother may be a risk to the baby_.

10. _Implying that the baby may be a risk to the mother_.

    Mother and baby must develop a mutually trusting, intimate relationship for breastfeeding to succeed.

11. _Suggesting that breastfeeding won't work_.

12. _Making breastfeeding sound complicated, painful, or stressful_.

13. _Implying that "normal" activities are difficult when the mother is breastfeeding_.

    Breastfeeding is sometimes treated as a convenient scapegoat for the normal inconveniences of infancy. This perspective ignores the concept that all baby care is time-consuming, regardless of feeding decisions.

14. _Focusing on any aspects of breastfeeding that could be approximated by artificial feeding_.

15. _Treating breastfeeding as the exception, thereby establishing artificial feeding as the norm_.

16. _Drawing attention to, or exaggerating, any possible drawbacks of breastfeeding_.

17. _Minimizing the role of the mother, by emphasizing the role of the father, grandparents, or other family members in feeding the baby_.

    When others are feeding the baby, the mother isn't breastfeeding. Without the mother, breastfeeding is impossible. Family members' help is beneficial to the breastfeeding mother in everything except feeding. See also #43.

18. _Implying that formula should be given to breastfed babies, that human milk and formula should be used together, or that formula should be used when breastfeeding is discontinued, without giving any real "reasons" why breastfeeding should stop_.

    When a baby is breastfed, formula is unnecessary. Formula is a replacement for breast milk, not a necessary addition to it. See also #6 and #19.

19. _Hinting that formula will eventually be necessary for all babies_. See also #18.

20. _Suggesting that breastfeeding is only for newborns; that babies should wean by age 12 months; or that longer nursing is abnormal, harmful, or inappropriate_.

    No documentation supports an arbitrary weaning age of 12 months. The American Academy of Pediatrics endorses breastfeeding for _at least_ 12 months; other health agencies concur and support breastfeeding for two years or more. A baby derives benefits from human milk regardless of his or her age. Normal acquisition of feeding skills occurs over time. Mandating feeding skill progression or overemphasis on the type and amount of foods consumed can lead to future eating disorders. See also #30.

21. *Presenting too many points in a given amount of space or time, causing sensory overload and confusion.* See also #49.

Errors in Visual Presentations/Portrayals

Note: These errors are especially detrimental because 85 percent of people are primarily visual learners.

22. <u>*Showing the baby poorly positioned at breast, usually with the mouth too close to the nipple tip, lips pursed or curled in, not open widely, or puckering.*</u>

    This positioning is typical of bottle-suck, and a primary cause of nipple pain, tissue damage, and inadequate milk transfer, which contribute to breastfeeding failure. See also #35–#41.

23. *Hiding details of the baby's positioning at breast, resulting in no useful information being conveyed.* See also #35–#41.

24. *Showing excessive or inappropriate nudity; mother is shown with much breast exposure.*

    Some cultural groups view breast exposure as offensive, which becomes a significant barrier to breastfeeding. Others view breast exposure as appropriate and beautiful. Cultural beliefs of the intended audience must be considered. If in doubt, avoid visual images with much of the breast exposed.

25. *Avoiding eye-to-eye contact between mother and baby; the baby is shown asleep, the mother's eyes are closed, or the mother is looking away.*

26. *Depicting the mother in a bathrobe or nightgown, suggesting that a limitation of lifestyle is necessary to breastfeed.*

27. *Dressing the mother in white clothing, suggesting "purity."*

28. *Depicting the mother as very beautiful, wearing a wedding ring, and/or shown in affluent settings.*

29. *Situating the mother and baby in overly romantic, sentimental settings that portray an unrealistic view of the early postpartum period.*

    Poor women and single mothers often feel they are not "good enough" to breastfeed. Seeing pretty women and beautiful settings may motivate some mothers, but impose a significant barrier for others. Few women feel pretty or beautiful in the early postpartum period. Cultural sensitivity is mandatory.

30. *Showing only very young babies breastfeeding, suggesting early weaning.* See also #20.

31. *Using colors that set a negative mood.*

32. *Showing the baby at breast without showing the mother, or cutting off part of her head.*

    This view minimizes the mother's importance.

Errors Specific to Moving Visual Images

Note: When reviewing videos or films, the visual track should be watched without sound, and then again with it. Discrepancies between the audio and visual images will create cognitive dissonance. (Linda Verlee Williams. *Teaching for the Two-Sided Mind.* Simon & Schuster, 1983.)

33. _Using video images that conflict with the narration_.
    The human brain retains visual images longer, and in preference to, auditory messages when dissimilar messages are received simultaneously. See also #45.

34. _Repeating incorrect techniques multiple times_.
    This error is particularly misleading when the audio track is fairly good while the visual track shows poor positioning. The incorrect image tends to invite imitation.

35. _Failing to show the baby going to breast easily and correctly_.

36. _Removing appropriate images very quickly, before retention is assured_.

37. _Failing to reassure new mothers that several tries may be necessary to correctly position the baby for nursing_.

38. _Failing to show the mother responding appropriately to baby's feeding cues_.

39. _Failing to show and comment on infant swallowing to confirm intake_.

40. _Failing to show long, pleasant breastfeeding interactions_.

41. _Failing to show close-up details of the baby at breast_.
    Detailed visual images of realistic babies nursing effectively and correctly are beneficial. Images must be shown long enough for retention. Incorrect technique or too-perfect images can interfere.

42. _Showing little or no mother-infant nonbreastfeeding comforting, communication, and interaction, implying that breastfeeding is the only way a mother can show affection to her baby_.
    Breastfeeding is one of many appropriate ways that a mother and baby can interact lovingly. This idea's presentation will be affected by the total length of the video. A long program should include nonfeeding interactions, while a short one should instead concentrate on details of the breastfeeding process.

43. _Showing many scenes of other family members with the baby, with the mother absent_.
    Mother-baby closeness is central to breastfeeding success. See also #17.

Errors Specific to Auditory Presentations (Sensory Faults)

44. _Narrating in a choppy, rushed, or excessively enthusiastic manner, creating a sense of anxiety_.

45. _Providing audio messages that conflict with the visual track_. See also #33.

46. _Using a female voice that is shrill, grating, or nasal_.

47. _Using a male voice that is too low in pitch, which may be intimidating_.

48. _Allowing the music to overpower the narration, or create a mood of tension, sadness, or anxiety_.

49. _Including too many points made in a given amount of time_.
    Too much information causes sensory overload and confusion. Presenting one idea per 10-15 minutes is enough. See also #21.

Errors Presented by Packaging of Materials

50. *Including formula samples in "breastfeeding" packets.*

51. *Including coupons for infant formula in "breastfeeding" packets.*

   Samples or coupons encourage the use of and imply the necessity of formula. See errors #1, #4, #6, #11, #18, and #19.

52. *Listing toll-free phone numbers staffed by sales representatives for competing products.*

   Breastfeeding information should be provided by unbiased, well-informed sources.

SECTION IV: RECOMMENDATIONS OF THE WORLD HEALTH ORGANIZATION

The World Health Organization's guidelines on educational materials for breastfeeding promotion as stated in the *International Code of Marketing of Breastmilk Substitutes* contain the following language:

(4.2) Informational and educational materials, whether written audio or visual, dealing with the feeding of infants and intended to reach pregnant women and mothers of infants and young children, should include clear information on ALL the following points:

1. the **benefits** and **superiority** of breastfeeding;

2. maternal nutrition, and the **preparation for** and **maintenance** of breastfeeding;

3. the **negative effect** on breastfeeding of introducing **partial bottle-feeding**;

4. the **difficulty of reversing the decision** not to breastfeed;

5. **where needed**, the proper use of infant formula, whether manufactured industrially or home-prepared. **When** such materials contain information about the use of infant formula, they should include the **social and financial implications** of its use; the **health hazards** of inappropriate foods or feeding methods; and, in particular, **the health hazards of unnecessary or improper use** of infant formula and other breastmilk substitutes. Such materials **should not use any pictures or text which may idealize** the use of breastmilk substitutes.

SECTION V: SELECTION CRITERIA

When selecting educational materials, consider the following factors in addition to the issues of reading level, esthetics, and layout design:

• Completeness
• Inclusion of supportive information
• Exclusion of errors
• Cost

Where circumstances necessitate the use of less-than-optimal resources, the professional should correct the deficiencies or errors. As better materials become available and budgets permit, replacement of deficient materials should be strongly considered to foster increased support for breastfeeding.

A Word on Guilt

Providing complete information on benefits *and* helpful techniques allows the mother to make an informed decision and successfully implement that decision. Lack of information on helpful techniques contributes to breastfeeding failure and the resultant grieving process. *The guilt of failed breastfeeding is caused by an insufficiency of information on techniques, not an abundance of information on the benefits.*

For more information on the *Score Sheet for Evaluating Breastfeeding Educational Materials*, contact Bright Future Lactation Resource Centre, 6540 Cedarview Ct., Dayton, OH 45459-1214. Phone (888) 235-7201 (BFLRC 01) or (937) 438-9458; fax 937-438-3229; e-mail lindaj@bflrc.com

NOTES

1. Prepared for Ohio Department of Health by Linda J. Smith, BSE, FACCE, IBCLC, 1992. These guidelines are now part of the ODH's "Policy on Breastfeeding Promotion and Support."

SCORE SHEET FOR EVALUATING BREASTFEEDING EDUCATIONAL MATERIALS

TITLE:_____DATE OF EVALUATION _____

AUTHOR:_____PRODUCER/SPONSOR:_____

AVAILABLE FROM _____

MEDIA: Pamphlet ( ) Video ( ) Book ( )OTHER _____ ( ) LENGTH _____PRICE _____

PURPOSE: Motivate ( ) Instruct ( ) Solve problems ( ) Collect/store milk ( ) OTHER_____

INTENDED AUDIENCE: Prenatal ( ) New Parents ( ) Professionals ( ) OTHER_____

POSITIVE FEATURES / CORRECT	✓	NEGATIVE FEATURES / ERRORS	✓	COMMENTS
SUPPLY *"Milk-making is easy"*		**SUPPLY** *"You might not have enough"*		
Breastfeed soon after birth		First feeds delayed, unimportant		
Stay together 24-hrs, no separation		Separation normal, expected		
Nurse often, no limits on frequency		Scheduled feeds expected, described		
Follow baby's cues, let baby end		Mother ends feed, prescribed length		
All sucking at breast, no pacifiers		Other sucking objects OK, expected		
Exclusive human milk feedings		Supplements encouraged, expected		
Reassuring signs of intake- stools, urine, satiation, weight gain		Absence of reassuring signs of intake, hints of insufficiency		
COMFORT *"Breastfeeding is pleasant"*		**COMFORT** *"Breastfeeding is unpleasant"*		
Correct Latch-on and positioning		Incorrect or no info on positioning		
Early intervention if painful		"Pain is normal" messages		
Diagrams, photos correct and clear		Photos, diagrams incorrect or unclear		
HEALTH *"BF protects baby and mom"*		**HEALTH** *"BF doesn't really matter"*		
Species-specific nutrition		Animal, plant milks "equivalent"		
Mom's diet fairly unimportant		Elaborate rules for mom's diet		
Lactation good for mother		Lactation unrelated to mom's health		
Specific protection from disease		No mention of protective aspects		
Good health presented as normal		Good health seen as an "advantage"		
Reduction in fertility		Fertility impact ignored		
Breastmilk safer than other products		Hints at "polluted" breastmilk		
Milk supports brain functioning		Cognitive issues ignored		

SOCIAL *"Baby and mom belong together"*	**SOCIAL** *"Baby is inconvenient to mom"*		
Baby can trust mother to meet needs	"Baby is manipulative" messages		
Mother can trust baby for cues	Mother has total control of feeding		
Closeness desirable and normal	Distancing expected, encouraged		
Mom's relationship with baby unique	Emphasis on other family members		
Clear message: exclusive BF 6 mos	Supplements expected		
Clear message: continue 2+ years	Early weaning expected		
Clear message: BF more than food	Emphasis on "nutrition"		
PRESENTATION *"BF is fun and easy"*	**PRESENTATION** *"BF is a hassle"*		
Visual and auditory congruence	Visual, auditory tracks dissonant		
Accurate, positive images at breast	Incorrect, negative images at breast		
Comfortable pace & amount of info.	Hectic pace, sensory overload		
Appropriate language, scenes	Inappropriate language, scenes		
Narration positive, clear & direct	Language "tricks," mixed messages		
PACKAGE *"We want you to keep BF"*	**PACKAGE** *"We profit if you stop"*		
No $$ profit if BF fails	Profit $$ if baby NOT at breast		
No product advertisements	Emphasis on products "needed"		
Reasonable price (not "free")	"Free" to user unless made with public funds		
Complies with WHO Code	Violates WHO Code		
OTHER	**OTHER**		
TOTAL POSITIVE FEATURES	**TOTAL NEGATIVE FEATURES/ERRORS**		

OVERALL IMPRESSION:_____

ERRORS NEEDING CORRECTION:_____

ESPECIALLY GOOD POINTS: _____

SUITABLE FOR:_____ **UNSUITABLE FOR**:_____

EVALUATOR _____ Title_____

EVALUATOR _____ Title_____

EVALUATOR _____ Title_____

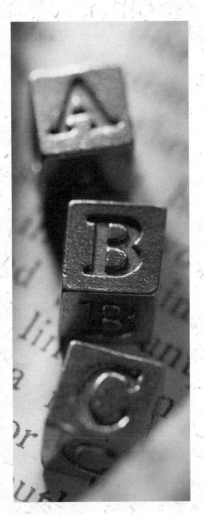

Clinical Forms and Handouts

Sample Charting Forms
Sample Client Handouts
Sample Reports to Primary Care Providers
Sources for Supplies and Equipment

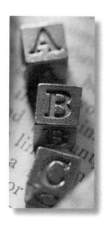

Introduction

Writing reports to the physician is one of the most important skills the PPLC must master. The major selling point of having an LC involved on a case is to save the doctor time. The physician generally cannot observe an entire feed or take a history that will tease out all the dynamics that contribute to a breastfeeding crisis. Thus the LC, via her more expanded interview/assessment, becomes the detective who reports back to the doctor. Her concise communication will facilitate strategic planning by the health care team.

The report should describe the problem and communicate a sense of its urgency (i.e., the baby needs to be seen immediately by a physician, the baby is stable and can be weighed tomorrow as follow-up, the baby is doing fine but mother needs antibiotics). A good report shares observations that will assist the physician in drawing conclusions and developing a treatment plan. As the doctor is the provider of medical care, protocol requires that the LC not dictate the treatment. She can, however, make recommendations based on her observations. Some physicians are particular about being the one to make further referrals; others are more casual and flexible if the LC suggests putting the mother in touch with other specialists such as physical therapists, occupational therapists, and the like.

A good report contains the baby's weight; observations about the baby's behavior, color, and tone; and feeding ability. It describes any infant or maternal signs of illness or trauma. The LC mentions her interventions and gives her plan for follow-up. Above all, the report should be brief—otherwise, it may not be read.

Several sample reports—real cases with the names changed—are provided in this appendix. Note that different PPLCs use different styles of reporting.

Bright Future Lactation Resource Centre

Linda J. Smith, BSE, FACCE, IBCLC • International Board Certified Lactation Consultant
6540 Cedarview Court • Dayton, Ohio 45459-1214 • (937) 438-9458 • Fax (937) 438-3229

Release/Consent Form

A lactation consultation usually includes visual and physical assessment of the mother's breasts, visual and physical assessment of the infant's mouth, observation of the mother and infant nursing, analysis of the data relating to the breastfeeding situation, demonstration of techniques for improving breastfeeding, and sometimes the use of breastfeeding equipment. I give permission for the lactation consultant to do all of the above.

I understand that all medical care is to be provided only by our physician(s). I give my permission for information about this and all additional consultations to be sent to my attending physician(s)/health care provider(s).

I understand that payment is due at the time services are rendered. I give my permission for information to be released to my insurance company to assist in evaluation of a claim.

I give my permission for information from this consultation/visit to be used to further the knowledge of breastfeeding. I understand that no specific names will be publicly used. I give permission to Linda Smith to photograph or videotape myself and/or my infant(s). I acknowledge that these images belong to Linda Smith and that she intends to use these images for the purpose of education and the promotion of breastfeeding and lactation counseling.

I understand that I have the right to refuse any or all specific techniques suggested, equipment to assist or remedy breastfeeding problems, and/or all recommended actions. Linda Smith will provide names of other qualified providers of lactation consultant services or equipment upon request.

_____   _____
Mother's Signature   Date

_____   _____
Lactation Consultant's Signature   Date

Bright Future Lactation Resource Centre

Linda J. Smith, BSE, FACCE, IBCLC • International Board Certified Lactation Consultant
6540 Cedarview Court • Dayton, Ohio 45459-1214 • (937) 438-9458 • Fax (937) 438-3229

Lactation Consulatation Intake and History

Mother's Name_____ Age_____ Today's Date_____

Address_____ City_____ Zip_____

Phone (Home) _____ (Work)_____

Baby's Name_____ Birth Date_____ Age Today_____

Reason for Visit

❏ Breast/Nipple Pain   ❏ Poor nursing   ❏ Slow gain   ❏ Other_____

Who else is helping with problem_____

Mother's OB/PCP_____ Baby's Ped/PCP_____ Hospital_____

Family/Personal

Other children, ages, duration BF _____

_____

Family BF	Mother _____	Sister(s) _____	Breast surgery___ ❏ _____
Allergy	Mother _____	Father _____	Siblings _____
Recent illness/injury/surgery other than births _____		Chronic illnesses _____	
Depression _____	Abuse _____	Eating _____	Abortion _____ ❏ _____
Smoke _____	Alcohol _____	Medications incl. vitamins _____ ❏ _____	
Caffeine _____	Dairy _____	Other dietary _____	

Birth History

Pregnancy	Planned _____	Surprise _____	Fertility _____	❏ Problems_____
Breast chgs _____	Yeast inf's _____	Toxemia/HBP _____	❏ _____	
Wt gain _____	Feelings about pregnancy_____			
Labor @Wks _____	Induced _____	AROM _____	Baby problems_____	
Epidural @ cm ____	Other meds _____		Quality/length _____	

_____

Birth	❏ Vaginal	❏ Vacuum	❏ Forceps	❏ Cesarean_____

Feelings about labor and birth_____

_____

Baby

APGARs _____   Birth weight _____   1st Nursing _____

First day pattern _____

Separation _____   Supplements _____   Pacifier _____   Jaundice _____

Copious milk _____   Engorged _____   Nipple pain_____

Baby sick _____   Circumcised _____ Pumped _____   Alternative fdgs_____

In-hospital BF _____

_____

_____

Current Pattern

❏ Exclusive BF   #/day _____   Avg length _____   Who ends _____   Time between _____

Quality _____   Longest sleep _____   ❏ EBM by _____   Amt _____

❏ ABM feeds _____   Amt _____   ABM by _____

Output: #wet/24 hrs _____   BMs/24 hrs _____   Color _____   Quantity _____

Moods   ❏ Fussy _____   ❏ Alert/calm _____   ❏ Sleepy _____   ❏ Other_____

❏ Baby meds _____   ❏ Pacifier _____

_____

_____

_____

Home/Social

Father's feelings _____   Home life: ❏ Calm   ❏ Chaotic   ❏ _____

❏ Help at home   ❏ Relatives/visitors   ❏ Mixed advice   ❏ $$ problems

❏ Back to work_____   ❏ BF supporter   ❏ LLL meetings

Mother's BF Goals

_____

_____

Comments

Signature _____
          Linda J. Smith, FACCE, IBCLC

Bright Future Lactation Resource Centre

Linda J. Smith, BSE, FACCE, IBCLC • International Board Certified Lactation Consultant

6540 Cedarview Court • Dayton, Ohio 45459-1214 • (937) 438-9458 • Fax (937) 438-3229

Breastfeeding Assessment

Mother's Name_____   Today's Date_____

Baby's Name_____   Age Today_____

Reason for Consult_____

Breasts/Areolas	Nipples
Size	Texture
Fullness	Elasticity
Lact. sinuses	Shape after
MER	Color after
Supply	Integrity
Amt pumped	

Physical Condition of Baby	At-Breast Behavior
Appearance/mood	Behavior
Skin/color	Position/alignment
Head	Latch
Posture	Organization
Oral structures	Suck/swallow bursts
Tongue motion/suck	Duration
Weight	

Birth date	Disch./low	Date	Date	Date
WT	WT	WT	WT	WT

Impression/Analysis: _____

_____

_____

Plan/Techniques: _____

Equipment Needed: _____

_____

Follow-up/Evaluation: _____   Send Report to:_____

Referral/Consult to: _____

Signature: _____

Bright Future Lactation Resource Centre
Linda J. Smith, BSE, FACCE, IBCLC • International Board Certified Lactation Consultant
6540 Cedarview Court • Dayton, Ohio 45459-1214 • (937) 438-9458 • Fax (937) 438-3229

Lactation Care Plan

Mother's Name_____ Today's Date_____

Baby's Name_____ Weight Today_____

Reason for Consult_____

- CORRECT POSITIONING at breast: Support breast well behind areola. Bring baby up onto areola so gums compress milk sinuses. Baby's lips should be turned outward. Lean back to assist with deeper grasp of areola. Support breast during entire feeding. IF PAINFUL, break suction and start over, bringing baby onto breast more quickly to avoid the nipple tip. If pain continues or increases, CALL.

- FREQUENT NURSING: Watch baby's cues and nurse at least 8-12 times per day, about every 2 hours when awake and every 4 hours at night. The baby should finish each side at his or her own pace. If baby falls asleep after less than 10 minutes of swallowing, DO NOT remove from the breast unless painful. Cluster nursings and more frequent nursing are fine.

- **FEED THE BABY** about_____ ounces per day. 10 minutes of swallowing is about 1 ounce. Breastfeed first. Use collected milk next. Use MD-recommended prepared formula only if needed.

- DO NOT USE PACIFIER OR ARTIFICIAL NIPPLES for at least the next two weeks. All sucking should be at the breast. Feed any supplement with dropper, small cup, spoon, or feeding tube device.

- BREAST CARE: Nurse, pump, and/or massage as often as needed until breasts are soft and no lumps are present. Use cool compresses and/or cabbage leaves around breasts to reduce swelling.

- BUILD SUPPLY: Express or pump at least _____times daily. Collect milk about every 2 hours during the day. Don't go longer than 5 hours without collecting milk. Save and use what you collect.

- INCREASE SKIN-TO-SKIN CONTACT with baby. Stay in bed with baby for 24–48 hours. Give baby at least two 20-minute massages daily. Wear baby in carrier at least 3 hours when NOT fussy and continuously if fussy.

- SEE PRIMARY CARE PROVIDER _____

- CALL if things are NOT improving, or are getting worse. Follow-up is planned for _____

- _____

Signature: _____
    Linda J. Smith, FACCE, IBCLC, Certified Lactation Consultant

Bright Future Lactation Resource Centre

Linda J. Smith, BSE, FACCE, IBCLC • International Board Certified Lactation Consultant
6540 Cedarview Court • Dayton, Ohio 45459-1214 • (937) 438-9458 • Fax (937) 438-3229

Breast Pumping Instructions and Milk Storage Information

• Pump about every 2-3 hours when you are awake, and every 4 hours at night, for a total of at least 6-10 times per 24 hours. Do NOT go longer than 5 hours without collecting milk. If your breasts feel full of milk before 2-3 hours, pump sooner. Save and use the milk that you collect.

• Pump each breast until the milk stops flowing, then another 2 minutes. This should take about 10-20 minutes. Even if you "get nothing," pump 10-20 minutes anyway. If you are double pumping, one side may continue flowing milk longer than the other.

• Depending on your breasts' storage capacity, you may be able to go longer between pumping sessions as time goes on. In the beginning, stick to this schedule until your daily total milk supply is 15-25% more than your baby needs.

• If you don't have time to pump the full length of time, at least pump SOME milk.

Milk Storage Times and Containers:

Air Temperature	How Long Milk Can Be Stored
Fresh—77°F (room temperature)	4 hours
Fresh—59°F (cooler)	24 hours in Styrofoam chest with blue ice "freezer pack"
Fresh—refrigerator	3-5 days
Thawed milk	24 hours in the refrigerator
Frozen	2 weeks to 6 months or more
Preferred containers	Glass with secure tops/lids
Acceptable containers	Rigid plastic (clear or cloudy) with secure tops
Less desirable containers	Soft plastic bags and "nurser bags"

• Start by putting 2-3 ounces in each container. Later, after you know your baby's eating pattern, you can match containers to his or her appetite. Keep a few 1-3 oz. containers of frozen milk on hand.

• Feed the collected milk to your baby in this order: Use fresh milk first, then refrigerated, then frozen.

• DON'T throw out extra frozen milk unless it has spoiled. Thawed milk is good for skin injuries, burns, and other uses. Many of the protective properties remain stable even when milk is frozen or heated.

Call if you have questions!

Bright Future Lactation Resource Centre
Linda J. Smith, BSE, FACCE, IBCLC • International Board Certified Lactation Consultant
6540 Cedarview Court • Dayton, Ohio 45459-1214 • (937) 438-9458 • Fax (937) 438-3229

Breat Pump Rental and Cleaning Instructions

Pump Use

Follow instructions in the booklet provided with your collection kit unless directed otherwise by your physician or lactation consultant. Pump about every 2–3 hours for 10–20 minutes or until the milk stops spraying, for a total of at least 100 minutes in 24 hours. For highest milk production, pump for 2 minutes after the flow of milk stops. Do not let milk remain in your breasts more than 5 hours without breastfeeding or pumping. Please don't stop abruptly—it's hard on you and your baby. **If you think your milk supply is dropping, you want to stop, or the pump is not working correctly, call a lactation consultant immediately (that day).**

If milk is drawn into your tubing, stop the pump! It means something is WRONG. If you continue to pump and milk is drawn into the pump body (inside the plexiglass cover), the pump is contaminated and must be sent back to the manufacturer for reservicing. YOU WILL BE CHARGED the $35 reservicing fee AND the shipping and insurance. Empty the collection container before it is overly full, and keep it upright during collection. If the filter membrane is intact, it is virtually impossible to draw milk into the tubing. If milk gets in the filter and the membrane gets wet, you will lose suction. Do not scrub the membrane, as it is delicate. Rinse it with warm water, shake off the excess, and air dry. You may use a blow-dryer to speed up the process.

Cleaning

The pump and case must be returned CLEAN. Clean the case and outside of the pump body with Windex™ or other mild cleaner. Do not scrub the plexiglass cover of the Classic pump. If the pump or case is returned soiled with milk or otherwise dirty, YOU WILL BE CHARGED a cleaning fee of at least $10.00.

Medela 015 (Classic) Pumps

Remove all of your tubing. Coil the cord under the handle and put the plug in one of the two circular openings. Carefully fit the pump into the case. When the motor is in the case correctly, the top closes easily.

Lactina Pumps

Remove your piston assembly. Carefully fit the pump into the case. When the motor is in the case correctly, the top closes easily.

Rental Fees

Daily rates will be charged unless the long-term rates are paid AT THE START of each rental period. At the end of a long-term period, daily rates will go into effect until a check or credit card authorization is received for the next rental period. All long-term rental months are "30-day" months. Refunds are not issued for early returns of long-term rentals. DO NOT WAIT to be billed! **Mark your "due dates" on your calendar.** If you are seeking reimbursement from your insurance company, a doctor's prescription for the pump and a personal letter from you stating the reason for rental will help. Insurance companies will not pay in advance of services rendered, so claims should be submitted at the end of a rental period. If the pump is rented for use during employment, check with an accountant or tax preparer as the rent may be deductible as a child care expense.

If You Absolutely Must Return the Pump When My Office Is Closed

CALL AHEAD. YOU ARE RESPONSIBLE FOR THE PUMP until I check in the pump and sign the receipt. If I'm unavailable, put your name inside the case and place the pump either inside the front doorway or just inside the gate to the yard, behind the garage. Call me at (937) 438-9458 and leave a message on my voice mail with the time and date of the call. I will mail you a bill or refund and the pump receipt.

Remember, you are responsible for the pump itself and all rent charges until you have a signed receipt for the pump.

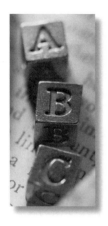

Client Handout Packet Suggestions

FROM LINDA J. SMITH

Every client gets copies of her consent form, assessment sheet, specific care plan, and arrangement for follow-up. She also receives an itemized receipt, my general price list, my business cards (which list my Web site and e-mail addresses), a list of good parenting books, local La Leche League contact information, and a copy of our local Coalition's *Services Directory*.

The *Directory* has some basic breastfeeding information (much of which I wrote), including sections on the following: The Importance of Breastfeeding, How to Get a Good Start, Tips for Pumping, Is Baby Getting Enough, Your Milk Supply, What to Expect in the Early Weeks, When to Call for Help, and What You Can Do to Help the Breastfeeding Mother (which includes the *Ten Steps to Successful Breastfeeding*). The *Directory* also lists local pump depots, classes, other PPLCs, hospital-based lactation programs, and public health and WIC clinics that provide breastfeeding services. I like giving out the *Directory* because it gives the mother additional resources for support besides me—it's part of my commitment to creating a community safety net.

FROM LIZ BROOKS

I use a brightly colored, two-pocket folder. On the left side are papers that I generate during the consult: the mother's copy of my consent form, my history sheet, any care plans, handouts such as logs to track feedings/diapers, and an HCFA form (for third-party reimbursement).

On the right side are items that do not need immediate attention: extra business cards (paper-clipped with a sticky note "for your friends"), my practice brochure, a "Consider Giving a Gift Certificate" form, breast pump information and rental rates, "For Fathers Only: Ways to Father a Breastfed Baby," "If Your Grandchild Is Breastfed," and other general how-to handouts. Some of it is marketing, including my handout "Why an IBCLC?", which highlights the benefits of seeking out an IBCLC for lactation issues.

I use the brightly colored folder so these documents are easier to spot and grab in the detritus of a home with infant feeding difficulties. ("Honey, where's the lactation consultant's number?" "I don't know. Look for that red folder.")

FROM DIANE WEISSINGER

Every client who has a full initial consultation receives a client packet—a two-pocket folder with Linda Smith's "Rules for Helping Breastfeeding Mothers" on the front along with my name, phone, e-mail, and Web site address. The left inside pocket is labeled "Papers on this side are for future use or general interest," and contains a LLL meeting announcement, a discount coupon for our local LLL group, sheets on starting solids and on working, and other handouts not immediately necessary.

The right inside pocket is labeled "Review these now. Insurance forms at back." Newborn and positioning information, and any sheets that will be of special importance to that mother's situation, are found here. When I fill out the mother's insurance forms at the end, I tuck them behind the other sheets.

Attached to the outsides of the pockets are my business card and a sticker that says, "Milk supply depends on frequent and effective milk removal." To avoid copyright issues and save money, most of the handouts in the folder are written by me, on standardized colors (the sheet on weaning is always purple, the father's sheet is always ivory, and so on). I tell the mother or her partner to look over the sheets on both sides when they get home, and often suggest that the partner do the reading, pulling for the mother any that seem especially important.

A great deal of thought and energy goes into the folders. Although I work with a highly literate population, I know mothers are often too stressed to make much use of them. On the other hand, I know that they have accurate information at their fingertips if they choose to make use of it; some sit right down and devour it all. It can only be reassuring for them to realize that their questions and uncertainties are so common that a handout has already been written about it.

Toward the end of a consultation, the mother and I make out a "cheat sheet" together—my version of a care plan. It is handwritten on triplicate paper. I write down anything of which she wants to remind herself, and anything of which I want to remind her. We review each phrase as it is written, to make sure it is written the way she wants it. The top copy goes in the front of the right-side pocket, the second goes in my file, and the third may or may not be mailed with my report to her physician.

Diane's handouts can be purchased from Common Sense Breastfeeding at www.wiessinger.baka.com.

FROM PATRICIA LINDSEY

My handout packet includes "instructions for patients filing for reimbursement." I developed a *Lactation Visit Receipt* that has helped many clients and PPLCs obtain third-party reimbursement.

Pat's *Lactation Visit Receipt* packet for professionals, including full instructions, may be purchased from Pat at www.patlc.com or e-mail at PatIBCLC@aol.com.

FROM MECHELL TURNER

My handout packet contains a Client Survey (in Appendix G) that was published in the *Journal of Human Lactation*.[1] As a result of surveying my clients, I now suggest fewer interventions, and I'm more patient in using one intervention at a time. It works better to have an uninterested third party read and compile the surveys and send the results to me, than if the clients respond directly to me.

NOTES

1. Turner, M. R. Twenty questions for the consumer: A quality assurance tool for the lactation consultant. *Journal of Human Lactation* 1996;12(1):50–53.

Pat Lindsey, IBCLC - Lactation Services
Board Certified Lactation Consultant - Registered Lactation Consultant
TAX ID/PROVIDER # 59-3579433

3849 Oakwater Circle, Orlando, FL 32806 - Telephone 407-859-7239 - Fax 407-850-9185 - Pager 407-596-4359

"Affordable Health Care Begins with Breastfeeding"

PATIENT INFORMATION

© 2002 Pat Lindsey, IBCLC

PATIENT'S LAST NAME	FIRST	INITIAL	PT'S BIRTHDATE	PATIENT: ☐ MALE ☐ FEMALE	RELATIONSHIP TO SUBSCRIBER

ADDRESS	CITY	STATE	ZIP	REFERRING PHYSICIAN

PHONE ( )	SUBSCRIBER	INSURANCE CARRIER

ADDRESS - IF DIFFERENT	CITY	STATE	ZIP	INS. ID	COVERAGE CODE	GROUP

☐ LACTATION ☐ ILLNESS
☐ ACCIDENT ☐ PREGNANCY
☐ INDUSTRIAL

DATE SYMPTOMS APPEARED:

OTHER HEATH COVERAGE? YES ☐ NO ☐ IDENTIFY:

ASSIGNMENT. I hereby assign my insurance benefits to be paid directly to the undersigned health care provider. I am financially responsible for non-covered services.

SIGNED: (Insured or Authorized Person)   Date:

RELEASE: I authorize the undersigned health care provider to release any information acquired in the course of my examination or treatment.

SIGNED: (Insured or Authorized Person)   Date:

NEW	ESTAB	OFFICE SERVICE	FEE
99203 30min.	99213 15min.	Hx Evaluation and Management	
99204 45min.	99214 25min.	Hx Evaluation and Management	
99205 60min.	99215 40min.	Hx Evaluation and Management	

NEW	ESTAB	HOME SERVICE	FEE
99342 30min.	99348 25min.	Hx Evaluation and Management	
99343 45min.	99349 40min.	Hx Evaluation and Management	
99344 60min.	99350 60min.	Hx Evaluation and Management	

NEW	ESTAB	HOSPITAL SERVICE	FEE
99221 30min.	99231 15min.	Hx Evaluation and Management	
99222 50min.	99232 25min.	Hx Evaluation and Management	
99223 70min.	99233 35min.	Hx Evaluation and Management	

NEW	ESTAB	TELEPHONE CONSULT	FEE
99371	99371	Brief	
99372	99372	Intermediate	
99373	99373	Lengthy/complex	

TRAVEL	# Miles @		

SUPPLIES				CPT/MOD	FEE
BREAST PUMPS					
Breast Pump Collection Kit	Single	Double	Conversion	A7002	
Pump In Style	Orginial	Traveler	Companion	E0603	
Purely Yours	with case	w/out case		E0603	
Nurture III	with case	w/out case		E0603	
Mini-Electric				E0603	
Hand Pump	Medela	Ameda	Avent	E0602	
Other Pump				E0603	
SUPPLEMENT NURSING		Starter	Regular		
BREAST SHELLS				99070	
NIPPLE SHIELD				99070	
BOOKS / PAMPHLETS				99071	
OTHER Feeding Supplies					
Baby Weigh Scale Rental		days @ $		E1399	
ELECTRIC HOSPITAL GRADE PUMP RENTAL				E0604	
Equipment Serial Number					
Rented Date		Return Date			
# days @ $		# months @ $			
Delivery / Extra Cleaning Charge on Rental Pump					
TOTAL SUPPLIES AND/OR RENTAL					
SALES TAX IF NO PRESCRIPTION					

LACTATION DX ICD 9 CM CODES

CHILD

BREASTFEEDING PROBLEM

783.21	Abnormal Weight Loss
775.5	Dehydration Newborn
783.41	Failure to Gain Weight
779.3	Newborn Feeding Problem
	Breast Refusal
	Latch-on Difficulties
	Regurgitation of food
	Slow feeding
	Vomiting
	Other
783.3	Infant Feeding Problem
	Breast Refusal
	Latch-on Difficulties
	Mismanagement of feeding
	Other
783.6	Polyphagia-Overeating
783.2	Under weight

SUCKING PROBLEMS

796.1	Suck Reflex Abnormal

JAUNDICE (V12.3)

774.39	Breastmilk Jaundice
774	Newborn - Physiologic
774.2	Newborn - Premature

ABNORMAL FUSSINESS/COLIC

777.8	Newborn - Colic
789.0	Infant - Colic
780.59	Sleep Disturbances Infant

DERMATITIS/INFECTION

691.0	Diaper Rash
693.1	Due to Food
691.8	Eczema
771.7	Thrush-Newborn
112.0	Thrush-Infant

OTHER

750.0	Ankyloglossia - Tongue Tie
530.18	GEReflux-NoInflam(V12.70)
530.11	GEReflux-Inflam(V12.70)
750.15	Macroglossia (V12.40)
750.16	Microglossia (V12.40)
520.7	Teething Syndrome

_____
_____
_____

CHILD DIAGNOSIS

PRIMARY DX_____
SECONDARY DX_____
SECONDARY DX_____
SECONDARY DX_____

MOTHER

NIPPLE/AREOLA PROBLEM

676.14	Cracked/Fissured
692.9	Dermatitis Contact
676.04	Dimpled/Folded/Creviced
676.34	Flat
675.9	Infection (unspecific/Thrush)
676.04	Inverted (Retracted)
676.34	Sore Nipples
676.3	Trauma
676.3	Ulceration
676.34	Unusual Shape

BREAST PROBLEM

676.3	Breast Pain
692.9	Dermatitis Contact
676.9	Disorder of Lactation
676.8	Galactocele
757.6	Hypoplasia of Breast
611.72	Mass (es) / Lump (s)

ENGORGEMENT, BREAST

676.20	After the Perinatal Period
676.24	Perinatal, Moderate/Severe

MASTITIS

675.14	Breast Abscess
675.04	Filled Duct
675.20	Non-Purulent Infection
675.24	Plugged Duct
675.14	Purulent Infection

MILK SUPPLY

676.44	Agalactia (No Milk)
676.64	Galactorreah
676.8	Polygalactia (Over Supply)
676.54	Suppressed (Reduced)

LACTATION

676.50	Induced (Adoption) (v61.29)
676.54	Relactation

OTHER

_____
_____
_____
_____

MOTHER DIAGNOSIS

PRIMARY DX_____
SECONDARY DX_____
SECONDARY DX_____
SECONDARY DX_____

NOTES

INSTRUCTIONS TO PATIENT FOR FILING INSURANCE CLAIMS:

COMPLETE THE PATIENT INFORMATION SECTION AT THE TOP OF THIS FORM. SIGN AND DATE. THEN MAIL THIS FORM DIRECTLY TO YOUR INSURANCE COMPANY. PLEASE ATTACH YOUR OWN INSURANCE CARRIER'S CLAIM FORM.

PLEASE REMEMBER THAT PAYMENT IS YOUR OBLIGATION. REGARDLESS OF INSURANCE OR OTHER THIRD PARTY INVOLVEMENT.

REC'D BY	
☐ CHARGE	
☐ CASH	
☐ CHECK	
# _____	

TODAY'S FEE	
OLD BALANCE	
TOTAL DUE	
AMT. REC'D	
NEW BALANCE	

NEXT APPOINTMENT	PROVIDER'S SIGNATURE	DATE OF SERVICE

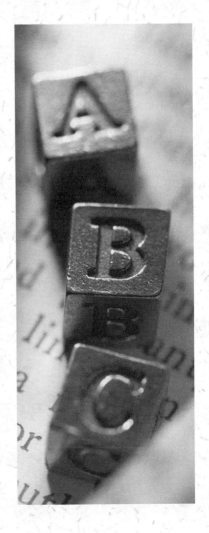

Sample Reports to Physicians

REPORT #1
Barbara Wilson-Clay, BSE, IBCLC

Reason for visit: Breastfeeding difficulty: Mother has inverting nipples—baby has broken clavicle.

The Consultation Included
Technique taught:

- ✔ Correct latch-on
- ✔ Correct positioning
- ✔ Milk supply support
- Hand-expression
- Milk collection and storage
- Other:

- Electric pump
- Periodontal syringe
- Hand pump
- Supplemental nursing system
- ✔ Nipple shield
- ✔ Baby weigh scale
- Other:

Referred to: Pediatrician for growth monitoring

Summary

Joshua weighs 8 lb.,15 oz. and appears alert with good tone and color. Watching the feeding, it is clear that the feeding position currently being used is awkward and uncomfortable for both mother and baby. I repositioned the baby in side-lying to relieve the pressure on his broken collar bone. Both of Belinda's nipples invert, the left more severely than the right. The baby is quite frustrated by the way they retreat when he attempts to latch-on. The hospital LCs had given Belinda a nipple shield. This intervention provided a good alternative to bottle-feeding, and has preserved the baby's interest in breast-feeding. Belinda's nipples are already beginning to increase in elasticity, and they draw up well under the shield once the baby starts sucking.

I performed a test weight, and documented a 70 g intake during a feed with the shield in place. The feeding was slow, however, and baby rested frequently between sucking bursts. He may have stamina problems that may be a result of the long and difficult birth. The broken clavicle probably is causing him to be more stressed during feedings. If the mother is willing to allow baby the time it takes him to complete a feeding, and continues to be willing to feed frequently, the baby should be able to maintain normal growth at breast.

Belinda was encouraged to briefly use her electric pump after nursing to ensure that she drains her breasts thoroughly. Pumped hind milk can be used as a supplement if needed. I've asked Belinda to log the diaper output carefully, and to use 1 oz. pumped hind milk following 3–4 of the daily feeds if the baby isn't making 3–4 stools per day. I advised Belinda to weigh the baby weekly during the time he's using the nipple shield to make sure his intake is appropriate. Joshua was willing to nurse briefly without the shield on the more everted right nipple. This was encouraging to Belinda. I explained how to wean baby off the shield as nipple elasticity improves, and will stay in touch by phone until this goal is accomplished.

Reason for visit: Mother has tender nipples—has been self-medicating for suspected candidiasis for 6 months.

REPORT #2
Barbara Wilson-Clay, BSE, IBCLC

The Consultation Included

Technique taught:

Correct latch-on
Correct positioning
Milk supply support
Hand-expression
Milk collection and storage
Other:

Electric pump
Periodontal syringe
Hand pump
Supplemental nursing system
Nipple shield
Baby weigh scale
Other:

Referred to: Consider consulting dermatologist.

Summary

The baby was diagnosed with thrush at two months postpartum. The pediatrician prescribed topical Nystatin for two weeks. Bella's nipples became tender at that time, and this soreness has persisted. In the past months, Bella has completed two courses of oral Diflucan, and baby has been treated with Diflucan elixir. In spite of no real change in her condition as the result of the antifungal therapy, Bella has continued to apply Nystatin, Lotrimin, and Gentian Violet almost daily. Today both nipple tips are slightly pink, and the skin, although unbroken, looks a little dry and scaly. I am concerned that Bella has been continuing to use a variety of medications on herself and baby for six months in the absence of a clear diagnosis. She tells me that her nipples feel somewhat better when she treats them with topical antifungals, and they also felt better when she used topical cortisone for a few days. Typically, however, shortly after applying the medications, she states that her nipples again feel irritated. It is possible that her nipples are irritated by the medications. She may now have contact dermatitis or may have a chronic condition such as eczema. I think it is prudent to discontinue all forms of self-medication and consult a dermatologist.

Additional Issues

The baby apparently reacted with patches of eczema when exposed to soy formula as a younger infant. However, Bella still gives soy formula and tofu to baby. I have suggested discontinuing soy for a while to see if this strategy changes anything. While rare, I personally have seen several cases, and read of one case, where a protein intolerance in the infant provoked irritated nipples (changes in saliva?).

Finally, Bella has noticed nipple blanching after feeds. She also reports sensitivity to thermal changes in her toes. Vasospasm (Reynaud's syndrome) can create nipple pain similar to what she describes. Bella washes her nipples with cold water and vinegar after feeds, which may provoke vasospasm. I've advised her to discontinue this practice and to try warm compresses to see if they reduce her discomfort. The literature describes oral therapy with Nifedipine (Hale, 1999) as safe for nursing mothers experiencing nipple vasospasm.

REPORT #3
Barbara Wilson-Clay, BSE, IBCLC

Reason for visit: Mother complains that nursing is difficult—baby is "frantic" at breast.

The Consultation Included
Technique taught:

Correct latch-on
✔ Correct positioning
✔ Milk supply support
Hand-expression
Milk collection and storage
Other:

Electric pump
Periodontal syringe
Hand pump
Supplemental nursing system
Nipple shield
✔ Baby weigh scale
Other:

Referred to:

Summary
Baby is 6 weeks old and weighs 11 lb., 11 oz. (birth weight, 7 lb., 2 oz.) and is alert and robust. Anne has a copious milk supply and a forceful milk ejection. She is concerned that the baby feeds only 5–8 minutes and averages only 6 feeds per 24 hours. This pattern is very different from what she expected. Anne has read a lot about breastfeeding, and her baby isn't following the rules. Additionally, it distresses Anne when the baby latches on, acts overwhelmed, gasps and chokes, gets mad, and pulls off. Anne tells me this is their typical feeding pattern. To prevent him from pulling away, Anne holds the baby very tightly.

I showed her how to allow milk to eject before latching-on the baby, which will decrease the initial force of the spray in his mouth. We then latched Drew to the breast with his head in a more upright position, which will help him cope with the rapid milk flow. He fed for 4 minutes and pulled off. I asked Anne not to force him to take the other side until we weighed him. Test weighing (on a digital electronic scale sensitive to within 2 gs) demonstrated a 3.7 oz. intake. Due to the shortness of the feed, Anne was shocked that the baby had taken in so much milk. I explained that baby was probably quite full, and to force him to take the other breast was part of the problem. Anne experimented with trying to latch Drew onto the other breast. His body language was eloquent. He averted his head and leaned away from her.

I have advised Anne to allow more baby-led control of feedings, and to be aware that he will not act as aversive if he is allowed to pull off to catch his breath, to burp, and so on. With a milk supply like hers, Anne will feed less often and in shorter feeds than would a mother with a different production standard. We discussed deliberately down-regulating her supply by only using one breast at a feed. I think Anne feels she now has some better insight into reading the baby's cues. She has been encouraged to call if she needs reassurance.

Client report: "Pat Jones" and baby "Joey" (DOB 4/25/2001)

Date of service: May 31, 2001, with follow-up phone calls on 6/1, 6/3, 6/5, 6/7, and 6/11

Chief complaints: Fussy baby; possibly due to allergy

Referred by: GSH North; requested pump information

Care providers: OB: "Heller"; Ped: "Youngberg" (group)

REPORT #4
Linda J. Smith, BSE, FACCE, IBCLC

Subjective/Relevant History

First baby; 5 weeks old; both parents have history of allergies. Early feeds "went well." Sporadic pacifier use; some supplementation with Alsoy. Pat reports she recently increased her smoking; wishes to resume use of an antidepressant. Pat's goal is to "feed when he's hungry with him happy afterward, and not be tired myself."

Objective

Mother: Breasts moderate size; soft bilaterally before and after feed; nipples firm and elastic, very slightly pink; no visible cracks or wounds.

Baby: Weight 10 lbs., 5.5 oz. in dry diaper. Skin appears dry and slightly yellow; dry pink eczema-like rash on both cheeks. Head is still slightly molded; prefers to curve (L). Palate is somewhat flat.

At Breast: Positioning good on a wrap-around pillow. Feed duration on L breast very long (>20 minutes) with habituation and disorganized suck-swallow-breathe coordination. Did not nurse on R breast during visit. Subsequent feeds on L breast similar in pattern to first observed feed.

Postfeed: Breasts soft; Pat attempted to feed about 1 oz. in bottle with Nuk nipple; Joey is disorganized with bottle, too. Pat reports that nipple is sometimes creased after feeds.

Assessment/Impression

1. Disorganized suck, which is likely playing a major role in Joey's fussiness because his suboptimal suck is limiting full milk transfer at breast, resulting in more frequent hunger cues.

2. Somewhat suppressed milk supply due to poor milk transfer by baby.

3. Possible allergic cause for facial rash is more likely due to supplements given directly than maternal dietary allergens transferred via breast milk.

Plan

1. Pat will pump after feeds for at least a week to increase her milk supply. This should reduce Joey's fussiness due to hunger.

2. Pat will begin a detailed diet and behavior diary to track down the source(s) of Joey's fussiness and facial rash.

3. Suggested use of a tie-on carrier for additional comforting while doing household chores.

Evaluation/Follow-up

Phone calls on 6/1, 6/3, 6/5, 6/7, and 6/11: Pat noticed an increase in her milk supply after beginning use of a rental electric breast pump on 6/5. She believes Joey's rash is better when she avoids dairy products; she is now taking Zoloft. On 6/11, Pat reports wanting to reduce or discontinue direct breast-feeding but may continue pumping milk for Joey.

Follow-up is planned by phone and e-mail over the next few days or weeks. Pat will read my "long-term pumping" and "rapid weaning" handouts.

Client report: "Juliana Jackson"; baby "Penny" (DOB 11/7/2000)

Date of service: Nov. 11, 2000

Chief complaints: Needs a breast pump; baby won't latch

Referred by: KMC pump list

Care providers: "Jane Doe," RN, IBCLC; Dr. "Pierce"; Dr. "Minolta"

REPORT #5
Linda J. Smith, BSE, FACCE, IBCLC

Subjective/Relevant History

Juliana's labor was induced at 40.6 weeks for postdates and elevated blood pressure. Juliana received Nubain to control twitching, and an epidural at 8 cm. Her labor was deliberately slowed until after midnight, and delivery was assisted with a vacuum extractor. Penny weighed 9 lbs., 11 oz. with APGAR scores of 7 and 9. She had some "raspy breathing" and first attempted nursing 3 hours postbirth; she "nibbled on and off." Since then, she has been increasingly unable to latch and feed well. Juliana is pumping milk and feeding it to Penny by bottle, supplementing as needed with Similac. Stooling and urination patterns are normal.

Objective

Mother: Juliana's breasts are large, moderately full, and with normal configuration of structures. Nipples are soft but with poor elasticity, possibly because of stored milk. Areolas are somewhat fibrous and/or edematous. The right nipple has a small crack in the center of the tip. Milk supply is beginning to increase; Juliana easily pumped 1 oz. from the right breast.

Baby: Penny appears calm, hydrated, and slightly yellow. Her head is asymmetrical, and she prefers to turn to the right. Her tongue humps, and her suck-swallow-breathe pattern is disorganized. Oral structures appear normal. She weighed 9 lbs., 5 oz., which is the same as her lowest/discharge weight and 6 oz. below her birth weight.

At Breast: Although she enjoys being in Juliana's arms, at breast Penny fights and only briefly latched on to the left breast. Using a Nuk silicone nipple, Penny took about 1 1/3 oz. of EBM in about 20 minutes, but with disorganized suck-swallow-breathe.

Postfeed: Penny self-detached appropriately from the feeding using EBM in a bottle.

Assessment/Impression

Penny's suck-swallow-breathe coordination is disorganized. The most likely explanation is residual facial asymmetry from the long, hard labor, epidural anesthesia, and vacuum extraction. Milk supply is rapidly increasing.

Plan

Juliana will pump and cup-feed or finger-feed for at least two days to allow her breasts time to heal, provide sufficient calories, and help organize Penny's suck. She will continue attempts at breast and document the most effective positions and strategies. Juliana plans to have her chiropractor evaluate Penny's situation.

Evaluation/Follow-up

Phone call in 2–3 days; in-person follow-up will be at Juliana's request unless Penny does not improve in 2–3 days, or she has further questions.

Today's date: «dateofconsult»   **Date of the consult:** «dateofconsult»

Mother's name: «momfirstname» «momlastname»

Baby's name: «babyfirstname» «babylastname»   **DOB:** «babydateofbirth»

Baby's birth weight: «babybirthwt» **Current weight:** «babycurrentweight»

At the time «momfirstname»'s concern was that «babyfirstname» «whyconsult».

My impression at the time was that «summary»

I instructed «momfirstname» in

 Hand-expression

 Use of an electric breast pump

 Positioning of the baby at breast

 Latch-on technique

 Suck training

 Finger-feeding with a feeding syringe

I gave her written instructions about

 Cleaning the feeding syringes

 Use and cleaning of the nipple shield

 Use and cleaning of the breast shells

 Pumping and storing human milk

I will remain in telephone contact over the next few days. It is my pleasure to provide lactation services to your patients. I will make every effort to give the support needed to meet their breastfeeding goals. If I can be of further assistance, please contact me.

Sincerely,

Kathleen L. Hoover

cc:

SAMPLE CLIENT REPORT SYSTEM
Kay Hoover, M.Ed., IBCLC

Filled-In Fields for Template

«momfirstname» «momlastname», «momstreetaddress», «momcitystatezip»

«referredbyname», «referredbyaddress», «referredbycitystatezip»

«pedname», «pedgroup», «pedstreetaddress», «pedsuite», «pedcitystatezip»

«obname», «obgroup», «obstreetaddress», «obsuite», «obcitystatezip»

«phone» «momlastname» «momfirstname»

«babylastname» «babyfirstname» «babydateofbirth» «sex»

«babybirthwt» «babycurrentweight»

«momstreetaddress», «momcitystatezip» Date of consult:«dateofconsult»

Referred by: «referredbyname»

«referredbyaddress»

«referredbycitystatezip»

Pediatrician: «pedname»

«pedgroup»

«pedstreetaddress»

«pedsuite»

«pedcitystatezip»

Obstetrician: «obname»

«obgroup»

«obstreetaddress»

«obsuite»

«obcitystatezip»

«whyconsult»

«dateofconsult»   «daysold»

«summary»

email: «email»

«other1»

«other2»

«other3»

«other4»

Today's date: 1/5/2003   **Date of the consult:** 1/5/2003

Mother's name: Jane Doe

Baby's name: Baby Doe   **DOB:** 1/1/2003

Baby's birth weight: 7 lb., 6 oz.   **Current weight:** 7 lb., 12 oz.

SAMPLE CLIENT REPORT—FILLED IN
Kay Hoover, M.Ed., IBCLC

At the time Jane's concern was that Baby Doe not latching.

My impression at the time was difficulty with latch secondary to Jane's flat nipples.

I instructed Jane in

   Hand-expression

   Use of an electric breast pump

   Positioning of the baby at breast

   Latch-on technique

   Cup-feeding

   Bottle-feeding

I gave her written instructions about

   Use and cleaning of the pump parts

   Use and cleaning of the nipple shield

   Use and cleaning of the breast shells

   Pumping and storing human milk

I will remain in telephone contact over the next few days. It is my pleasure to provide lactation services to your patients. I will make every effort to give the support needed to meet their breastfeeding goals. If I can be of further assistance, please contact me.

Sincerely,

Kathleen L. Hoover

cc:

Filled-In Fields for Template

Jane Doe, 100 Doe Street, Everywhere, OH 22334

Lactation Center, Everywhere General Hospital, Everywhere, OH 22334

John Smith, MD, Pediatric Associates, 666 Young Highway, Suite 100, Everywhere, OH 22334

Mary Jones, MD, OB/GYN Associates of Everywhere, Everywhere General Hospital, Suite 400, Everywhere, OH 22334

888-777-6666   Doe   Jane

Doe   Baby   1/1/2003   F

7 lb. 6 oz.   7 lb. 12 oz.

100 Doe Street, Everywhere, OH 22334   Date of consult:1/5/2003

Referred by: Lactation Center

Everywhere General Hospital

Everywhere, OH 22334

Pediatrician: John Smith, MD

Pediatric Associates

666 Young Highway

Suite 100

Everywhere, OH 22334

Obstetrician: Mary Jones, MD

OB/GYN Associates of Everywhere

Everywhere General Hospital

Suite 400

Everywhere, OH 22334

Baby not latching

1/5/2003   4 days

difficulty with latch secondary to Jane's flat nipples

e-mail: jane.doe@aol.com

APPENDIX E

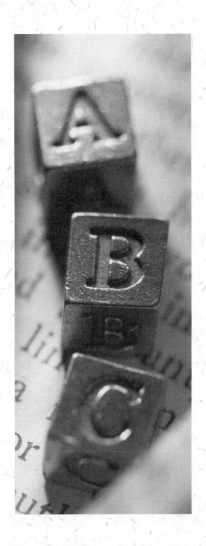

Sources for Supplies and Equipment

DIGITAL INFANT SCALES
- Medela, (800) 435-8316 or www.medela.com
- MedTech Source, (888) 888-8077, fax (508) 833-9933
- Seca, www.seca.com
- Tanita, (800) 826-4828 or www.tanita.com

BREAST PUMPS AND BREASTFEEDING EQUIPMENT/PRODUCTS
- Bailey Medical Engineering (Nurture III), www.BaileyMed.com
- Hollister (Ameda-Egnell), www.Hollister.com
- Medela, www.Medela.com
- Whittlestone, www.whittlestone.com

PROFESSIONAL MALPRACTICE INSURANCE FOR IBCLCS

Interstate Insurance Group/Maginnis & Associates, (800) 345-6917

GLOVES (LATEX AND NONLATEX)

Local pharmacies, drug stores, medical supply catalogs

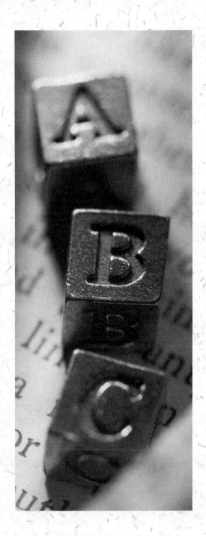

Gift Pack Generic Letter

January 26, 2001

Dear <Lactation Consultant>,

Thank you for seeking input from the Greater Miami Valley Breastfeeding Coalition regarding <Your Hospital's> possible distribution of <any formula company> "gift" packages for new mothers.

First, distribution of commercial products is an ethical issue. The *Healthy People 2010* goals for the nation include "increase the proportion of women who initiate breastfeeding to 75 percent." Breastfeeding is one of the top 10 specific goals in the DHHS Title V MCH Block Grant. Many experts consider it unethical and a conflict of interest for any health care facility and/or employee/provider to advertise a product or service from a for-profit company. Additionally, ethics committees in numerous hospitals consider the formula-containing discharge packs to be unethical and a conflict of interest. "Gift packs" are a classic and highly effective form of advertising.[1] The World Health Organization's *International Code of Marketing of Breastmilk Substitutes* specifically prohibits advertising of infant formula, bottles, and teats (nipples) to the public.[2]

Second, this is potentially a legal issue. Some hospitals refuse to hand out any formula-company materials on breastfeeding because they recognize their responsibility to provide accurate parent education materials. Because manufacturers of formula cannot legally promote a competitor (breastfeeding), these materials could be challenged for accuracy. Risk management departments in some hospitals raise concerns about the potential for provoking allergies and diabetes in susceptible families.

Third, the facility incurs additional costs to distribute these materials. Every minute that a nurse spends handling these items takes away from other assigned patient care responsibilities. Distributing free samples is a very effective marketing technique designed to promote brand loyalty. Unless "salesperson" is part of the staff nursing job descriptions, any such activity could compromise patient care. No other unit in the hospital gives its patients products that could alter their health status and cause them to return.

The danger in the gift packs is the marketing tactic that they are sanctioned by the hospital and given to cause a breastfeeding mother to supplement with formula. The repercussions that follow include insufficient milk, necessitating the purchasing of the product and altering of the infant's gut flora at a time before gut closure has occurred, which increases the risk of both allergy and gastrointestinal disease. Health care professionals would also need to ascertain if the parents could afford to buy the formula.

Finally, numerous studies have documented a decrease in breastfeeding initiation and reduction in duration related to "gift" pack distribution.[3] The *Blueprint for Action on Breastfeeding* recently released by the Surgeon General's Office on Women's Health states, "The marketing of infant formula negatively affects breastfeeding" and refers to the *Code* for specific guidelines. Individually and collectively, the items in the pack send the message that mothers will not have enough milk, breastfeeding is uncomfortable or painful, and formula is "just as good." The packs are designed to sell formula, and overtly and covertly undermine the *Healthy People 2010* goals and the health of women and children.[4]

In conclusion, we urge <Your Hospital> to discontinue distribution of "gift packs" from formula companies to maternity patients for ethical, legal, financial, and clinical/health reasons.

Linda J. Smith, BSE, FACCE, IBCLC
On behalf of the Greater Miami Valley Breastfeeding Coalition

NOTES

1. Blake, R. L. Jr., et al. Patients' attitudes about gifts to physicians from pharmaceutical companies. *Journal of the American Board of Family Practice* 1995;8(6):457-464.

    Chren, M. M., Landefeld, C. S., and Murray, T. H. Doctors, drug companies, and gifts. *Journal of the American Medical Association* 1989;262:3448-3451.

    Greer, F. R., et al. Physicians, formula companies and advertising. *American Journal of Diseases of Children* 1991;145(3):282-286.

    Howard, F. M., Howard, C. R., and Weitzman, M. The physician as advertiser: The unintentional discouragement of breastfeeding. *Obstetrics and Gynecology* 1993;81(6):1048-1051.

    Margolis, L. H. The ethics of accepting gifts from pharmaceutical companies. *Pediatrics* 1991;88(6): 1233-1237.

2. Article 7.4: "Samples of infant formula or other products within the scope of this Code, or of equipment or utensils for their preparation or use, should not be provided to health workers. Health workers should not give samples of infant formula to pregnant women, mothers of infants and young children, or members of their families."

3. Ajl S. "Free" infant formula also does harm in the U.S. *New York Times*, March 31, 1992.

    Bergevin, Y., Dougherty, C., and Kramer, M. S. Do infant formula samples shorten the duration of breast-feeding? *Lancet* 1983;1(8334):1148-1151.

    Bliss, M. C., Wilkie, J., Acredolo, C., Berman, S., and Tebb, K. P. The effect of discharge pack formula and breast pumps on breastfeeding duration and choice of infant feeding method. *Birth* 1997;24(2):90-97.

    Frank, D. A., et al. Commercial discharge packs and breastfeeding counseling: Effects of infant feeding practices in a randomized trial. *Pediatrics* 1987;80:845-854.

    Howard, C. R., et al. Infant formula distribution and advertising in pregnancy: A hospital survey. *Birth* 1994;21(1):14-19.

    Snell, B. J., Krantz, M., Keeton, R., Delgado, K., and Peckham, C. The association of formula samples given at hospital discharge with the early duration of breastfeeding. *Journal of Human Lactation* 1992;8(2):67-72. Published erratum appears in *Journal of Human Lactation* 1992;8(3):135.

    Sullivan, P. CMA supports breastfeeding, "condemns" contracts between formula makers, hospitals. *Canadian Medical Association Journal* 1992;146(9):1610-1612.

4. Kramer, M. S., Chalmers, B., Hodnett, E. D., et al. Breastfeeding in Belarus. *Journal of the American Medical Association* 2001;285:463-464.

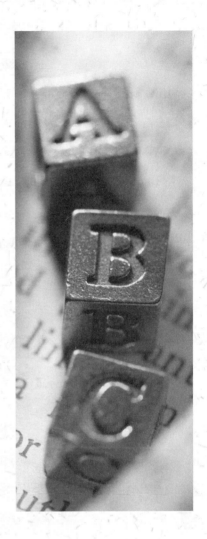

Client Satisfaction Survey

Appendix 2. Lactation client satisfaction survey*

Circle the answer given by the client.

A Excellent or yes	B Above standard	C Standard	D Somewhat Inadequate	E Inadequate or no

	A	B	C	D	E
1. Was the service you received punctual and timely?	—	—	—	—	—
2. Was follow-up available/given?	—	—	—	—	—
3. Was follow-up timely/adequate?	—	—	—	—	—
4. Were teaching materials available and understandable?	—	—	—	—	—
5. Were breastfeeding goals set?	—	—	—	—	—
6. Were options given to meet your goals?	—	—	—	—	—
7. Did the lactation consultant answer your questions satisfactorily?	—	—	—	—	—
8. Were risks and benefits of treatments, supplements, and devices explained?	—	—	—	—	—
9. Was teaching of breast pump and kit given?	—	—	—	—	—
10. Was the teaching and use of other devices clear and concise?	—	—	—	—	—
11. Did the lactation consultant refer you to another specialist/ group if necessary?	—	—	—	—	—
12. Did the lactation consultant help you meet your breastfeeding goals?	—	—	—	—	—
13. Did the breast pump or other devices help you meet your breastfeeding goals?	—	—	—	—	—
14. Did you consider the lactation consultant's charge a reasonable fee?	—	—	—	—	—
15. Did you feel the lactation consultant was honest?	—	—	—	—	—
16. Did you feel you received good care?	—	—	—	—	—
17. Would you recommend this lactation service to a friend?	—	—	—	—	—
TOTAL COLUMN RESPONSES:	—	—	—	—	—
TOTAL OF ALL RESPONSES (TIR):	———				

18. Are you still breastfeeding now?   ___ Yes ___ No
   If 'yes,' how long have you been breastfeeding?"_____
   If 'no,' how long did you breastfeed? _____

19. How were you referred to this lactation consultant?
   __ doctor or hospital staff
   __ advertisement
   __ friend
   __ other (specify) _____

20. What was the reason you contacted a lactation consultant?
   __ work
   __ illness
   __ other (specify) _____

*If a response is "not applicable," write 'NR' or 'NA.'

———

Index

Also available from Jones and Bartlett Publishers by Linda J. Smith:

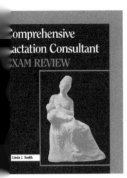

Comprehensive Lactation Consultant Exam Review

ISBN: 0-7637-0920-4
Price: $54.95 (U.S. List)*
Cover: Paperback
Pages: 384
Copyright: 2001

Comprehensive Lactation Consultant Exam Review will help you prepare for the IBLCE exam. The text parallels the 13 content areas of the IBLCE examination and is perfect for candidates of the IBLCE lactation consultant examination and recertification. The companion CD-ROM contains 240 full-color clinical pictures.

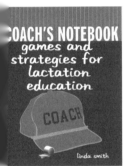

Coach's Notebook: Games and Strategies for Lactation Education

ISBN: 0-7637-1819-X
Price: $36.95 (U.S. List)*
Cover: Paperback
Pages: 172
Copyright: 2002

Coach's Notebook: Games and Strategies for Lactation Education contains a wide variety of games and activities for teaching breastfeeding and human lactation. For each tried and tested game you'll find goals, ideal audiences, playing times, and specific instructions for making teaching and learning human lactation fun and informative.

Order online or see more of our breastfeeding and lactation titles at http://womenshealthsource.jbpub.com

- -

Order Information:

Name: _____

Institution: _____

Address: _____

City: _____

State: _____ Zip: _____

Country: _____

Phone: _____

E-mail: _____

Mail Orders to:

Jones and Bartlett Publishers
40 Tall Pine Drive
Sudbury, MA 01776

Phone orders to: 800-832-0034
Fax orders to: 978-443-8000
E-mail orders to: info@jbpub.com

Payment Information:

Note: Please include $5.50 shipping and handling. When ordering more than one book, please include $1.00 for each additional book ordered. U.S. only.

❏ Payment Enclosed (make checks payable to Jones and Bartlett Publishers)
❏ Charge my:
❏ Visa   ❏ Mastercard   ❏ Amex   ❏ Discover

Card Number: _____

Expiration Date: _____

Signature: _____

Tax applicable for CA 7.25%, FL 6%, MA 5%, SC 5%, TX 6%

❏ Please send me e-mail updates on nursing and other related fields.

E-mail address: _____

Prices are subject to change   Source: NF2